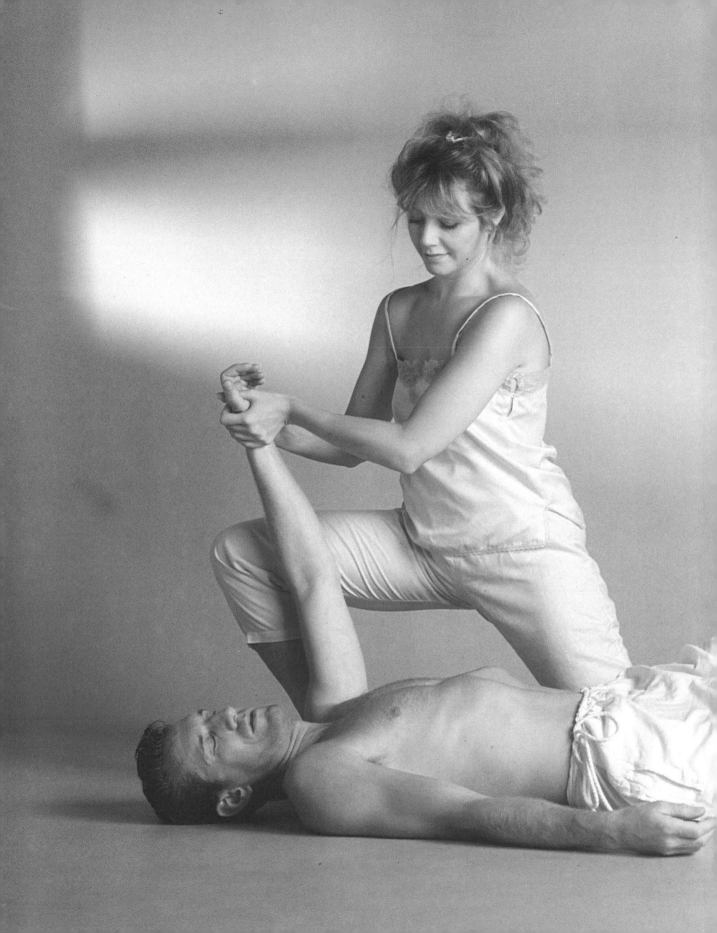

MASSAGE
—FOR—
COMMON
AILMENTS

Sara Thomas

Photography by Fausto Dorelli

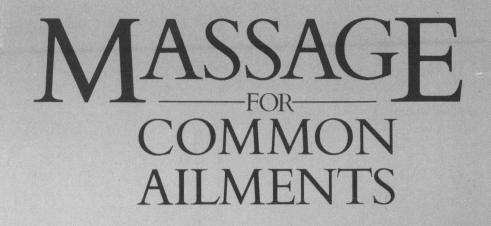

A GAIA ORIGINAL

A Fireside Book
Published by Simon & Schuster Inc.
New York London Toronto Sydney Tokyo

Written by Sara Thomas

with Jane Downer and Chris Jarmey
of the Shiatsu School of Natural Therapy, London

Photography	Fausto Dorelli
Editorial	Joanna Godfrey Wood Susan McKeever
Design	Lynn Hector
Illustration	Sheilagh Noble
Production	Susan Walby
Direction	Lucy Lidell Patrick Nugent Casey Horton

A Fireside Book
Published by Simon & Schuster Inc.
Simon & Schuster Building
Rockefeller Center
1230 Avenue of the Americas
New York, New York 10020

FIRESIDE and colophon are registered trademarks
of Simon & Schuster Inc.

Published in Great Britain in 1989
by Sidgwick & Jackson Limited, London

Printed and bound in Spain by Artes Graficas Toledo S.A.

10 9 8 7 6 5 4 3 2 1

Library of Congress Cataloging in Publication Data
D.L.TO.: 1650/1988

Thomas, Sara.
    Massage for common ailments.
    "A Gaia original."
    "A Fireside book."
    Bibliography: p.
    Includes index.
    1. Massage — Therapeutic use. I. Title.
    RM 721. T445   1989   615. 8'22   88-18554

ISBN 0-671-67552-4 (pbk.)

About this book

Two separate, but overlapping, therapies are introduced in Massage for Common Ailments – massage and Shiatsu. All the sequences for treating ailments are derived from massage unless the heading states Shiatsu. You can use them individually or together to help the healing process.

Before you start treating an ailment, take time to study Basic Strokes (see pp.22-7) and When Massage Should Not Be Used (see p.93). The main part of the book, Common Ailments (pp.28-89), is divided into separate sections that deal with different parts of the body, starting with the head and working down to the feet. The charts on pp. 30-1 show you where in the body the various ailments occur.

Note Always consult a doctor if you are in doubt about a medical condition, and observe the cautions given in the book.

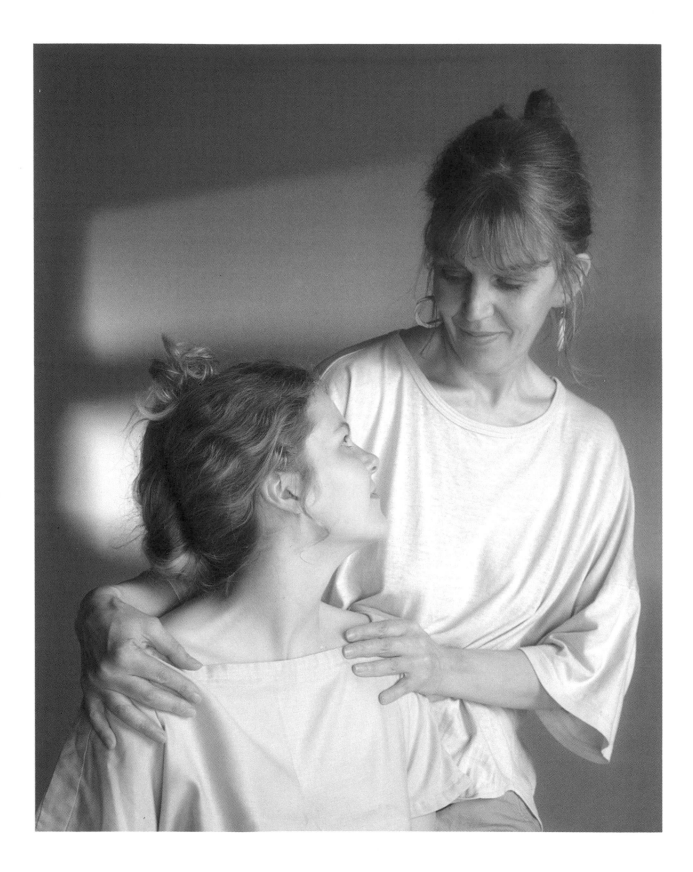

The use of the hands
as a means to convey friendship
to comfort and heal the sick
to express love and tenderness
to quiet and titillate the child
is as old as life

Bernard Gunter

Touch affects the body's vital forces

Jerome Liss

To permit simple contact is to permit,
and necessarily to experience,
the natural reinforcement
that the living has for the living.

Charles Brooks

CONTENTS

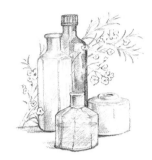
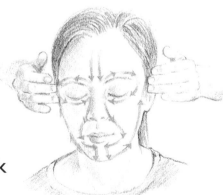

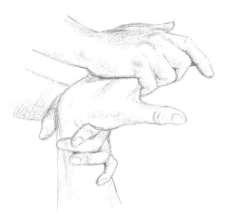
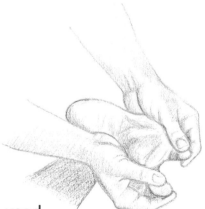

INTRODUCTION

Throughout history we have used our hands to impart comfort and healing to one another. Touching is contact, warmth, reassurance that we are not alone, affirmation of our sense of being and self-worth. It is a simple way of communicating, something we all do naturally. And with a little willingness and commitment we can turn this natural talent into a creative healing skill, by learning the basic strokes and techniques of massage and widening our vocabulary in the language of touch.

Our sense of touch is registered by our skin – our largest and most sensitive organ. In the developing embryo, the skin arises from the same cell layer as the nervous system and can thus be seen as the external portion of the nervous system – able to receive and register a vast quantity of varied signals, and to make a wide range of responses to them. Also, touch is the first sense to become functional in the embryo.

The value of massage

The intent that goes with touch makes all the difference to its effect. When we lay our hands on another with compassion and good-will many subtle changes take place. Gentle holding and stroking, touching given with tenderness and care, cause transformations both physically and psychologically.

In the 1920s in Philadelphia the anatomist Frederick Hammett and other American researchers in the 1950s and 60s conducted experiments with groups of rats to investigate the effects of touch. Some were consistently handled and stroked and others were not. The rats that were regularly touched showed faster growth rates, better immunity to disease and higher fertility and were less subject to stress than those that were not. It is well known, too, that for infants, fondling and tender touch that go beyond the basic needs for food and cleanliness are vital for life. In America, between 1910 and 1935, studies of babies in institutions were conducted by Drs. Chapin and Knox and J. Brennemann. They found that many babies died in infancy and others showed clear signs of disturbance and poor physical and emotional development as a result of too little tactile stimulation.

Physiologically, caring touch and massage help the flow of blood and lymph in our bodies. Touch can also decrease our blood pressure and heart rate, soothe our nerves and decrease tension, producing relaxation and a state of well-being. It has been suggested that massage may aid the production of endorphins

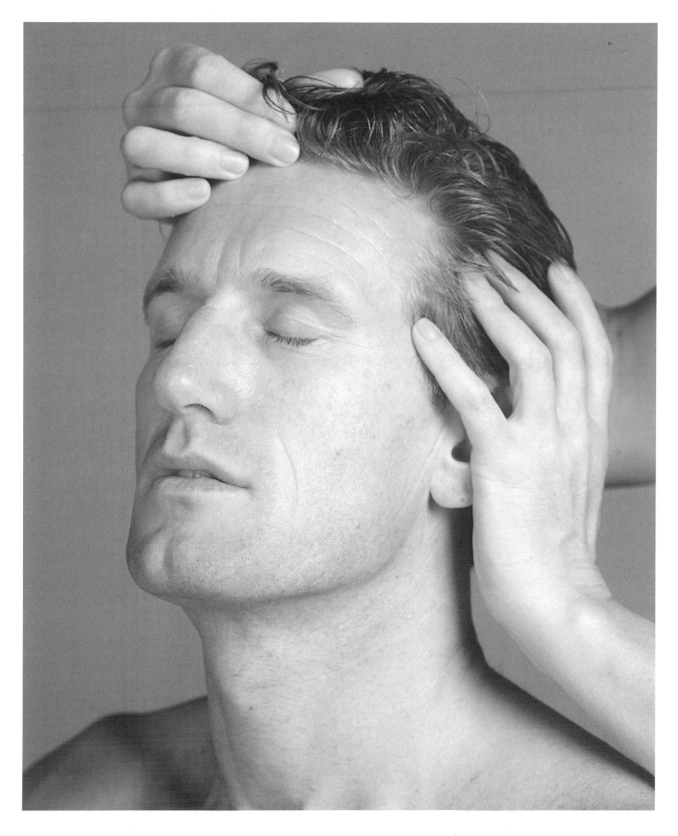

(meaning "morphine within"), the brain chemicals that function as natural pain-killers. One of these, enkephalin, has the ability to reduce pain and produces a state of mind akin to euphoria.

The experience of being nourished and cared for and allowing ourselves to receive healing touch affirms our self-esteem, creates trust and openness and can sometimes facilitate the release of blocked emotions as tense muscles relax. Touch can make us feel valued, peaceful and more aware of our whole body and being.

It is not only receiving touch that is beneficial, however. Giving massage is also highly rewarding. There is pleasure in the physical contact and in feeling the contours and undulations of the body as you begin to develop a sense of the muscles, bones and other tissues. There is enjoyment in knowing the body, in being alive to its different tensions and energies, and in realizing that you can care for and help another. There is also satisfaction in experiencing the results of your massage as you feel muscles relaxing and realize that your concern and your touch can help to stimulate the receiver's own healing process. Often the interaction between the giver and receiver induces a similar state in both – a state that is very similar to meditation.

The Chakras

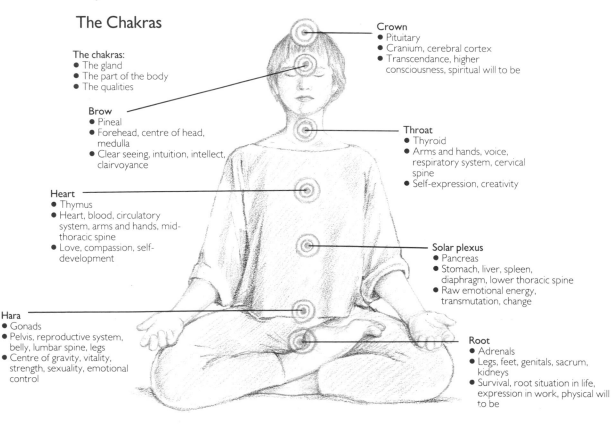

The chakras:
- The gland
- The part of the body
- The qualities

Crown
- Pituitary
- Cranium, cerebral cortex
- Transcendance, higher consciousness, spiritual will to be

Brow
- Pineal
- Forehead, centre of head, medulla
- Clear seeing, intuition, intellect, clairvoyance

Throat
- Thyroid
- Arms and hands, voice, respiratory system, cervical spine
- Self-expression, creativity

Heart
- Thymus
- Heart, blood, circulatory system, arms and hands, mid-thoracic spine
- Love, compassion, self-development

Solar plexus
- Pancreas
- Stomach, liver, spleen, diaphragm, lower thoracic spine
- Raw emotional energy, transmutation, change

Hara
- Gonads
- Pelvis, reproductive system, belly, lumbar spine, legs
- Centre of gravity, vitality, strength, sexuality, emotional control

Root
- Adrenals
- Legs, feet, genitals, sacrum, kidneys
- Survival, root situation in life, expression in work, physical will to be

Balancing the flow of vital energy

Wholeness goes beyond the body, mind and emotions. In wholeness is health, and in any kind of healing touch technique you are treating more than just the physical body; you are also affecting a person's "subtle" body and restoring balance to the flow of energy. This subtle body includes the energy field or "aura", in and around the body, and the major centres of subtle energy or vitality known as the *chakras*. The aura is composed of interpenetrating fields of subtle or vital energy that emanates from the body, out beyond the periphery of the skin, and is constantly in motion. Within the aura and along the midline of the body are the seven main *chakras*, whose function is to relay vital energy between the physical body and the subtle body. The word *chakra* is a Sanskrit word meaning wheel, which indicates the circling movement of energy in these centres. Five are situated on the spine and two in the head. They relate to different parts of the body – to glands, organs, and nerve plexii, and also to areas of our psychological and spiritual development. With practice you can learn to sense the energies of the aura and *chakras* with your hands.

Using Shiatsu as a healing tool

In this book, we have chosen to teach not only massage but also Shiatsu to give you a wider range of effective techniques for the relief of everyday health problems.

Shiatsu has its origins in Oriental medicine. The word literally means finger or thumb pressure, although other parts of the hand and body are also used. In Japan Shiatsu has traditionally been practiced as a simple remedy to promote health, alleviate pain and prevent sickness. Its techniques are based on the understanding that the body functions as a whole, linked by vital energy, or *ki*, which flows along channels, or meridians, which interlace as a network throughout the body, mostly on the skin's surface. Discomfort, pain, stress and illness are caused by *ki* energy stagnating and "blocking" the meridians, making the internal organs either deficient in or overloaded by energy. By holding and applying pressure to points, or *tsubos*, on the meridians, you can stimulate the *ki* energy, helping it to rebalance itself. This affects the physical body and can help to relieve pain and alleviate the causes and symptoms of illness.

Shiatsu should not be painful. Although some *tsubos* and meridians may be tender, pressure can be applied gently and slowly, so that it always feels comfortable. Shiatsu is a form of communication, and its effectiveness is dependent on a willingness to be open and receptive to your partner.

Shiatsu Meridians

Key to the meridians

Bl	Bladder	Ht	Heart	TH	Triple heater
Ki	Kidney	Lu	Lungs	HP	Heart protector
Liv	Liver	GB	Gall bladder	GV	Governing vessel
St	Stomach	SI	Small intestines	CV	Conception vessel.
Sp	Spleen	Ll	Large intestines		

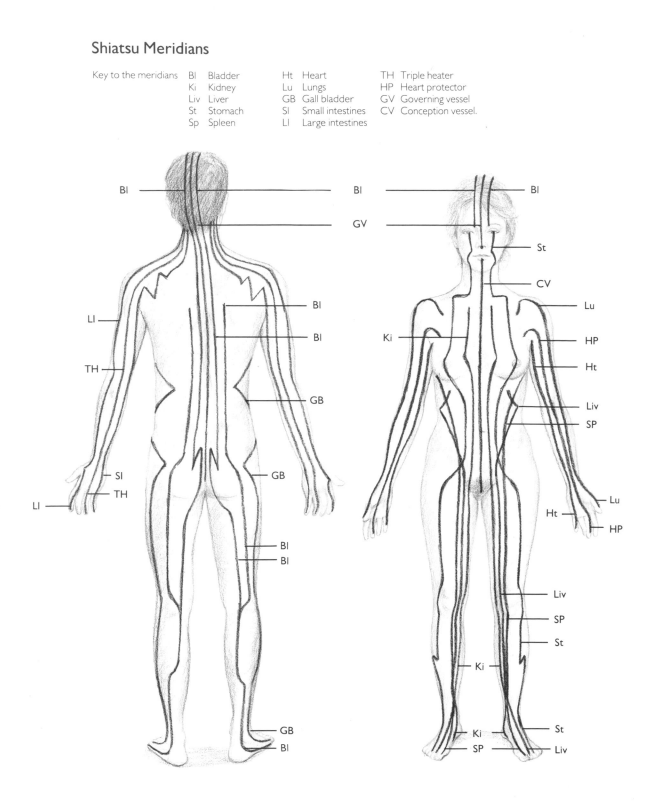

N.B. All the meridians are mirrored on the other side of the body.

Preventing and treating ill health with massage

When you already have the gift of health you need to maintain it. Touch does not just have to be used as a way of healing and hastening recovery – it can also be a way of preventing sickness. In today's "civilized" cultures it is only too easy to get caught up in striving, accomplishing, and conforming to society's mores. In the process you can become overly head-orientated and out of touch with your body. This also means being out of touch with reality, however, for it is through your body that you receive sensory messages that let you know what you need, what you are feeling emotionally, and what is happening around you in the immediate environment. This is all vital information for self-regulation, in the sense of giving your body what is best for health and balance. In order to be truly healthy you need to stop thinking that ideas and concepts are the only reality and wake up to the information that your whole body can give you. As Fritz Perls, the founder of Gestalt therapy, said "lose your head and come to your senses".

Massage is a way of getting back in touch with your body and finding trust in what it has to say. When you become more aware of yourself as a whole being, physical, mental, emotional and spiritual, you can start to respond more to fulfilling your real needs. Eating a healthy and balanced diet, exercising daily and breathing more freely can all be done with a sense of pleasure and rightness rather than as chores or acts of grim will-power.

Nevertheless, everyone gets sick from time to time, and illness is often a manifestation of the body's attempt to heal itself and to eliminate toxins and clear the system. This book is about how to use touch to help the body's natural healing process when you or your family or friends do succumb to any of the common ailments. It is not about miracle cures, but about giving warmth and support to another by a variety of caring touch techniques, which can help to speed recovery. As many illnesses result from stress and strain in daily life, the touch therapies are particularly effective, for they calm and soothe tension and bring balance to your being. Both massage and Shiatsu work with and for the body's healing energies; in contrast to states of stress and effort they create the conditions for healing to take place. As well as learning how to do a whole body massage, which you can use when an ailment is more general and affects the whole body – such as insomnia or fatigue – you will also learn strokes and techniques to aid more specific conditions, such as headaches, backaches, constipation and cramp. Use the book wisely. Don't try to take over a doctor's role – give where you can and seek medical advice where you can't. Your hands have healing in them. Use them.

BEGINNING

In order to help another by our touch we need to be caring, willing to give some time and to focus our attention fully on our partner. Just ten minutes of touch given by someone who is really present and caring can be far more beneficial than an hour of mechanical massage by someone whose mind is absent or distracted. So it is important to prepare yourself before beginning by centring yourself (see p.19). With a little practice you will become familiar enough with this centred state to be able to let go of your busy mind and come into the here and now at short notice. By staying centred you are able to tune in more fully to the areas of your partner's body that need a special touch or movement.

While giving massage and Shiatsu, "grounding" is also very important. This means being fully aware of your own body and its movements and position and letting these movements emanate from your pelvis and *hara* (see p.19), not just from your shoulders and arms. When you use your *hara* you use your relationship with the ground to get in touch with your strength. You save yourself from fatigue as strength comes from your whole body and all your movements are more gracefully controlled and more effective.

When doing massage or Shiatsu to alleviate common ailments you may find you have to improvise in situations or places that are not ideal. But even in unconducive environments, healing touch can bring welcome relief. However, if you have planned a massage in advance you will be able to set the scene and create an environment that is as warm and nurturing as possible. Without too much difficulty you can turn a room into a cosy space with everything you need at hand.

Once your environment is prepared there are a few guidelines for both giver and receiver to remember. When giving either massage or Shiatsu you should wear loose light clothing, as the room will be warm and your clothes should allow freedom of movement. You need to remove your watch, any bracelets and rings and your fingernails should be short to avoid scratching and you should wash your hands thoroughly. Throughout the treatment you need to remain receptive to what you are feeling with your hands. Avoid chatting but by all means communicate when necessary about pressure and discomfort. Shiatsu is done with the receiver fully clothed, but for massage the receiver should remove whatever clothes are necessary, plus watches and jewellery, and once lying down should relax and yield to gravity. The role of the receiver is not entirely passive. He or she needs to keep aware of the giver's touch and of the sensations being experienced.

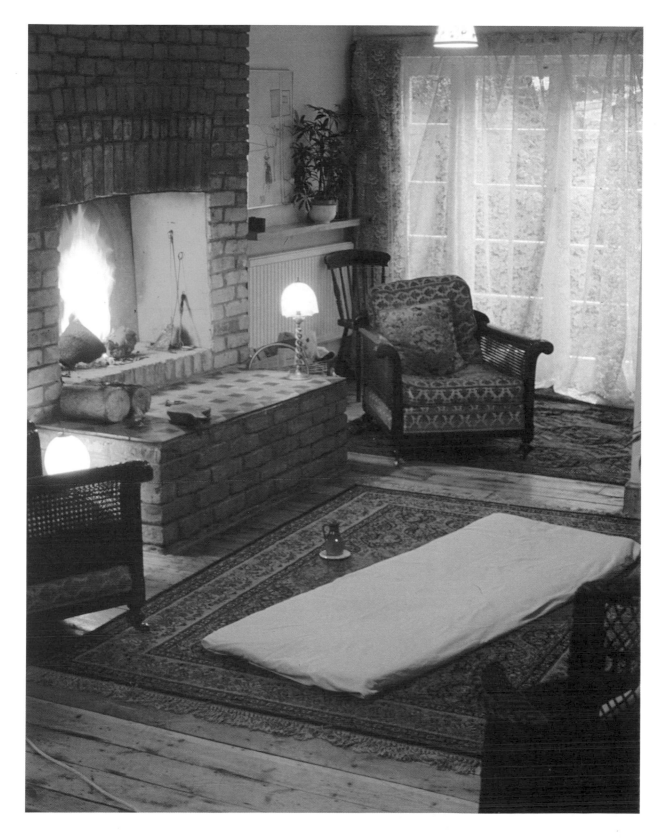

Creating the environment

When making a conducive environment in which to do either massage or Shiatsu there are several elements to consider. First, the room needs to be warm, as we tense up when chilled. For oil massage this is especially important, so have an extra heater on hand. A selection of small towels and pillows is also useful if you need to pad under any area of your partner's body, such as the ankles, belly or upper chest, when he or she is face down, or the knees when face up. Shiatsu is always done on the floor – on a pad or futon covered with a sheet or towel. This is fine for massage too, but if you are uncomfortable working on the floor, it is worth investing in a massage table. Avoid ordinary beds as they are usually too soft and the wrong height. However, for both massage and Shiatsu, many of the strokes and techniques can be given while the receiver sits in a chair. Lighting should be very gentle as our eyes cannot fully relax in glaring light. Some people like to work to a background of peaceful and unobtrusive music, others prefer quietness. In any case make sure you won't be disturbed. Finally, have a large warm towel ready to place gently over your partner's body at the end of massage. For Shiatsu, use a blanket and allow your partner to relax for several minutes.

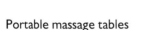

Portable massage tables
Ready-made folding massage tables are useful for those who find working on the floor difficult. Those with cross-over central legs are the most secure. Some tables, like the one shown here, also have face holes for people whose necks are too stiff to turn easily when lying on their fronts. The table should be about the same height as your palm if held parallel to the floor when your arm is hanging at your side.

Improvising with a chair
If your partner cannot get down on to the floor or up on to a table, you can use an ordinary chair. Your partner can either sit normally, so that you can work on neck, head, shoulders, hands, knees and feet. Or he or she can sit astride, as shown, resting head and arms on the back. Like this you can treat back, shoulders and neck very effectively.

Centring and the *hara*

In both massage and Shiatsu centring and grounding, or being focused and aware in the present, are of great importance. For it is by being wholly in the here and now that you can be of greatest help to your partner when you attempt to heal or help through touch. The *hara* (see also p.12) is situated in the belly, an inch or so below the navel, and is the centre of strength and vitality as well as the centre of gravity in the body. It links also with your legs and your connection to the ground, which gives you stability, hence the importance of using this centre for massage, and of letting the body move from here as you work. By directing your energy from this area your whole body becomes involved in the movements and you avoid fatigue and work more effectively. The meditation and exercise that follow will help you to centre yourself in your *hara*. If you have the chance, you should use it before any massage.

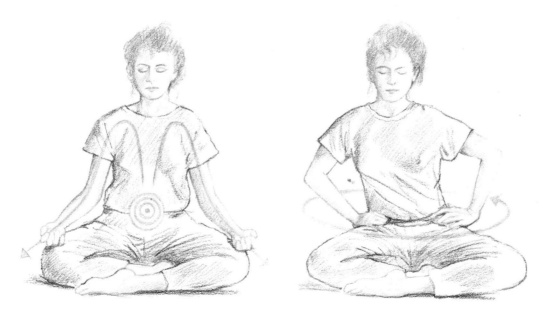

Centring and grounding meditation
Kneel or sit comfortably. Close your eyes and go inside yourself. Become aware of your legs, your feet and your buttocks, and where they make contact with the surface beneath. Try to feel your legs and pelvis as a firm base for your body, and then feel your spine rising gently up from it. Become aware of your trunk, shoulders, arms and hands and relax any tensions you might find. Then move slowly to your neck and head, letting go of any tightness around your eyes or in your jaw. Now let your attention turn to your breath and watch it coming in and out, like the waves on a beach. As you breathe in, let the breath sink more deeply into your *hara* and imagine it as light or energy filling your belly. Then, as you exhale, imagine the energy travelling down your arms and out through your hands. Notice the feeling in your hands as you do this.

After a few minutes place your hands lightly on your hips and begin to rotate your whole body slowly from the pelvis. Be aware of your legs and pelvis as a strong foundation and let your back and spine remain straight but not rigid. Having circled in one direction for a while, change and go the other way. Finally, rest and open your eyes.

Beginning an oil massage

You can use a variety of oils for massaging and will need to experiment to find out what suits you best. Suitable oils range from vegetable oils, such as sunflower, safflower or almond oil, to baby oils, which are mineral-based, or ready-mixed massage oils. If you enjoy scents and wish to enhance the effects of your massage with the therapeutic benefits of aromatherapy essences, you can add drops of these to a base of vegetable oil (see p.21).

At the start of a massage, before applying oils, you can make an initial acquaintance with your partner's body by means of a gentle touch, as shown below. You should apply oil only to the area that is to be worked on, rather than oiling the whole body at once. Oiling is done with long, smooth gliding strokes (see p.23), which spread a thin film of oil over the skin and also serve to warm and energize it. Don't overdo the amount of oil, but be more generous with areas such as hairy chests.

Throughout a massage, the way in which you make and break contact is extremely important, for if you suddenly "dive" on to the body it can be a shock to the receiver, and likewise, if you leap rapidly away with your hands, the harmony can be broken. It is not necessary to maintain a constant contact during a massage, however. Gentle breaks in touch, made with sensitivity, are like spaces of quietness within a passage of music.

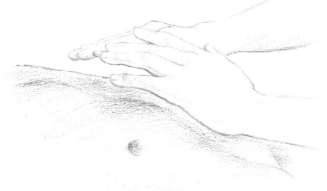

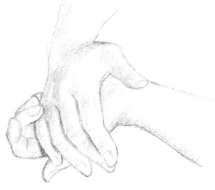

Applying oils
When you are ready to apply the oil (see below), hold your hands well away from your partner's body to avoid drips and pour a small amount of oil into one palm. Then rub your palms together, warming and spreading the oil, before bringing your hands gently to the body to start the oiling strokes.

Making contact
Centre yourself and allow your hands to float slowly down to a part of your partner's body, such as the head or back, and then rest lightly there for a few moments (see above). When you feel you have established the initial contact, lift your hands very gently away in order to begin oiling.

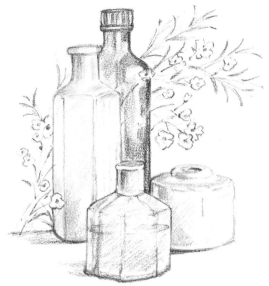

Useful amounts:
For full body: 5 drops of essence in 2 eggcupsful of carrier oil.
For body parts: 2-3 drops of essence in 1 eggcupful of carrier oil.
For small, localized areas: 1 drop of essence in one teaspoonful of carrier oil.

Aromatherapy essences

These essences (also known as essential oils) are obtained from the distillation of plants, flowers and herbs that have different therapeutic effects on the body. They also add the dimension of fragrant variety to enhance your massage and make it more healing and pleasurable. These essences have many different properties, ranging from effects on mood (i.e. antidepressant) to physical effects, such as anti-inflammatory and antibacterial. As they are very concentrated, aromatherapy essences always need to be diluted in a carrier oil before being applied to the skin, where they are absorbed quite quickly and enter the bloodstream. The best carrier oils are those of vegetable origin, such as soya, almond, or avocado. It is best to blend fairly small amounts of oil and essences as vegetable oil oxidizes and smells somewhat rancid after a while. A teaspoon of wheatgerm oil in a mix acts as an antioxidant. In the book, various essences are mentioned and suggested for different ailments.

Some aromatherapy essences

BERGAMOT	Antiseptic, antidepressant – uplifting and refreshing	Helps: depression, bronchitis, sore throat, digestive problems	LAVENDER	Antidepressant, antiseptic, sedative – refreshing and relaxing	Helps: depression, insomnia, flatulence, indigestion, asthma, bronchitis, menstrual pains, skin problems
CAMOMILE	Sedative – calming, refreshing and relaxing	Helps: aching muscles, headaches, menstrual pains, inflammations, stress, digestive problems	MARJORAM	Sedative, antiseptic – warming and strengthening	Helps: muscular pains, digestive problems, painful joints, sinus congestion
CARDAMOM	Antiseptic, tonic – refreshing	Helps: ease wind and digestive problems, painful joints, nausea, headaches, general debility	MELISSA	Antidepressant – uplifting and refreshing	Helps: headaches, migraine, menstrual pains, lowers high blood pressure
EUCALYPTUS	Antiseptic – head-clearing, stimulating	Helps: coughs, colds, bronchitis, aching muscles	ROSEMARY	Antiseptic – refreshing and stimulating	Helps: headaches, migraine, colds, bronchitis, muscular pains
FENNEL	Diuretic, laxative, tonic	Helps: ease wind and digestive problems, colic, constipation, bronchitis			

Because there are many aromatherapy essences, some of which are very expensive, we have selected a basic group that has a wide range of effects. As you become more familiar with the essences you can gradually add to your collection.

BASIC STROKES

In massage, the whole range of different strokes fall into four main groups: light gliding strokes; medium depth strokes; deep tissue, or friction strokes; and percussion. Once you have mastered these, you can begin to improvise and use them in a variety of different ways and combinations, developing your own personal style. Before using the massage strokes on a partner, practice them on your legs, so that you have some idea of how they feel and what their effects are. Make sure you are warm enough and sitting comfortably, and spend a few minutes centring yourself before you start (see p.19). Work very slowly at first and keep your awareness both in your hands and in the sensations you are receiving. Try to put your whole body behind your movements, not just your hands, and let them come from your *hara* and pelvis. See, also, if you can develop a rhythmical flow to the strokes as you practice. At a different time, try out the basic Shiatsu techniques (see p.27), which provide the essentials you need to learn before using Shiatsu as a healing tool.

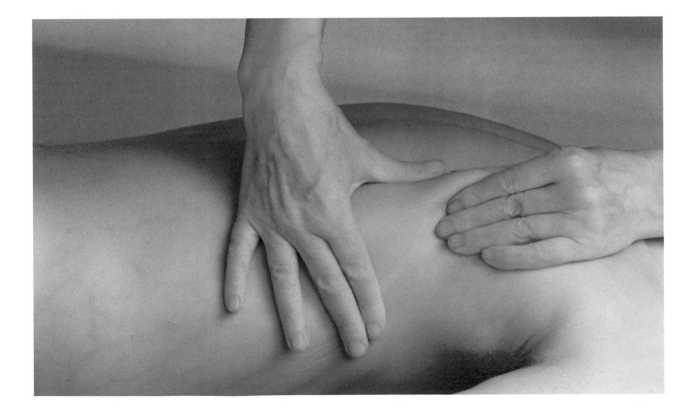

1 Long oiling strokes

Rest your oiled hands on the part of your partner's body you are about to work with. With your hands side by side and fingers together, glide smoothly away from yourself, reaching as far as you can go. Then divide your hands and draw back along the sides of the limb or torso, enfolding the area. Flow back to the original starting position and continue the cycle.

Gliding strokes

The long, light gliding and feathering strokes are used both at the beginning and at the end of a massage. With them you make the initial acquaintance with your partner's body. As you caringly spread the oil, you warm and energize an area of the body prior to working more deeply into it. The gliding strokes vary from light to firm, but should always be done slowly and with the whole of your hands flowing and moulding over the forms of the body. You can come back to these strokes at any time during a massage. The feathering is a long light trusting stroke that can connect a whole area – ideal for bidding farewell to a part of the body you have just worked with.

2 Circling

To spread oil more thoroughly or to stroke and soothe a wider area, make slow broad circles with your hands, using them simultaneously or alternately. Work slowly and rhythmically as you explore the terrain of your partner's body. Let the circles flow into each other in gentle spiralling movements.

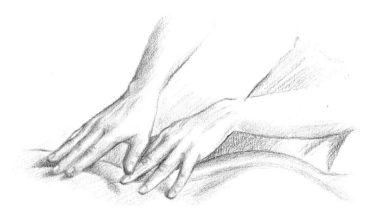

3 Feathering

Relax your hands and begin the lightest of brushing strokes with your fingertips, drawing your hands toward you, one after the other, with this stroke, which feels like feathers gently caressing the skin. Use it to connect a whole area as you prepare to take leave of it, or to change to a different stroke.

Medium depth strokes

These moderately deep strokes work more directly with the muscle masses. Sometimes circular, sometimes back and forth, they help to stimulate the circulation, which assists in clearing waste products more quickly from the muscles. They are also relaxing. Use a fairly bold and generous approach, allowing your body to rock gently behind the kneading, pulling or wringing. If you let the movements come from your pelvis rather than shoulders and arms it will be less tiring for you and more effective for your partner.

1 Kneading

Use the whole of your hand to grasp and lift a bunch of flesh or muscle in a circular squeezing motion. Work your hands alternately with a rocking rhythmical movement, very much like kneading dough. Your hands can maintain a constant contact with the skin while doing this stroke.

2 Pulling

With one hand over the far side of the torso or of a limb, as shown right, slowly pull upward, lifting the muscle firmly as your hand follows the curve of the part and gently breaks contact. Before the contact is broken, start pulling a little further on with your other hand. Let your hands pull in a flowing movement, overlapping as they travel along.

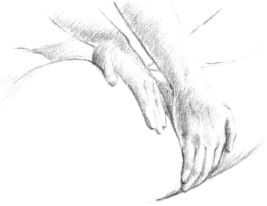

3 Wringing

Kneeling beside your partner, with your hands cupped over a limb, as shown left, slide the fingers of one hand right over to the far side, while the heel of your other hand comes down on the near side. Keeping your hands close together, repeat in the opposite direction. Continue in a steady back-and-forth movement, wringing either up or down the limb.

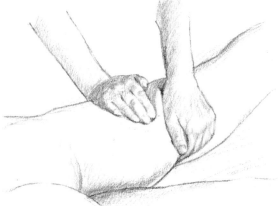

1 Thumb pressing

Place your thumbs on the soft tissue next to the bone at the edge of a joint. Keeping your arms straight, slowly lean forward from your hips so that your body weight builds up a gradual pressure on your thumbs. Hold, release, then move your thumbs a little and repeat. Continue to press all around the joint.

Deep tissue or friction strokes

The aim of these strokes is to penetrate into the deeper layers of muscles, into the connections of tendons and ligaments to bones and around joints. Thumbs and fingers are most commonly used for the friction strokes. Though appearing to circle or slide on the skin surface, they actually push in and direct pressure to the deeper levels below. The heel-of-the-hands stroke is a broader deep-tissue movement with quite a lot of power behind it. Go steadily and slowly, always staying very present. Never continue beyond the pain threshold.

2 Finger friction

With your fingers in the soft tissue between the bones of a joint, as shown right, apply fairly deep pressure to penetrate to the deeper structures within, and rotate your fingertips as you do so. Circling on the skin rather than sliding over it, try to focus your movement at a deeper level below the surface. Move all around the joint in this way.

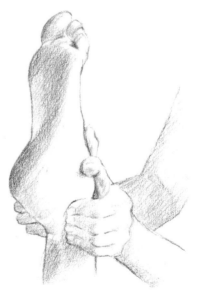

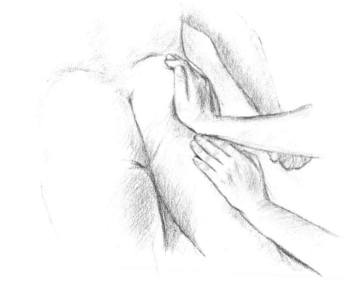

3 Deep pressure with heel of hand

With the heels of your hands pressing into the flesh, as shown left, push slowly and firmly away from you, one hand behind the other. Create a deep rhythmical movement in which you alternately push away, lift off and come down again with the heel of one hand behind that of the hand in front.

Percussion strokes

This group of pounding or drumming strokes stimulates the skin and circulation and can relax tight muscles. But because of the vigorous and noisy nature of these movements they are often more appropriate if you want your massage to be stimulating rather than relaxing. You will need to experiment and decide this for yourself. Before beginning, shake your hands up and down for a few moments to relax your wrists. The blows themselves are light and bouncy – as if you are striking a rubber ball. Don't use percussion strokes on the spine or any other protruding bony area.

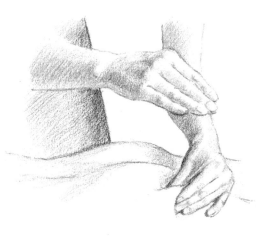

1 Hacking

With the first three fingers of each hand together and your little ones slightly apart to act as shock absorbers, start a rapid up-and-down movement, keeping your wrists relaxed. Practice in the air, then let your hands come down in a series of light quick blows, travelling up and down along muscled areas.

2 Cupping

With your fingers fairly straight, cup your hands, as shown below, closing the sides with your thumbs, and begin to do the same brisk and rhythmically alternating sequence of strokes described in Step 1. The position of the hand creates a slight vacuum with each blow, which results in a rather loud clapping noise on the skin.

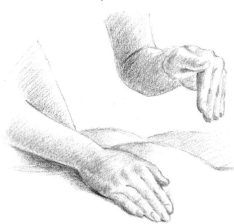

3 Plucking

Gently pluck small portions of flesh between thumbs and fingers, as shown above, lifting and letting them slip from between your fingers in quick succession.

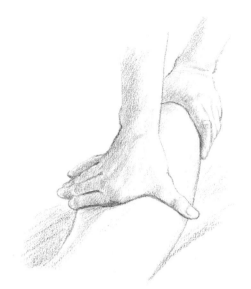

1 Shiatsu "Dragon's mouth" technique

Extend your thumbs and forefingers to stretch the connecting skin. Holding this shape place both hands over one of your partner's arms or legs, and apply pressure down through this part of your hands, keeping your arms straight and fingers and shoulders relaxed. You can also use this technique on the back of the neck (see Step 3, p.48).

2 Shiatsu palm and heel-of-hand pressure

Rest the palms of your hands on your partner's body, as shown below, and apply pressure as in Step 1. Lean into your hands to increase the pressure. For more precision of pressure, focus your body weight through the heels of your hands, while still keeping the rest of your hands in soft contact with your partner's body.

Basic techniques: Shiatsu

The application of pressure and stretching backed up by support forms the basis for most of the techniques used in Shiatsu. You create variety by using different parts of your body. We show three commonly used methods. Keep your shoulders relaxed, and your knees apart for stability. Focus on using your body weight in a controlled yet relaxed way, letting movements come from your hara. You should apply pressure as you both exhale. Keep both hands in contact with your partner – if one hand is active, let the other, the "mother hand", rest on the body. For clarity we have shown the receiver naked, but Shiatsu is normally done clothed.

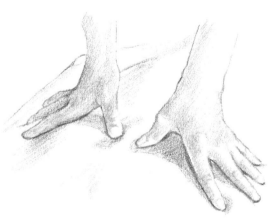

3 Shiatsu thumb pressure

Place the pads of your thumbs on your partner's body, as shown above, your fingers spread and resting there lightly to balance you and to reassure your partner. Slowly lean your body weight over your thumbs to increase the pressure. Keep your arms straight, but not rigid. Build up pressure gradually, hold then release.

COMMON AILMENTS

This section consists of a series of strokes and techniques that can help bring comfort and healing to a variety of common ailments. Most of the techniques shown are massage strokes, but where we feel that they are especially effective, we have also included some Shiatsu techniques. The body chart on pages 30 and 31 will help you to locate specific problems and lead you to the respective treatment, where you can try the strokes suggested. It is a good idea to start by practicing the whole body massage (see pp.32-43) as this will familiarize you with the basic strokes and accustom you to using your own body correctly.

When working on the floor and moving around your partner stay aware of your own posture and be careful not to jolt him or her. Be sure to work in positions that are comfortable to you, as any discomfort in your own body will be transmitted to your partner. It may be worth investing in a table (see p.18), as this makes it easier to move freely around your partner.

Always begin by centring and then making a gentle contact with your partner's body (see pp.19-20), before starting to work slowly and sensitively with the strokes. Pleasure is conducive to healing, and a caring touch gives both encouragement and reassurance.

When you move on to strokes and techniques for ailments in specific parts of the body you should always begin with the basic oiling stroke for that part of the body, unless you are doing Shiatsu or clothed massage, when of course you won't be using oil. In Shiatsu you can begin by briefly making contact to allow the body to open to your touch before beginning the technique.

A certain degree of pain can feel welcome during a massage, especially when treating stiff or tense muscles. But you should always let pain be a guideline and never exceed your partner's pain threshold. Encourage your partner to tell you what feels particularly helpful and to let you know immediately if anything you do feels too tender. If any aches and pains are severe or persist in spite of the massage, encourage your partner to consult a doctor. This book is not intended to help you to diagnose ailments or offer instant "cures". You should only treat ailments that are not serious or those that have already been professionally diagnosed, and before beginning any of the following treatments you should read the advice on pages 90 to 93, on arthritis, sprains, strains and times when you should not massage. If you can bear these simple points in mind, caring touch can provide many physical and psychological benefits and help to mobilize your partner's own healing energies toward a quicker recovery.

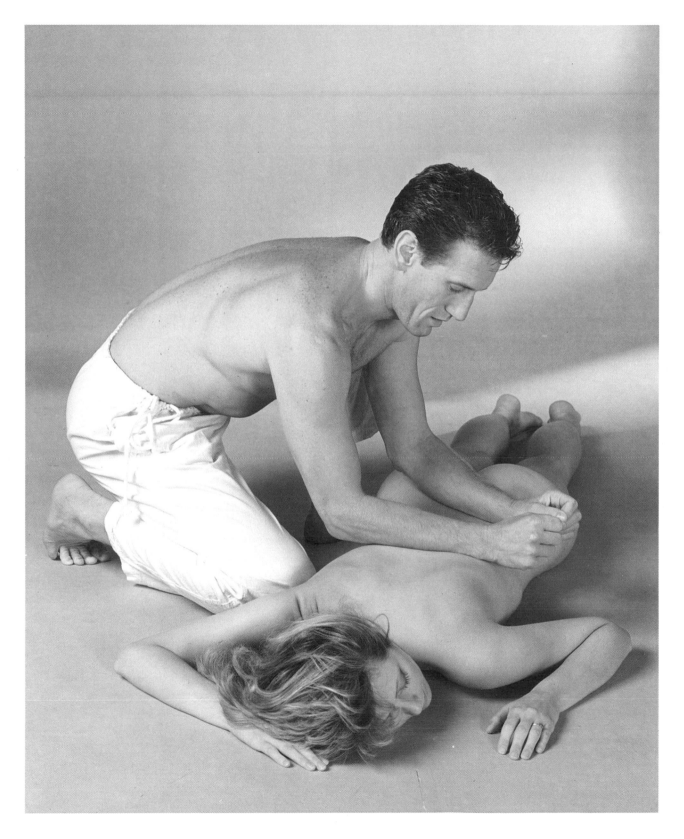

Where does it hurt?

To make it easier for you to find the relevant strokes and techniques, ailments are grouped under the part of the body chiefly affected. The parts of the body run in a sequence starting at the head and working down the body to the legs and feet.

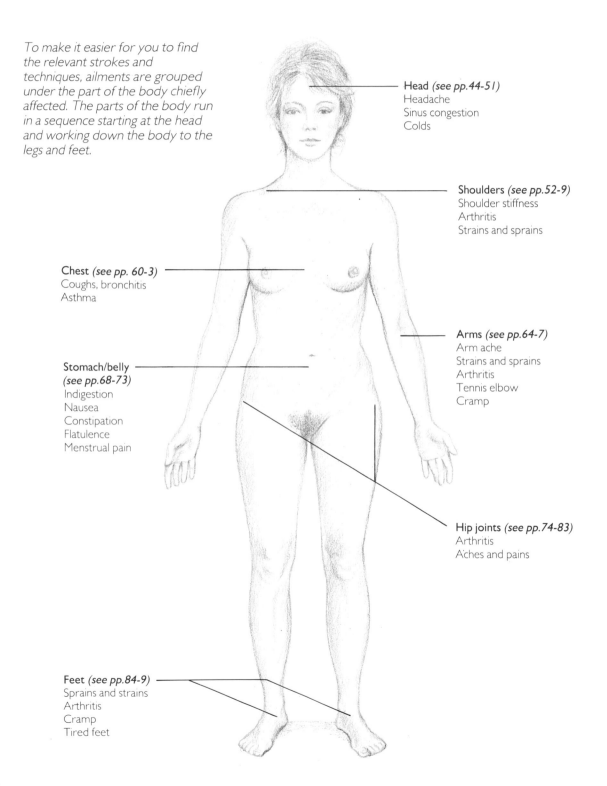

Head *(see pp.44-51)*
Headache
Sinus congestion
Colds

Shoulders *(see pp.52-9)*
Shoulder stiffness
Arthritis
Strains and sprains

Chest *(see pp. 60-3)*
Coughs, bronchitis
Asthma

Arms *(see pp.64-7)*
Arm ache
Strains and sprains
Arthritis
Tennis elbow
Cramp

Stomach/belly *(see pp.68-73)*
Indigestion
Nausea
Constipation
Flatulence
Menstrual pain

Hip joints *(see pp.74-83)*
Arthritis
Aches and pains

Feet *(see pp.84-9)*
Sprains and strains
Arthritis
Cramp
Tired feet

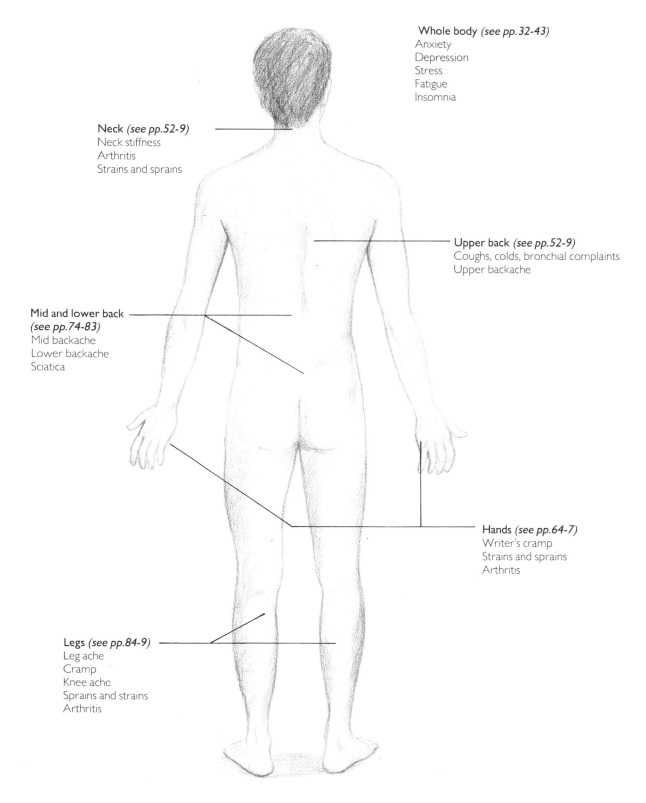

Whole body *(see pp.32-43)*
Anxiety
Depression
Stress
Fatigue
Insomnia

Neck *(see pp.52-9)*
Neck stiffness
Arthritis
Strains and sprains

Upper back *(see pp.52-9)*
Coughs, colds, bronchial complaints
Upper backache

Mid and lower back
(see pp.74-83)
Mid backache
Lower backache
Sciatica

Hands *(see pp.64-7)*
Writer's cramp
Strains and sprains
Arthritis

Legs *(see pp.84-9)*
Leg ache
Cramp
Knee ache
Sprains and strains
Arthritis

WHOLE BODY

A whole body massage can be a wonderfully nourishing and relaxing experience, good for body and soul. The overall benefits of massage, such as improved circulation, soothed nerves and relaxed muscles, and the general sense of well-being that results, make it a great way to maintain good health. Massaging the entire body also enhances body awareness, giving us a more complete body image and making us feel more whole. When we do succumb to the stresses and strains of life, then often a massage can help to restore the harmony that we have lost. The following sequence, which should take about one hour, takes you step by step through the whole body. It is just one possible way of doing a massage. As you become more familiar with the strokes and with giving massage you will develop your own sequences and discover many other techniques. Stay aware with your hands, and use them to "listen" to your partner's body. See if you can put your whole body behind your movements, and let them come from your *hara* (see p.19) and pelvis. Try, also, to regard the massage as a kind of dance or a piece of music. As you go, flow from one part of the body to another and develop your own natural rhythm.

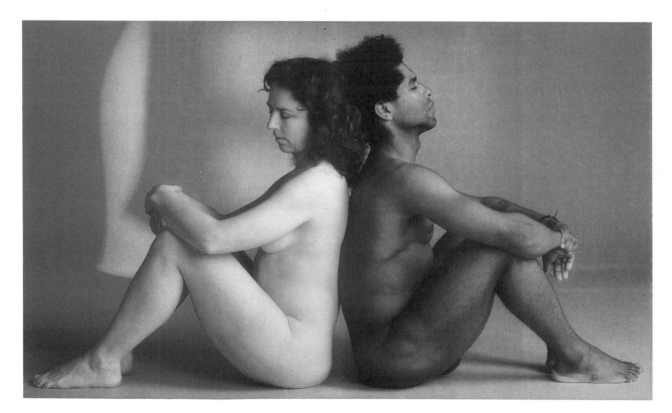

Insomnia, fatigue, anxiety and depression

Mental and physical over-activity can lead to any or all of these complaints. They are our body's "warning signals". A caring massage, combined with essential oils, can supply the relaxing space that is needed. For insomnia you can use camomile essence (see p.21), for fatigue use bergamot, and for anxiety and mild depression use lavender. Before starting the massage, read the section on contraindications (see p.93).

Caution: *If you have deep depression or anxiety you should consult your doctor.*

1 Spreading oil on back

With your partner lying on her front, kneel at her head, oil your hands and let them rest on the centre of her upper back. Glide down alongside her spine with your fingers together and hands relaxed. Go forward from your hips, not just your shoulders. At the end of your reach divide your hands and glide back up her sides. Repeat several times.

2 Sliding up curve of shoulder

Choose the shoulder opposite to the way in which your partner is facing, as shown right, and glide one hand slowly across her upper back, then along the curve of shoulder and neck up to the base of her skull and off at the hairline. Let your other hand follow behind, alternating your hands in a continual rhythmic movement.

3 Working shoulder in strips

Place your thumbs on the side of your partner's neck, your fingers resting on her back, as shown left. Now glide your thumbs along the shoulder, in the channel between bone and muscle, and out toward the shoulder joint. Repeat, but each time work a little higher, covering the shoulder top in strips. Help your partner to turn her head and repeat from Step 2 on the other side.

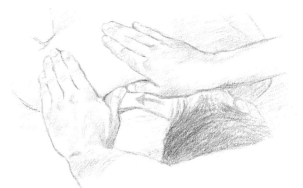

4 Oiling buttocks
Sit at one of your partner's sides facing up toward her head. Oil your hands and let them come to rest on the sacrum (base of spine). Now glide up the centre of the lower back and circle your hands out and down to the sides of the body, draw back across the hips and circle around the buttocks and back to the sacrum. Repeat this stroke several times.

5 Circling lower back
Still facing up toward your partner's head, begin to make counter-clockwise circles with your right hand around the lower back while your left hand makes clockwise circles. Allow both to overlap. Apply more pressure as you pull in toward the centre of her back and down toward the buttocks. Let your hands move slowly.

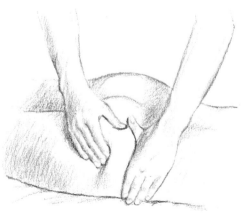

6 Kneading buttocks and sides
Turn to face across your partner's side and reach over to the opposite buttock. With both hands, begin to knead the muscles with firm generous squeezing and lifting strokes. Continue kneading right up the side of the body to the shoulder and back down again. Repeat on the other side.

7 Oiling backs of legs

Sit or kneel at one of your partner's feet and rest your oiled hands at the back of her ankle and lower calf. Then gliding slowly up the leg to the top of her thigh, divide your hands, one branching out around the hip joint and the other down the inside of the thigh. Avoid going too close to the genitals. Then, with both hands enfolding her leg, draw right down to the foot, across the sole and off at the toes. Repeat.

Caution: Avoid using any of the leg strokes on varicose veins (see p.93).

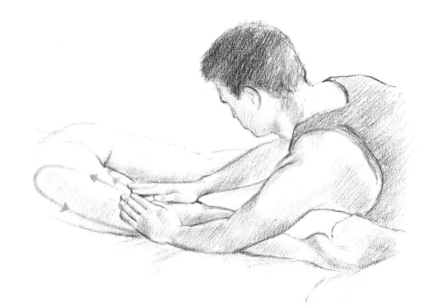

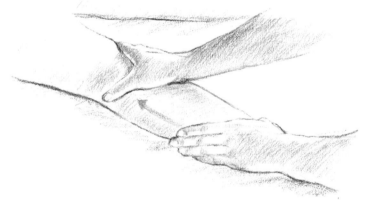

8 "Draining" back of leg

With both hands cupped, start an alternating stroke that pushes slowly up the back of the whole leg from ankle to thigh. Keep all your fingers in contact with the sides of the leg, and let your hands glide upward in a series of rhythmical strokes. Check with your partner for pressure and make sure you "drain" both back and sides of the thigh thoroughly.

9 Wringing down back of leg

Move around to kneel beside your partner's thigh and rest both your hands at the top of the thigh. Then wring your hands slowly and firmly back and forth in opposite directions (see p.24), stretching the tissue in between them. Let each of your hands simultaneously touch the work surface on either side of the leg before wringing across again. Move down the leg to the ankle.

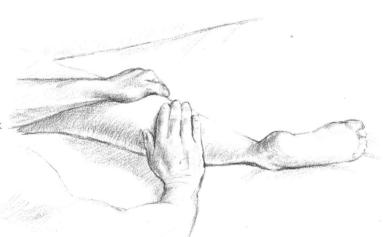

10 Lifting lower leg

Sit or kneel facing sideways on to your partner's leg and, with one hand just above the back of her knee, lift the lower leg with the other hand to a vertical position.

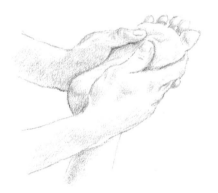

11 Loosening ankle joint

Using both your fingers and thumbs, start to work with slow sensitive strokes on either side of the ankle, as shown below, pushing into the soft tissue between the bones with small stroking and circling movements. Stay focused, and travel right around the joint in this way.

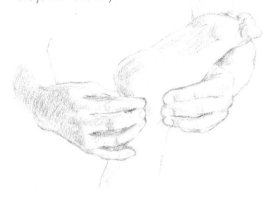

12 Thumbing sole

Clasp both hands around the foot, as shown above, and let your thumbs rest on the sole. Using your thumbs, push and slowly circle all the way along the sole from the heel to the toes, exploring every hill and hollow as you go. Repeat from Step 7 on the other leg.

13 Neck and shoulder cycle

Ask your partner to turn over, and kneel at her head. Turn her head to rest on one of your cupped hands, her cheek upward and her chin toward her collar bone. Let your free hand rest on the upper chest, fingers toward the centre, heel of the hand facing out toward the shoulder. Draw slowly out toward the shoulder joint and curve your hand around it . . .

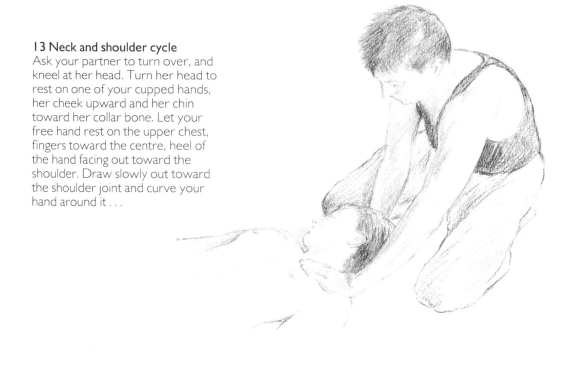

. . . then, with a firm slow pressure push in with the flats of your fingers along the curve of shoulder and neck, as shown left, drawing your hand slowly right up the back of the neck to the base of her skull. Let your fingers slide along the rim of bone until only the tips are in contact . . .

. . . then rotate your hand so that your fingers point down toward the centre of your partner's chest again, and slide your whole hand down, as shown right, into the "V" shape made where the collar bone joins the long neck muscle, and then on to the chest. Avoid the throat. Then repeat the whole cycle several times. Turn your partner's head and work the sequence on the other side.

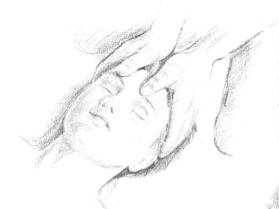

14 Stroking forehead

Sit at your partner's head and rest your thumbs on the centre of her forehead. Now with your hands supporting the sides of the head, slowly draw your thumbs away from the centre, as shown left, to the hairline, and off. Repeat this stroke several times.

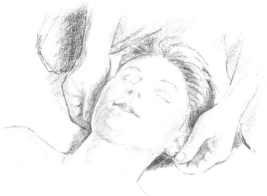

15 Massaging cheeks

With the heels of both your hands resting on the cheeks close to and on either side of the nose, and your fingers pointing down toward the ears, slide your hands slowly out across the sides of the face until you reach the ears, as shown right.

16 Stretching and squeezing ears

Now gently grasp the ears between fingers and thumbs and stretch them slightly outward and downward. Then spend some time squeezing and massaging the ears, exploring all the little crannies and crevices, as shown left.

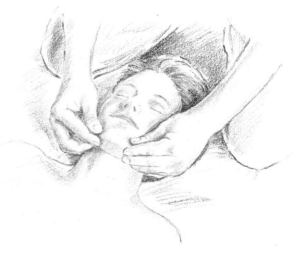

17 Clearing along jaw bone

Gently squeeze the tip of the chin with your thumbs and fingers and then slowly draw them out along the jaw bone in a long firm stroke, tracing the whole length of the rim of the bone to the ears, as shown right.

18 Oiling arm with gliding strokes

Sit or kneel by your partner's hand, facing up her arm. Oil your hands, and, keeping your fingers together on the centre of her arm, glide upward to her shoulder. Here, curve your outer hand around the joint and your inner hand down toward the armpit. Then enfold the arm with both hands and draw right back to the wrist, across the hand and off. Repeat a few times.

19 "Draining" arm

With her palm facing upward, hold one of your partner's wrists, and with your free hand begin to squeeze her arm between your thumb and fingers all the way along from the wrist as far as you can reach. Break contact at the top and start at the wrist again. Try to cover a different strip each time.

20 Spreading thumbs down arm

Clasp your partner's upper arm with both hands, your thumbs together in the centre. Squeezing with your whole hand, draw your thumbs outward to spread the flesh. Now slide a little way down and bring your thumbs together again to squeeze out once more. Continue like this all the way down the arm to the wrist.

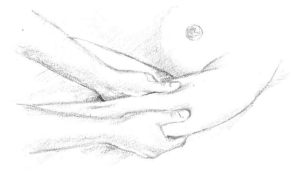

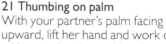

21 Thumbing on palm
With your partner's palm facing upward, lift her hand and work on it with your thumbs, making slow circles and squeezing and pressing into the whole of the palm area.

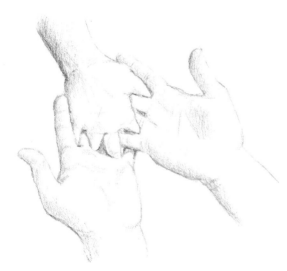

22 Spreading palms and fingers
Interlock your fingers between your partner's, as shown left, then gently open out the hand, spreading and stretching both the palm and fingers. Ask your partner to let you know when the stretch feels enough.

23 Stretching fingers
Hold your partner's hand palm downward in one hand, as shown right. Now take hold of one of her fingers at the point where it joins on to her hand and, squeezing the sides firmly, slide slowly down the finger, stretching it as you go. Let the pressure ease off as you reach the tip and slide off. Repeat on each finger and also the thumb. Repeat from Step 18 on the other side.

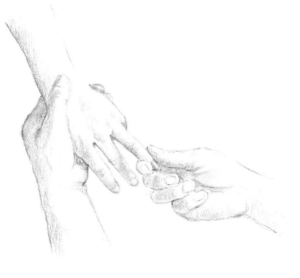

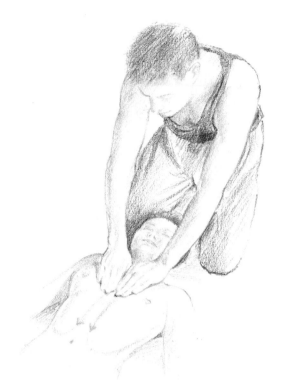

24 Oiling torso with gliding strokes

Sit or kneel at your partner's head and let your oiled hands float gently down to rest on her upper chest. With your hands together glide slowly down the centre of the body, divide your hands, then glide back up the sides and back to where you started. Repeat. (When working on the front of the torso, work around the breasts, not directly on them.)

25 Pulling up side of ribs

Start with one hand on the base of one side of your partner's ribcage. Glide up the side of the ribs, and on up the front of the chest. Let both your hands follow each other in this flowing stroke, each time starting higher up. Finally, pull up the side of the torso beneath the breast to the armpit. Repeat on the other side.

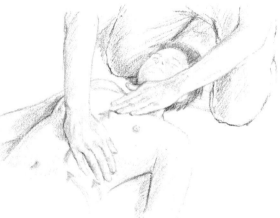

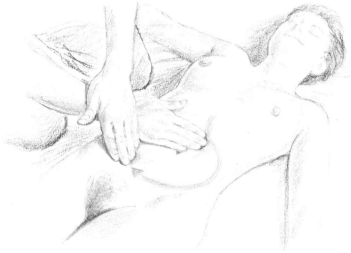

26 Circling around belly

Moving to your partner's side, let both hands come to rest very gently on the abdomen and pause there for a moment or two. Then, using both your hands, start to make slow, broad circling movements in a clockwise direction. One of your hands remains constantly on the body while the other gently breaks contact once in each cycle.

27 Oiling legs with gliding strokes

Kneel at your partner's feet and place your oiled hands on the front of her leg at the ankle. With your fingers together in the centre, glide up the leg to the top of the thigh and divide your hands outward, letting one go around the hip joint and the other curve down the inside of the thigh. Then enfold her leg and draw right down to the foot and off at the toes. Repeat.

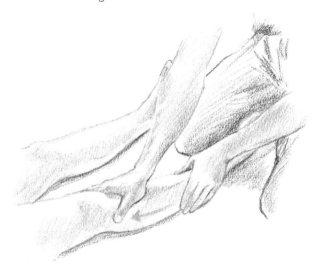

28 "Draining" leg

With your fingers and thumbs curved over the leg in a "V" shape, push upward with alternating strokes, pressing the muscles on either side of the shin bone, around the knee joint, and along the sides and front of the thigh right to the top of the leg.

29 Enfolding foot

Place one of your hands on your partner's sole and the other on the top of her foot. Now slide your hands in a warm enfolding stroke slowly along top and bottom until your fingertips slide off the tips of her toes. Repeat a few times and then move to the other leg and repeat the whole sequence from Step 27.

Connecting

At the end of a massage it always feels good to the receiver to have some long flowing strokes that link together all the parts of the body and give a sense of wholeness. Keep your touch light, but don't skip little bits as this will detract from the sense of completeness. Also, make sure that you travel to the very ends of the extremities of your partner's body. Another way of connecting is to link up any two parts of the body your hands feel drawn to. Finally, slowly break contact, gently cover your partner with a large warm towel, and leave her to rest and enjoy the feeling of relaxation for a while.

1 Connecting two parts

Sitting or kneeling at your partner's side, let one of your hands come to rest lightly on the belly and the other on the forehead. With your eyes closed just stay quietly in contact as you link body and head. Focus on your hands and the rhythm of your partner's breath. After a time, very slowly take your hands away.

2 Connecting strokes

Using middle and ring fingers of each hand, rest them on your partner's forehead. Then glide over the top of her head, down the back of her neck, along the shoulders, down the arms to the fingertips and off. Return to the forehead and repeat, but from the back of her neck come around to the front of the upper chest and then glide down, dividing at the belly and travelling down the legs to the tips of the toes and off.

HEAD

The head is the main control centre of the body, and in the protective cave of the skull lies the amazing brain – a vastly complex and mysterious organ. The head is also the seat of two of the *chakras*, or energy centres (see p.12), found along the centre line of the body. The Crown *chakra*, at the top of the head, is related to our essence and spirituality, and the Pineal or Brow *chakra*, at the centre of the forehead, is related to clear seeing, intuition and intellect. In a head-oriented culture, we sometimes find our mind racing and overloaded. Instead of clarity of thought we experience confusion and weariness. The result of this is often a headache. There are a variety of other causes for headaches – one of the commonest is stress, which can create tension in the muscles of the neck, shoulders and scalp. Other types of headache include those resulting from sinus congestion, colds or flu; menstrual-related headaches; headaches following whiplash or neck injury; and migraines – recurring, throbbing headaches, which may be accompanied by nausea or vomiting. Both massage and Shiatsu have effective treatments for headaches and head congestion, so in the following pages we have included helpful sequences from both.

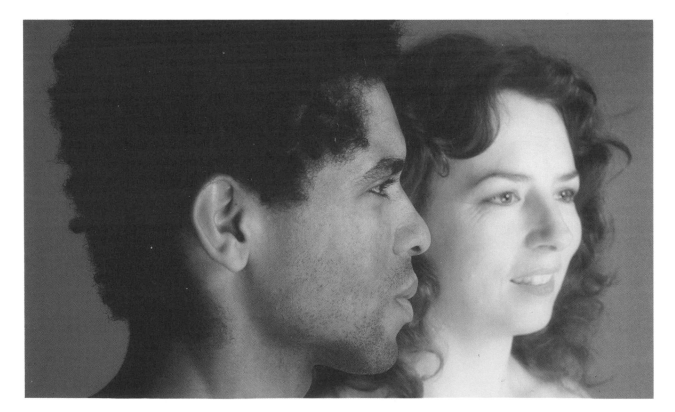

Headaches: massage

Since it is hard to distinguish between the different types of headaches, several massage sequences are given in the following pages and it is a good idea to try all the different strokes, focusing on those that seem to give your partner most comfort. On this page the receiver is lying down, and on pages 46 and 47 sitting up. The series of strokes on page 47 is a soothing and relaxing sequence taken from an ancient Indian healing massage. Camomile and lavender essences are both helpful for headaches (see p.21). Melissa is good for migraines and

Continued overleaf

1 Working forehead in strips

Kneel at your partner's head and rest your thumbs in the centre of her forehead just above her eyebrows, with your fingers around the sides of her head. Slowly and firmly draw your thumbs away from the centre, out toward the temples, the hairline and off. Work like this in strips right up the forehead until you cover the whole area.

2 Pressing and circling temples

Begin by pressing on your partner's temples, for ten seconds or so, with the flats of your fingers. Then slowly release the pressure and make slow circles over both the temples. Check with your partner whether she'd like a deeper or lighter touch.

3 Base of skull pressure

Turn your partner's head to rest comfortably on one hand, with her cheek facing upward. Using the fingertips of your free hand, push up and under the bone of the skull base. Hold, letting the pressure build up, then slowly release. Work right along the rim, searching out tense spots, then turn the head to the other side and repeat.

Continued from p.45

the stroke in Step 2 which circles the temples, may be particularly beneficial. It is also helpful to lie in a darkened room and apply a cold compress (see p.91) to the forehead. Many headaches will also respond well to the sequence given in Shoulders, Neck and Upper back (see pp.54-9). If you have had a whiplash injury and keep getting headaches, or if you have pain in your arm, it would be wise to see an osteopath or doctor to check for joint damage.

Caution*: If a headache comes on suddenly, is severe, and is accompanied by a very stiff neck or back, a fever, weakness in a limb, drowsiness or confusion, loss of vision and/or epileptic fits, seek medical help and advice at once.*

4 Massaging scalp along hairline

Stand behind your partner, allowing her head to rest against your body. With your hands in a "spider" shape, use the tips of your fingers to massage the scalp right along the hairline, from the top of the forehead around to the base of the skull. Travel slowly, using as much pressure as your partner needs.

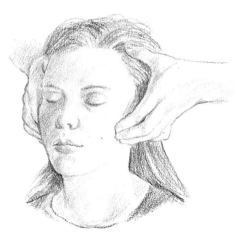

5 Pressing and circling jaw muscles

Rest the pads of your fingers on the jaw muscles. If you have difficulty finding them, rest your fingers on the cheeks and ask your partner to clench and unclench her teeth, which causes these muscles to rise and fall. Now begin to press and circle your fingers over the whole area of the jaw muscles. Work slowly and thoroughly to release tension.

6 Fingertip healing

Ask your partner to focus on her breath and let your fingertips come to rest very lightly in two vertical lines on either side of her forehead, above the middle of her eyebrows. Keep your shoulders relaxed, focus on your *hara* and maintain a light steady contact for a few minutes.

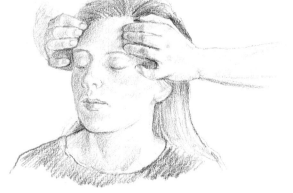

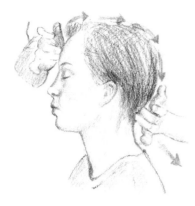

7 Stroking over top of head
Rest the middle and ring fingers of one hand on the middle of the forehead and those of the other in the hollow at the centre base of the skull. Now lightly stroke your fingers from the forehead up and across the centre line of the skull and down to meet the fingers at the base. Then pull both hands out and away from the body as if draining tension away from the back of the head. Repeat.

9 Stroking around hairline
Begin as before, your fingers touching at the centre of your partner's forehead. Then stroke gently straight up to her hairline. Divide your hands and draw your fingers right along the hairline, curve above the ears and around the rim of the skull to the centre base. When your fingers meet at the centre, pull them back away from the head as before. Repeat several times.

8 Stroking head to shoulders
Stand behind your partner and gently rest the same fingers of each hand on the centre of her forehead. Draw your fingers lightly up to the top of the head then divide your hands, coming down the sides of the head behind the ears, down the sides of the neck, along the tops of the shoulders, and off. Repeat the movement several times.

10 Face massage sequence
Starting at the centre of the forehead, and using the same fingers of each hand, stroke down and then out and right around each eye, down alongside the nose, then around the mouth, letting your fingers meet under the lower lip. Continue down to the chin tip then along the jaw bone, up and over the ears, along the rim of the skull to the centre base and off. Repeat a few times.

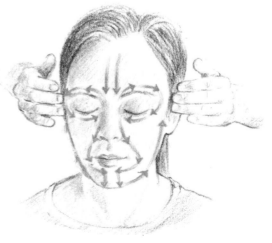

Headaches: Shiatsu

Headaches are frequently caused by poor digestion and inadequate elimination of toxins. Most of the meridians concerned with these functions run through the neck, shoulders, and upper back and any imbalances can affect different parts of the head. Working around the upper back, shoulders and neck, as shown here, will release stagnant energy in the appropriate meridians and help relieve headaches. Pressing tsubos on the meridian lines in other parts of the body, such as feet, legs, hands, arms and shoulders, can also help to relieve pain in the head, as in Step 6. If the tsubos are painful, hold them with light pressure, and agitate the point slightly in a comfortable way.

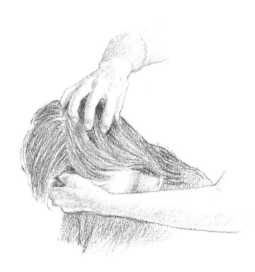

1 Shiatsu scalp massage
Bring your partner's head forward and support her forehead in your cupped palm. With your free hand begin to massage the whole of the scalp, using your thumbs and fingers in a slow shampooing motion that travels over the whole area. Focus your attention on the parts of the scalp that feel most tender to her.

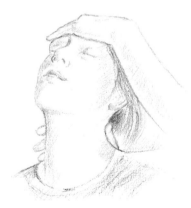

2 Shiatsu neck stretch
Support your partner from behind, with your elbows resting on the front of her shoulders, ease them slightly back. Place your hands on the back of her head while her head sinks forward to the point of resistance. Hold for up to 30 seconds, while she breathes deeply. Do not apply strong pressure.

3 Shiatsu neck side roll
With your partner's head still forward, cup her forehead with one hand and let the other support the back of the neck between stretched thumb and forefinger. Now slowly tilt the head back to rest on the hand supporting the neck and begin to roll it gently in a semi-circle from side to side. Finally return the head to an upright position.

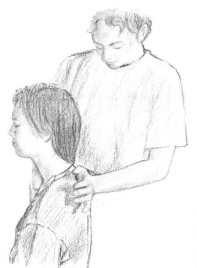

4 Shiatsu heel-of-hand massage
Stand beside your partner and place one of your hands on her upper chest. With the heel of your other hand, make firm circling and vibrating movements all over the area between the spine and the shoulder blade and up on to the muscles at the top of the shoulder. Reverse your position and repeat on the other side.

5 Shiatsu pressing top of shoulders
Stand behind your partner and place the balls of your thumbs on top of her shoulders, near to the neck, as shown below right. Use your body weight to apply pressure gradually, hold for a few seconds, then release slowly. Repeat the technique, moving outward along the shoulder, working the soft tissue between the bones.

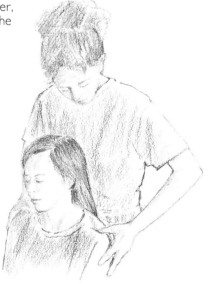

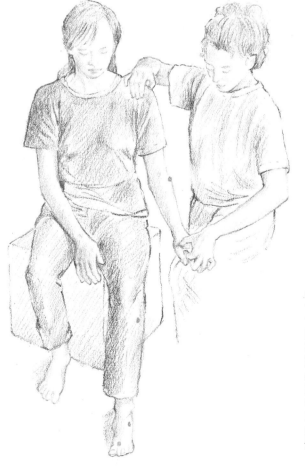

6 Shiatsu connecting points
Kneel, with one knee up, beside your partner. With one hand on her shoulder, use your other thumb and forefinger to squeeze gently into the fleshy part between the bones of her thumb and her forefinger. Meanwhile, press into the small indentation on the outside of the shoulder bone with your thumb. Hold for up to 30 seconds. Continue, using your thumbs, with light pressure, to connect up any points that are tender, as indicated in the illustration left.

Sinus congestion

The sinuses are air spaces in the skull that connect with the cavity inside the nose, and when the mucous membranes of the nose are inflamed or congested, the tiny passageways into the sinuses become blocked. This can lead to discomfort and inflammation in the sinuses, and may cause aching in the face or a headache. The following sequence works around and across the bones where the sinuses are located and should be done slowly and sensitively, with your partner lying down. Check that the amount of pressure you are using feels right. Use either marjoram or lavender essence here (see p.21).

1 Pressing around eye socket
With your partner lying down, rest the tips of your forefingers under the rims of her upper eye sockets, by her nose. Now push up and under the bones, build up pressure, hold and release. Move a step outward and repeat. Circle both eye sockets, using your thumbs to press the lower sockets.

2 Clearing cheek bones
Begin with your thumbs on the cheek bones, just below the eyes and next to the nose. Slowly and firmly sweep out in a curving line that travels out to the hairline and away. Move down a little way and repeat the stroke. Work in this way in strips down the cheek bones from side of nose to hairline, until you reach the base of the cheek bones.

3 Pressing under cheek bones
Using the tips of the first two fingers of each hand, start close to the sides of the nose, and press up under the rim of each cheek bone. Gradually build pressure, hold, then release. Move a step outward on each side and repeat the pressure. Continue along the edge of the bone until you get to the ears.

Colds

The common cold is a virus infection, and the probability of catching colds rises when your natural resistance is lowered. All you can really do is let a cold run its course. A face and head massage can help to clear congestion; any of the sequences in this section on the head may be useful. The two Shiatsu techniques shown work on the tsubos, *which help to clear congestion and aid elimination of mucus, and the In-Do point on the forehead, which relieves heaviness in the head caused both by colds and sinus problems. Rosemary or eucalyptus essences may be helpful (see p.21).*

1 Self-help oil rub
Use eucalyptus or rosemary essence (see p.21). Gently massage the oil into the whole area around your nose and sinuses. If you have a chesty cold, apply it to your upper chest as well. Use small, deep circling movements to rub the oil quite thoroughly into the skin.

3 Shiatsu In-Do point
Kneel and ask your partner to lie down, supporting her head on your knees. Place your middle fingertips, one resting on the other, between and very slightly higher than the eyebrows. With light pressure, move the skin sensitively in tiny circles over this *tsubo*. Use your lower fingertip to "sense" while the upper one subtly creates the movement.

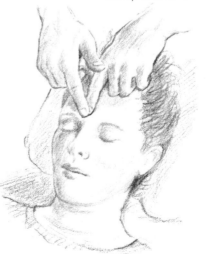

2 Shiatsu lung *tsubos*
Stand behind your partner, and let her lean against you. Curve both your hands over her shoulder joints so that your fingertips rest in the valleys between her shoulders and chest. Now move your fingers slightly forward on to the muscles and massage in small circles, applying pressure with your fingertips.

NECK, SHOULDERS AND UPPER BACK

Bridging the head and the shoulders, the neck is a busy junction where a huge amount of activity takes place. Major blood vessels in the neck link the body to the head. The spinal nerves travel through the vertebrae of the neck and on down the spine, carrying messages between the brain and all other parts of the body. And the throat houses the voice-box, as well as the passages for food and air. The shoulder joints have the widest range of movement in the body, and the whole shoulder and neck area can be easily strained by overuse, unwise lifting or sudden jarring movements. When we are under stress, it is the shoulder and neck muscles that tend to hold tension the most. This area also links with the Throat *chakra* (see p.12), which relates to the expression of feelings via arm or body movements, or through the voice. "Heart" feelings (see Heart *chakra* p.12) are also expressed through the arms. When we bottle up our feelings we actually tighten muscles in the throat, shoulder and chest area to hold them in. Tense raised shoulders can reflect fear, being the posture of the "startle reflex" when we galvanize ourselves to meet some real or imagined threat. For all these reasons this area often causes us discomfort.

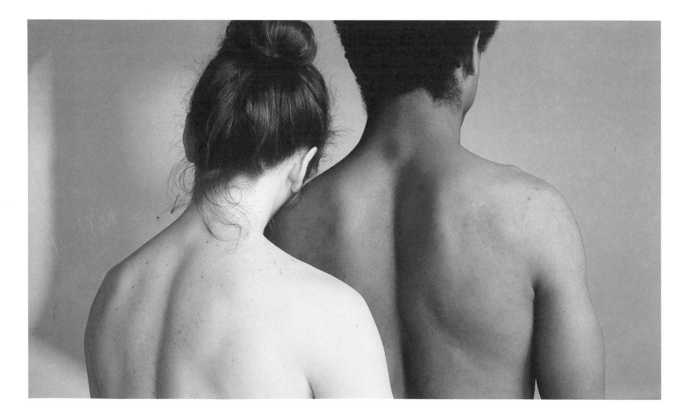

Neck stiffness, arthritis and strain

Stiffness in the neck may be caused by sleeping in an awkward position, or from getting very cold, from straining muscles or ligaments, by sudden jarring movements, or simply from being anxious. When applying the following massage strokes, keep your touch gentle but firm, always remain within the threshold of pain, and go slowly. If your partner has arthritis of the neck (see p.92) omit Steps 4 and 8, p.54-5. Try rosemary essence (see p.21). Compresses (see p.91) can also be helpful for neckache.

I Stroking and stretching back of neck

With your partner lying on her back use both hands alternately to stroke up the back of the neck from base to skull. Then cup your hands under the back of the head and pull toward you, stretching the neck. Make sure your thumbs don't drag on the ears. Now glide your hands along the back of the head and slide off at the top.

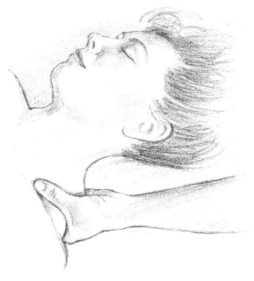

2 Turning head and circling back of neck

First cup both your hands around and under your partner's skull, with your thumbs resting in front of the ears. Then slightly lift and gently turn the head to rest on one of your cupped hands. Check that the position feels comfortable. Now use your free hand to massage the back of the neck in slow firm circles, moving right up to the skull base.

3 Kneading muscle at base of neck

Slide your hand down one side of the neck and grasp the muscle at the top of the shoulder between your fingers and thumb. Slowly squeeze and knead the muscle, pushing your fingers underneath it with circling movements to reach different parts. Ask your partner to say what feels particularly good. Repeat from Step 2 on the other side.

4 Stretching side of neck
Cup one of your hands under your partner's skull and draw her head sideways toward her shoulder. Now use your free hand, fingers pointing toward the floor, to glide down the side of the neck and along the shoulder to the top of the shoulder joint, as shown. Press firmly down toward her hand, stretching the side of the neck between your two hands. Then glide back up the shoulder and neck and repeat the stretch twice more. Now reverse your hands and stretch the other side of the neck.

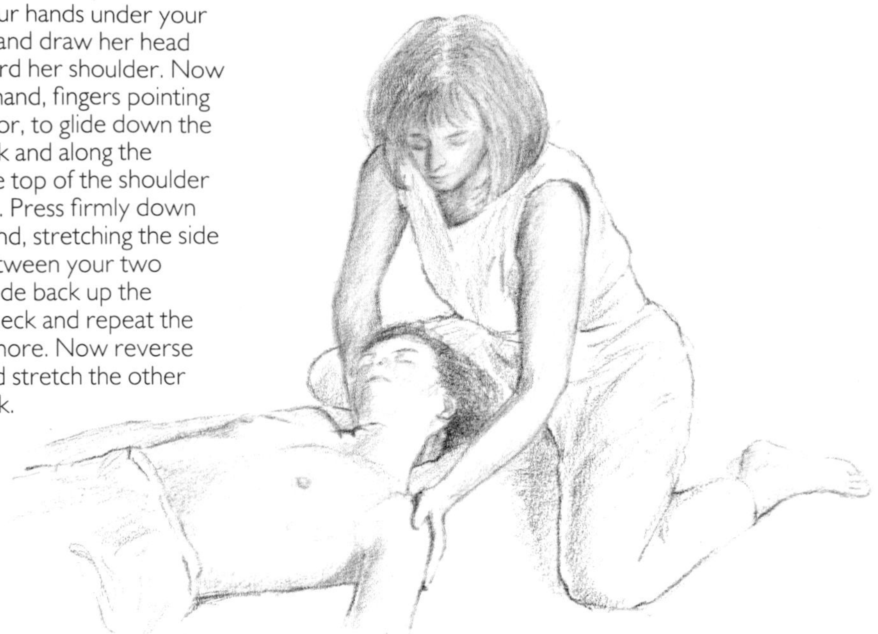

5 Stretching neck forward and backward
Cup both your hands under your partner's skull and slowly lift her head forward, chin toward chest, to the point of resistance, as shown left. Bring her head down again and repeat. Now cup one hand under the skull, the other on top of her head, fingers pointing toward the floor, as shown below. Tilt the head right back so the chin comes up as high as possible. Release and stretch again. Then bring her head gently back to rest.

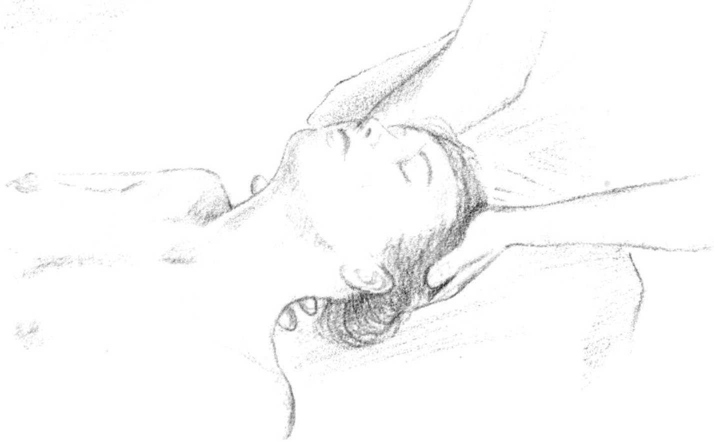

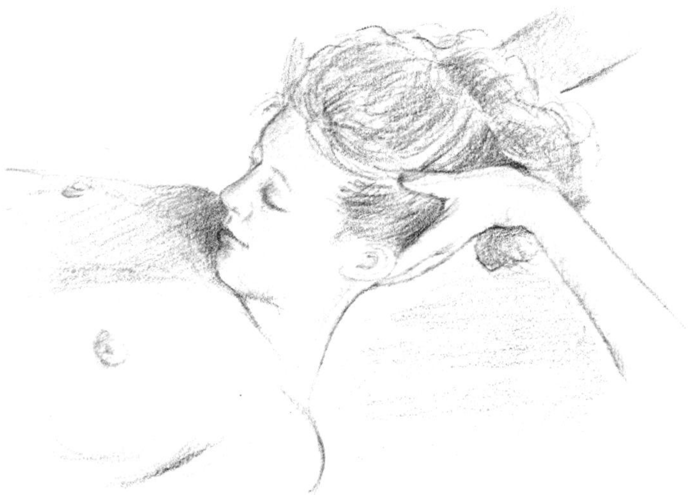

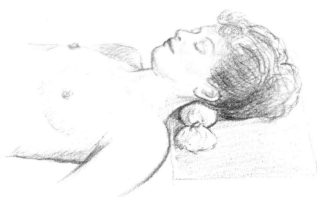

6 Self-help for arthritis and aching neck

Put two tennis balls into a sock and knot the end. Lie down with the balls at the top of your neck, just below the rim of your skull, one on each side. Do this for about five minutes a day. It can be very soothing for aching necks or osteoarthritis.

Caution: If you feel dizzy or experience pain, stop at once.

7 Neck massage with partner sitting

Let your partner sit at a table, supporting her head with her hands. Gently squeeze and stroke the back and sides of her neck with rhythmical movements. Move slowly, letting your partner be your guide for the amount of pressure needed. Try also massaging the upper shoulders and base of the neck with slow, firm kneading strokes, as this is a continuation of the neck muscle.

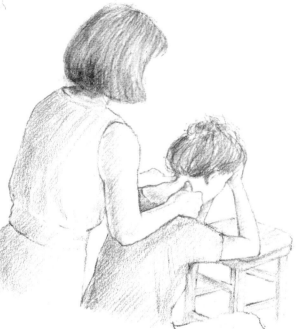

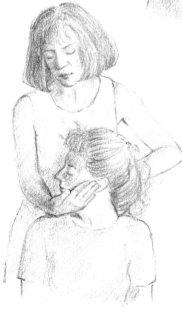

8 Rotating the neck

Stand behind your seated partner and put your wrist under her chin, your hand cradling her cheek. Cup the opposite side of her head with your other hand. Now slowly turn the head by simultaneously pulling the cheek and pushing against the side of the head until you reach the point of resistance. Release the head a little, and then take it back to the resistance point two more times. Then reverse the positions of your two hands and repeat the stroke on the other side.

1 Circling shoulder blade

Kneel at your partner's side, facing her head. Lift her hand on to her lower back and cup your outermost hand under her shoulder. Now cup your free hand over the top of the shoulder, close to the neck, and firmly lift the muscle. Then continue down along the edge of the shoulder blade, pushing in under the rim. Circle around the blade and back to the top of the shoulder. Repeat several times.

Upper back and shoulder stiffness or pain

Stiffness in the upper back can be caused by muscle strain or arthritis. Emotional stress can also cause tightness in the muscles, as can spending long hours sitting at a desk or making repetitive arm movements. In Shiatsu, the upper back relates to the lungs and heart, so by working here you can influence these organs and help treat such ailments as asthma or bronchial complaints. Try bergamot or rosemary essence here (see p.21). *Muscular pain in this area can also be eased using compresses (see p.91).*

Caution: *Before treating arthritic or injured joints see pp:90-3.*

2 Pressing flat of blade and squeezing along ridge

With the heel of your free hand, push slowly and firmly up the flat of the blade from base to top until your hand meets the ridge of bone running along the top of the blade. Clasp your fingers around the top of the ridge and squeeze your hand out toward the shoulder joint. Repeat the whole movement several times.

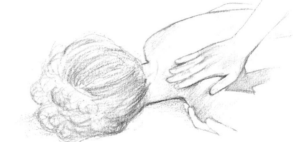

3 Rotating shoulder joint

Cup your outermost hand under your partner's shoulder joint, while your other hand holds her upper arm just above the elbow. Now start to lift and rotate the shoulder joint in a large slow circle, going to the point of resistance all the way around. After several circulations change direction and rotate the shoulder the other way. Repeat on the other side from Step 1.

4 "Sandwiching" out to shoulder joint

With your partner lying on her back, sit at her side facing toward her shoulders. Place one hand under her upper back at the base of the neck and the other hand on the centre of her chest, just below the collar bone. Slowly and firmly draw your hands toward you, squeezing out toward the shoulder joint. Repeat the stroke several times.

5 Kneading top of shoulder and joint

Begin to do some broad strokes from the neck along the top of the shoulder toward the joint. Use both hands alternately to squeeze and stroke along the muscle, and then spend some time working slowly around the joint, pressing into the soft tissue between the bones with your thumbs and fingers.

6 Stretching shoulder joint

Kneel by your partner's side, facing toward her head. Take hold of her wrist and hand between both of yours, with your thumbs in her palm. Now lift her arm and stretch it away from you up and out above her head. Release the pressure and then stretch again two or three times. Let the arm down to rest by the side and then repeat the stroke on the other side from Step 4.

7 Pulling up along spinal muscles
Sit at your partner's head and push both hands about a hand's length under the back on either side of the spine. Press up with the pads of your fingers into the muscles close to each side of the spine, then slowly draw your hands up along these muscles to the base of the neck, ironing out knots of tension. (See vertical arrows below.) Repeat several times.

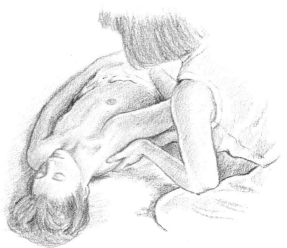

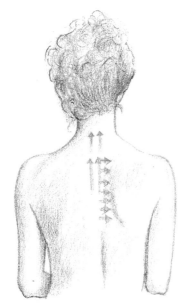

8 Pressing near spine and shaking shoulder
Sit facing your partner's side, at shoulder level. Push both hands under the shoulder blade until your fingertips reach the spine, as shown below left. With the pads of your fingers slowly press up into the muscles close to the spine. Press different areas alongside the upper spine. Now pull your hands toward you, to the rim of the shoulder blade (see horizontal arrows left) and lift and shake the whole shoulder quite vigorously, as shown below right. Repeat on the other side.

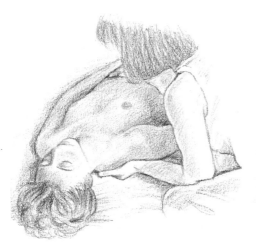

1 Shiatsu thumb pressure down bladder meridian

With your partner lying on her front, sit at her head and place the pads of your thumbs on either side of her spine, at the top of her upper back. Gradually apply pressure by moving your weight on to your thumbs. Hold for a moment or two, then release slowly and move in this way down her upper back. Repeat this technique three times.

Upper back stiffness and pain: Shiatsu

Deep pressure down the bladder meridians in the upper back will relax this whole area and will affect the functioning of the lungs and heart. Weakness in the front of the shoulders often causes tightness in the upper back meridians and muscles. These stretching techniques will open the upper chest and help relieve this stiffness. The back needs to be seen as a whole, however, since pain in the upper back can also be caused by lumbar problems. Whenever possible treat the mid and lower back areas too.

2 Shiatsu upper back stretch

Ask your partner to sit back on her heels and stretch her arms over your thighs. Encourage her to relax her neck and back and place the sides of your hands either side of her spine at the base of her neck. Move from your *hara* to increase the pressure through your hands and work slowly and carefully down the muscles of her upper back.

3 Shiatsu elbow stretch

With your partner sitting cross-legged or on her heels, ask her to put her hands behind her head, with fingers interlaced. Standing behind her, place the side of one of your legs against her back and cup her elbows in your hands. Ask her to breathe out and gently stretch her elbows back as you brace her back with your leg. Hold, then release. Repeat two or three times.

CHEST

The chest is the emotional centre of the body, housing our Heart *chakra* (see p.12), which relates to compassion, love and self-development. It is also the centre of breathing and if our chest is not constricted by tension, the ribcage expands and contracts freely as we inhale and exhale. Any tension in the chest area will restrict the breath and hence limit the amount of oxygen that we take in and use. Chest problems are often due to bottling up feelings – hence the expression "get it off your chest". Asthma attacks, though often an allergic reaction, may also be triggered by anxiety and upset. Those who suffer from chest problems can try cutting down dairy produce (thought to create mucus) and those who smoke should give it up. The following pages contain strokes that will help loosen mucus from the chest, and others that will aid and deepen the breathing. When massaging this area, bear in mind that the front of the body is more vulnerable and "open" than the back. Before beginning, rest both hands gently on your partner's chest and tune in to the breathing rhythm. If your partner is undressed, oil and soothe the chest first, using the strokes from the whole body massage (see p. 41).

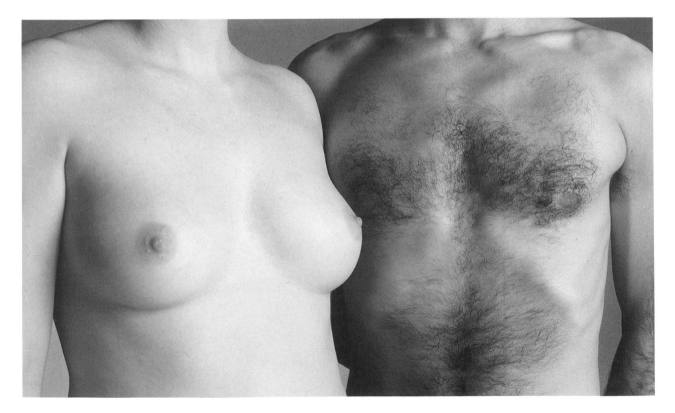

Chest congestion

*These strokes will help to relieve
any tension in the chest caused by
bronchial infections and asthma.
Easing the muscles alongside the
spine will affect the nerves leading
to all the organs of the chest. Try
bergamot or eucalyptus essences
here (see p.21). The percussion
strokes create vibration in the
chest cavity and lungs and can help
to loosen mucus and phlegm from
the bronchial tubes. For these
(Steps 2 and 3) your partner needs
a cushion under his belly so that his
upper body is lower than his hips.*

1 Pushing muscles at side of spine

Kneel up, facing your partner's side.
Leaning from your hips, place the
heels of your hands just beyond the
far edge of the spine at the top. Let
your weight press down as you slide
your hands outward across the ridge
of muscle. Repeat this stroke, moving
slowly down to the base of the ribs.
Repeat on the other side.

2 Cupping on ribs

Put your hands into a cupped
position (see p.26). Then, with loose
wrists, begin a rapid alternating
clapping stroke over the whole far
side of your partner's ribcage, from
bottom to top and back again. Avoid
working directly on the spine itself.
Cupping on the upper back area
affects the upper lobes of the lungs.
Change sides and repeat on the
other side of the chest.

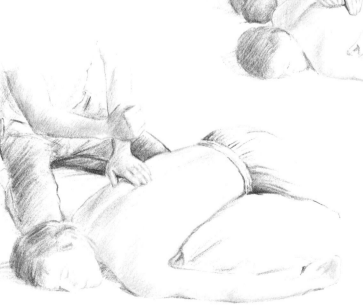

3 Thumping alongside spine

Place the flats of your fingers on the
ridge of muscle nearest to you, at the
side of the spine. Starting at the mid
back, thump the back of your fingers
quite rapidly, with your other hand
in a loose fist, while sliding your
fingers up alongside the spine (not
directly on it), until you reach the
base of the neck. Then thump down
to the start again. Adapt your
pressure to your partner's wishes.
Repeat on the other side.

Breathing exercise for chest problems

This is a breathing exercise that derives from bioenergetics, and although it is accompanied here by a partner, it can be equally effective done by yourself. Rocking the pelvis as you breathe helps to exaggerate healthy respiratory movements. The movement also helps you to fill and empty the lungs fully. Here we give instructions separately for giver and receiver, but it is up to the giver to keep time with the receiver, and not the other way around.

1 Breathing exercise with pelvic movements (for receiver alone)

Lie on your back, with your knees up and feet shoulder-width apart. Inhale, rocking your pelvis back so that your sacrum presses into the floor and your lower back hollows (see receiver in illustration above). Then exhale fully, letting your pelvis swing forward in the opposite direction, so that your tail bone lifts a little way off the floor (see receiver below). Repeat several times, then rest.

2 Co-ordinating stroke (for giver)

Sit at your partner's hips and watch his breathing pattern. Place your hands on his belly. As he inhales, glide up the centre of his body to the top of the chest and over the shoulders (see above), and as he exhales slide your hands down the sides of his chest, applying some pressure as air is expelled (see below). Repeat several times.

Coughs, bronchitis and asthma: Shiatsu

Circulatory and respiratory functions take place in the chest and Shiatsu will increase the energy to these two vital systems, encouraging the elimination of toxins and mucus. Rounded shoulders and a hunched back are indications that the person is protecting a weak chest. Work with care and respect as this area is the centre of emotions and can be vulnerable in many people. The technique shown in Step 2 should not be used on asthma sufferers.

1 Shiatsu pressing down on shoulders
Kneeling at your partner's head, cup the tops of his shoulder joints and rest the heels of your hands in the valleys between shoulders and chest. With straight arms bring your body over your hands and lean some of your weight down on to his shoulders. Hold for five seconds and release. Repeat twice more.

2 Shiatsu chest release
Kneel at your partner's head and place the heels of both hands beneath his collar bone. As he takes a deep breath in, apply pressure against the rise of his chest. Then suddenly release your pressure before he reaches full inhalation. To encourage full exhalation, gently lean your body weight through your hands on to his chest. Repeat the sequence twice.

3 Shiatsu centring technique
Support your partner's head on your knees and stroke through his hair, resting your fingers on top of his head. Place the fingers of your other hand softly on the base of his breast bone and pause. Now move your fingers slowly up the bone, pausing as he exhales and moving only with his inhalation.

ARMS AND HANDS

Our arms are crucial for our survival and how we relate to the world. Ever since we stood upright during the process of evolution we have been able to use our arms for a whole variety of activities, aided especially by our "opposable" thumbs. These thumbs probably make our hands the most skilful biological organs to have evolved. Our arms and hands are also vehicles of self-expression. They relate to the Throat and Heart *chakras* (see p.12) and with them we are able to express a huge range of feelings – from reaching out tenderly in love and affection, to expressing hatred and rage by beating or hitting, to warding off danger. As the arms, wrists and hands are so mobile and are used constantly in everyday activities, the joints and muscles can be subject to sprains or strains if they are stressed or overstretched (see p.90). These injuries can respond well to massage in their recuperative stages. Tennis elbow is a common strain of the arm for which we have given a massage sequence here. Hands and arms can also sometimes suffer from cramps, and the joints from rheumatic complaints such as arthritis (see p.92). Careful working with massage around the joints of the hand can bring relief and comfort.

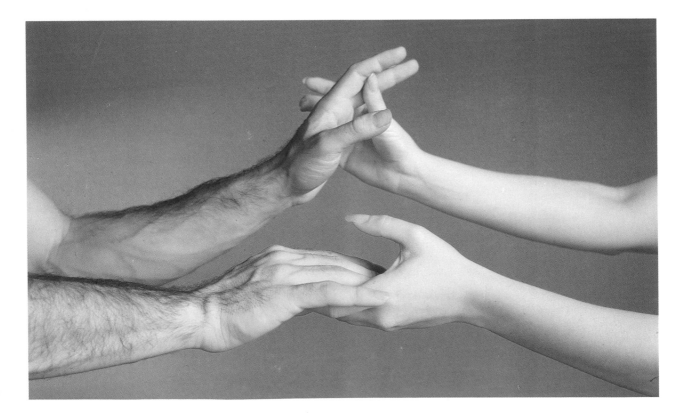

Tennis elbow, cramp, strains

Tennis elbow is a strain caused by overstretching the muscles and tendons of the forearm at the outer side of the elbow, and pain is felt when the person grips or bends the arm when lifting heavy things. This strain can also happen after overuse in such activities as sawing. This sequence can be particularly helpful after an initial rest period and ice treatment (see p.91). Wait for one to two days before massaging. The sequence can also be helpful for cramp (see also p.85) or aching arms. Use rosemary essence here (see p.21).

Caution: *Before treating arthritic or injured joints see pp.90-3.*

1 Kneading arms
With your partner lying down, face his side and begin to knead his upper arm with firm, rhythmical squeezing strokes. Travel right down to his wrist, giving special attention to the muscles of the forearm, just below the elbow. Knead thoroughly up and down the arm two or three times.

2 Massage around elbow joint
Support your partner's arm on your knee, so that his elbow is slightly raised. Now begin to work slowly with your thumbs and fingers around the whole joint, paying special attention to the outer (lateral) part of the elbow. Stay focused on the underlying structures, but if there is soreness, work with sensitivity.

3 Thumbing across fibres of forearm
Slightly raise your partner's lower arm and work first up the back, and then the front, of his forearm from the wrist with slow, firm thumb movements that push alternately upward and outward, crossing the fibres of the muscles that run down the arm. Give extra attention to the area just below the elbow.

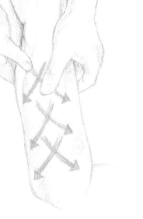

Hand and wrist problems

Arthritic hands can benefit from gentle and sensitive massage around the joints. The sequence on these two pages may be useful and your partner can either lie or sit. Writer's cramp is muscle fatigue arising from any sustained, repetitive movement of the hand. Try out the strokes shown here, along with the hand massages from Whole Body (see p.40), to see which feel best. Fingers and thumbs can suffer from sprains or strains (see p.90) and massage can help healing and mobility in the recovery period.

Caution: *Before treating arthritic or injured joints see pp.90-3.*

1 Wrist rolling

Support your partner's forearm in an upright position, with your palms on the back and front of his wrist. Now move your hands rapidly back and forth, rolling his wrist between them as you go. His hand should flop loosely as you do this stroke.

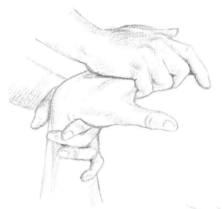

2 Flexing wrist

With his arm still upright, next stretch the back of the wrist. Support his hand by holding his wrist. With your free hand press down with your palm on the back of his hand. Do this slowly and carefully as you can reach the point of resistance quite quickly.

4 Opening the palm

Let your partner's palm face the floor and place the heels of your hands on the back of his hand and your fingers in his palm. Now press down with the heels of your hands and firmly lift with your fingers so that you open and spread the bones of his palm.

3 Extending wrist

With his arm in the same position, now stretch the front of his wrist by pushing down on his palm with your own palm. Press slowly to the point of resistance, then release. While you are doing this support his lower arm with your other hand.

5 Squeezing along channels
Holding your partner's hand in one hand, use the thumb and first finger of your other hand to squeeze along the channels between the bones. Press in firmly from both sides and work slowly along the groove from wrist to web of finger. It is easier to work two channels with one hand and two with the other.

6 Extending fingers
Stretch the inside of his knuckle joints by pressing your thumb on the back of his knuckle, with your other hand pushing the fingertip slowly backward till you reach the point of resistance. Ask your partner to say "when". Extend each finger in turn.

8 Stretching fingers
Begin, as before, by clasping the whole of your partner's finger, but this time begin to squeeze, wring, and stretch down the whole length of the finger to the tip and off, as shown below. Give firmest pressure on the root and especially along the ligaments at the sides of the finger.

7 Circling knuckle joint
Holding your partner's hand with one hand, clasp and isolate one of your partner's fingers by wrapping all the fingers of your other hand firmly around it, as shown above. Use your thumb to slowly circle around the knuckle joint, pushing into the softer tissue. Work each knuckle in this way, including the thumb.

STOMACH AND BELLY

The stomach and belly are a soft, sensitive, muscle-covered area of the body, unprotected by encircling bones (though the lower abdomen is in part protected by the bowl of the pelvis). Long ago, when we first became upright, we exposed our tender bellies to the world. This made us more vulnerable, but also able to relate more sensitively to one another. The stomach is also linked to the Solar Plexus *chakra* (see p.12), which is the seat of raw emotional energy, often of fear, but also of change and transmutation. Also on this level is the diaphragm, which separates chest from abdomen. Our breathing pattern is a vital gauge of our physical and emotional health. Stomach problems, such as indigestion, are often linked to anxiety and emotional causes; a surge of adrenalin can provoke a sudden sick feeling in the stomach. The belly houses the gut and also our "gut feelings". The *Hara chakra*, just below the navel, is our centre of gravity, strength and vitality. This is the centre from which we "ground" ourselves through our legs (see p.19). It is also closely linked with our sexuality. Tension and congestion here may cause constipation, flatulence or menstrual pain. Both massage and Shiatsu can help to ease complaints in the abdominal area.

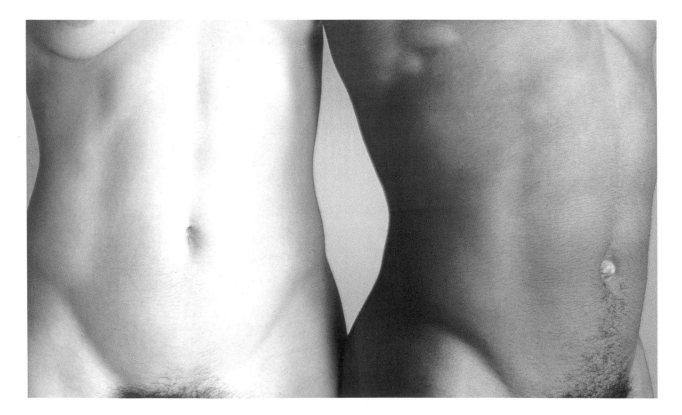

Indigestion and nausea

Indigestion can be the result of acid over-production due to stress, or eating too much, or foods that don't agree with us. The following strokes and techniques can help to soothe the discomfort. The vulnerable stomach must be worked on slowly, with great sensitivity. Camomile or cardamom essences (see p.21) can be helpful. Step 5 works by increasing the energy flow by linking the stomach with the stomach meridian. Step 6 is specifically for nausea and releases tightness in the area caused by stress.

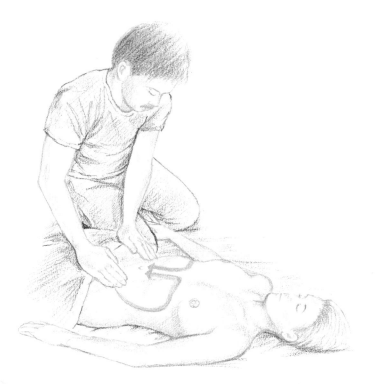

1 Light circling on sides and stomach
Kneel beside your partner's hip, facing her head, and rest your hands gently just inside her two hip bones. Now very lightly stroke up the sides of her torso, then across the lower ribs under her breasts. Stroke especially lightly down the centre, ending at the hip bones. Repeat the circling several times.

2 Gentle stroking down from ribs
Start at one side of your partner's ribcage and begin to glide your hands smoothly downward, one after the other. Move over the lower ribs, the base of the ribs, and on to the abdomen, with very light, slow strokes. Work right across the lower ribcage and repeat several times.

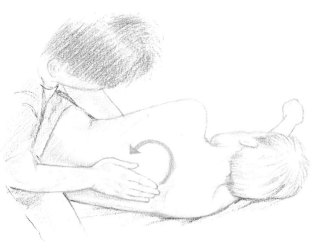

3 Holding stomach and circling back
With your partner lying on one side kneel by her back and rest one hand on her stomach just below her breast bone. With your other hand circle the mid back opposite your holding hand, in a counterclockwise direction. As you circle, relax your hand and stay present. Move your hand slowly, flowing over the forms.

4 Working under ribs
Kneel at your partner's right side and begin to press gently, but also fairly deeply, under her ribs on the left side. Keep the whole of your hands in gentle contact, and use your thumbs and the flats of your fingers to circle and press along under the bony ridge from left to right across the body. Keep your massage slow, smooth, and very sensitive here, remaining always within the threshold of pain.

5 Shiatsu pressing down stomach meridian
Kneel by your partner and turn her leg inward by holding her foot with your foot. With your "mother hand" placed over the stomach area above the navel, palm down the front of her thigh with your active hand by leaning in with your body weight. Move slowly and repeat three times.

6 Shiatsu stroking along base of ribs
With your partner standing up stand behind her and bring your arms around her sides, letting your fingertips meet at the solar plexus. Now very lightly sweep both hands slowly out and away below the ribs and off the sides of the body. Repeat the technique several times.

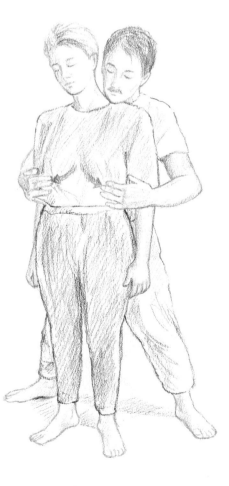

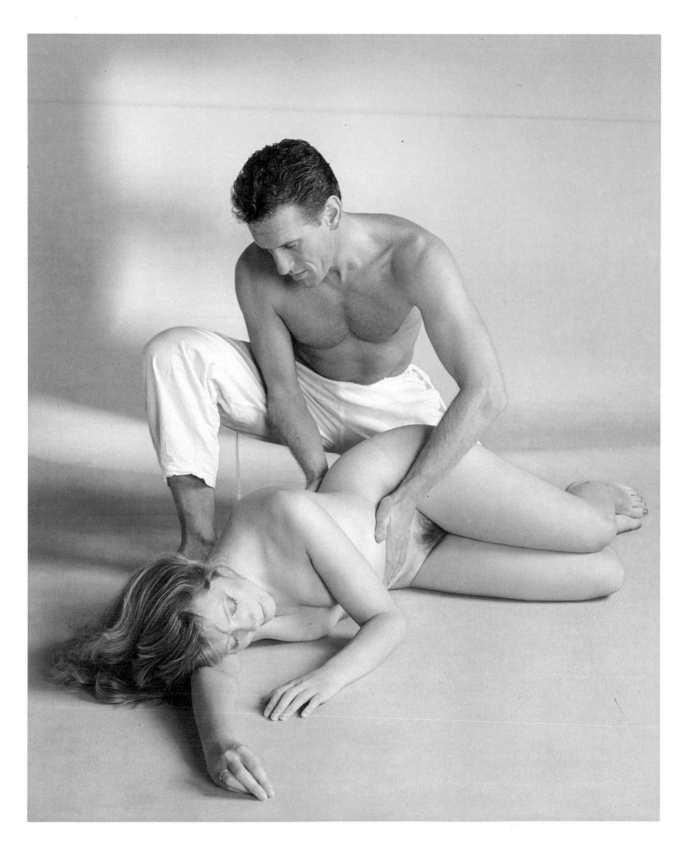

Constipation and flatulence

Constipation can be caused by lack of fibre in the diet, by emotional factors or by an inadequate fluid intake. Flatulence is a buildup of gases resulting in distention and discomfort. The first stroke (Step 1) works specifically with the colon and follows the direction of its wavelike muscular movements, which help to pass digested food along inside in a clockwise direction. With all these strokes on the belly area you should start lightly and gradually work in more deeply, with care and sensitivity. Always move slowly and stay aware of what your hands are sensing. Marjoram or fennel essences are suggested (see p.21).

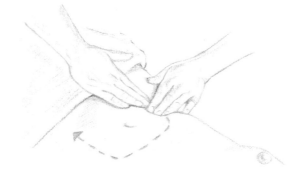

1 Working around colon
Kneel at your partner's right side and rest both your hands on the right of her lower abdomen. Start to work slowly upward with small firm circling strokes. Follow the direction of the colon, up to the right lower ribs, across to the left and then down to the inside of the left hip bone. Slide lightly across to the right side again and repeat.

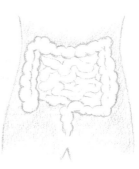

2 Pulling up sides
Reach across to your partner's far side and begin to pull up the side with slow generous strokes, your hands alternating and overlapping as they cover the area between ribs and hips. The movement should slightly lift and rock your partner. Let the stroke come from your pelvis. Repeat on the other side.

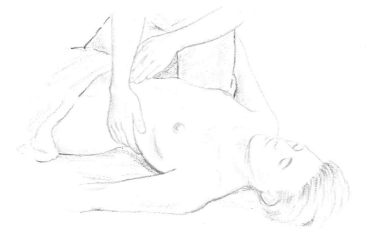

3 "Wave kneading" of belly
Lightly rest your hands on the centre of your partner's belly, one on top of the other. Using the heels of your hands push away across the belly and then let your hands curve over like a wave, so that your fingers come into contact and begin to pull back toward you. Continue to rock slowly back and forth rhythmically in this way for a short time.

Menstrual pain

Painful periods usually result from hormonal imbalances in the body, and you might find it helpful to use some of these techniques to relieve tension in the area. Begin with slow circling on the sacrum, as this is very soothing. The sacral bone contains several pairs of holes from which nerves issue, and pressing these will help to relieve congestion. Rocking the pelvis relaxes the whole body and loosens the pelvic area. Massaging the legs can also help to relieve menstrual pain. Try using either camomile or jasmine essence (see p.21) for this problem.

Caution: *Seek medical advice if menstrual pain is persistent and/or severe.*

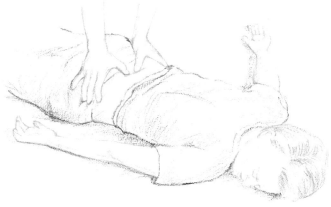

I Holding belly and circling sacrum

With your partner lying curled on her side, kneel behind her and rest one hand gently on her lower abdomen, below the navel. With your other hand circle slowly, counterclockwise, over the sacrum and lower back area. Keep your hands and shoulders relaxed and stay centred and aware.

2 Pressing into sacrum

With your partner lying on her front, kneel on one side of her thighs and place your thumbs at the top of her sacrum, keeping your fingers in contact with the body. Locate the two upper indentations and, coming forward from your *hara*, lean in with your thumbs. Hold for a moment and move on down the sacrum to the base, pressing in the same way.

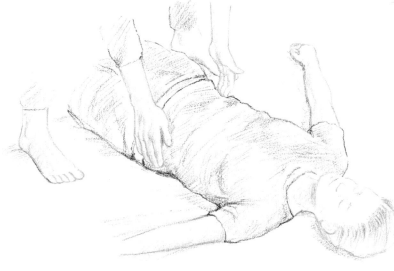

3 Rocking pelvis

Ask your partner to lie on her back and stand with one foot either side of her legs. Bend your knees and drop forward from your *hara*. Using your palms, start to rock her hips rhythmically from side to side. Once you have found a comfortable rhythm the rocking motion needs only a light touch to maintain it.

MID AND LOWER BACK

The back is the strength area of the body. Yet despite its strength more people have a back problem at some time in their lives than any other ailment. Lack of regular exercise, poor posture, tension and stress all contribute to our backs' proneness to aches and strains, and sometimes to more serious problems. One of these, the "slipped disc" occurs when the pad of cartilage between two vertebrae ruptures and some of the gel-like nucleus protrudes and presses against a nerve. Yet this is not always the cause of back pain. The large muscles of the back can suffer from strains that massage can often ease. The mid-back area relates to the Solar Plexus *chakra*, which is linked with emotion and change, and the lower back connects with both the *Hara* (strength, vitality and sexuality) and the Root *chakra* (our work, grounding and basic life situation – see p.12). Many back problems, and particularly those located in the lower back area, seem to have emotional causes, often linked to energy blocks and withheld mobility in the pelvic area. Since it is so vital to your back's health to have sufficient flexibility in the joints and muscles, we have included exercises to help your back to regain or retain its suppleness.

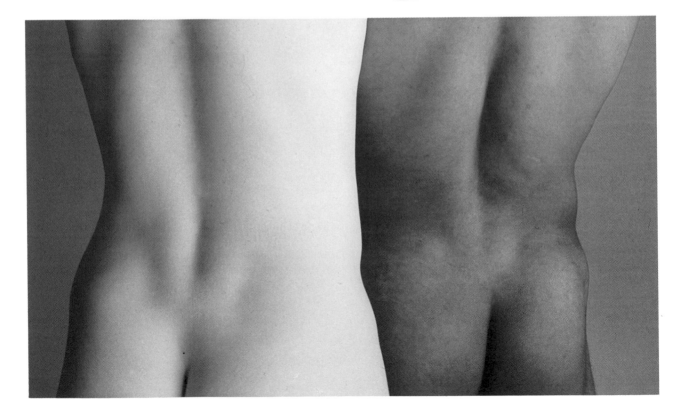

Mid backache
Aching in the mid back is often caused by tightness in the vertical bands of muscle on either side of the spine. Begin with slow gliding strokes and then move on to Steps 1 and 2, which work directly on the spinal muscles, Step 1 pushes up along the grain of the muscle and Step 2 works out across the fibres with the heels of your hands. Step 3 is performed with the soft inner parts of your forearms, and stretches the whole area with broad comforting movements. Try marjoram essence here (see p.21).

1 Pushing along spinal muscles
Kneel beside your partner's hips and rest one hand on his sacrum. Using the heel of your other hand, begin to push up very slowly along the ridge of muscle on one side of the spine, covering the whole mid-back area. Repeat several times along both sides of the spine, using your body weight to push up along the muscles.

2 Pushing across spinal muscles
Kneeling at your partner's side, knees apart, rest the heels of both your hands on the muscles at the far side of his spine, just below his shoulder blades. Lifting your hips up and forward, use some of your weight to push slowly out across the ridge of muscle. Move down the mid back in this way, then change sides and repeat the stroke.

3 Forearm stretch
Kneeling by your partner, rest the insides of your forearms on his mid back. Then glide them apart, one to the top of the neck and the other to the bottom of the sacrum. Start again at the mid back, but now glide your arms apart diagonally, so that one goes over one shoulder, the other over the opposite buttock. Repeat the stroke over the other buttock and shoulder.

Lower backache

Lower back pain is one of the commonest of all the ailments treated in this book. As well as these massage strokes, which can be done in combination with lumbar circling (see Step 2, p.34), we show some useful stretching techniques. In Step 3 the receiver curls up in the yoga "child's pose" – if this is not comfortable you can achieve a similar effect by pressing down on your partner's knees (see Step 2, opposite page). Try rosemary essence (see p.21) for pain in this area.

Caution*: If back pain is severe and acute or if there are any other medical symptoms, consult a doctor, osteopath or chiropractor.*

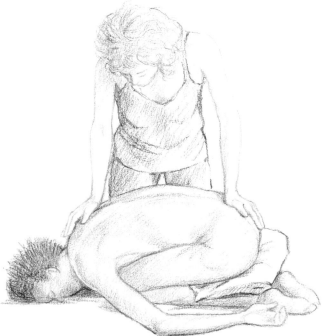

1 Circling sacrum
Kneel by your partner and rest both hands, one on top of the other, on his sacrum, as shown above. Now, transferring some of your weight forward on to your hands, start slow counterclockwise circles on the sacrum. Gradually extend them upward on to his lower back area, returning each time to the sacrum. Check how much pressure your partner prefers.

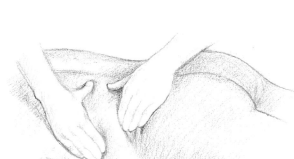

2 Kneading lower back
Now, using large, rhythmical rocking movements, knead the whole of your partner's lower back area on the opposite side, from work surface to spine. Use generous grasping and squeezing movements, with the whole of your hands, to work into the muscles slowly and thoroughly. Repeat on the other side.

3 "Child's pose" and back stretch
Ask your partner to kneel down with his forehead on the floor in the yoga "child's pose". If this is difficult, place a cushion between his buttocks and heels. Kneel by his side and rest one hand on the upper spine and the other on the base. Now press down so your hands push in opposite directions, stretching the spine.

1 Shiatsu back swing

With your partner lying on his back, stand astride his legs and raise his knees. Your feet should be shoulder-width apart and your knees bent. Now, using your forearms, lift his lower legs below the knees, resting your elbows on your own bent knees. Feel yourself firmly rooted on both legs, and sit back slowly on to your partner's feet. This will lift his pelvis an inch or two off the floor. Now swing his whole lower body gently from side to side.

Lower backache: Shiatsu

Shiatsu of the lower back aims to relax distorted muscles and so allow realignment of vertebrae. Pain in the lumbar area can be the effect of imbalance in the functioning of the kidneys, small intestines and the organs in the pelvis. Tight hamstrings also put extra stress on lower back muscles and techniques that stretch and loosen the back and legs as well as strengthening the hara will be beneficial. The lower back is an area that is weak in many people, so work slowly, with care, synchronizing your breath with your partner's and with your own movements, exhaling as you apply pressure.

2 Shiatsu pressing knees to chest

Begin as above, but this time rest your hands on the fronts of both your partner's knees, keeping your own knees bent and your shoulders relaxed. Use some of your weight to lean gently down, pressing his knees slowly toward his chest. Do not force past the point of resistance. Hold for a moment or two then release slowly.

3 Shiatsu holding *hara* and lower back

Kneeling beside your partner, slide one hand beneath his lower back, palm upward, and rest the other on his lower abdomen, or *hara*, just below the navel. Relax and tune in to your partner's breath. Imagine your hands are channels for healing energy that flows effortlessly through them. Hold for up to three minutes.

Sciatica

Sciatica is a sharp shooting pain felt in the legs and/or buttocks and back (usually on one side only), sometimes accompanied by a tingling in the corresponding leg or foot. It is caused when a disc bulges out between the vertebrae and presses against the sciatic nerve. Most disc protrusions heal themselves, given enough time and rest, and some of the strokes shown here may help to assist the healing process. Try the different movements and focus on those that afford most relief. Work slowly and be guided by your partner for the amount of pressure to use. Camomile or lavender essences (see p.21) may be helpful.

Caution: *If sciatic pain is persistent and severe and/or on both sides seek help from your doctor or an osteopath.*

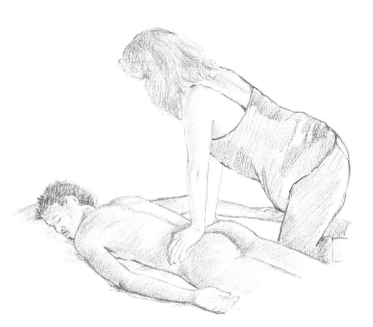

1 Stretching to sides of sacrum
With your partner lying face down kneel by one thigh, facing his head. Place the heels of both your hands on his sacrum, with your fingers pointing outward. Now raise your pelvis and lean slowly forward on to your hands. Then gradually slide your hands away from his sacrum, out across the sides of his buttocks and off. Return to the sacrum and repeat a few times.

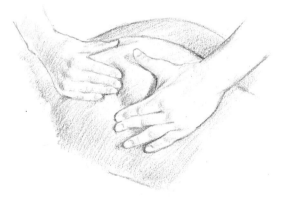

2 Kneading buttocks
Facing your partner's side at hip level, reach over to his opposite buttock and start to knead it with slow, firm circling movements, as shown above, using your whole hand. Focus with your fingers and thumbs, searching into the soft tissue between bones. Avoid areas of sharp pain – work around them, not directly on them, and always stay within the threshold of pain. Move around and repeat on the other side.

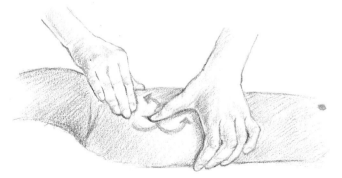

3 Circling down back of leg
With the fingers of one hand and the thumb of the other, trace small overlapping circles down the back of one thigh. Ease the pressure at the back of the knee, then pause to press gently on the Shiatsu *tsubo* (marked) with your thumb. Then continue to circle down to the lower calf. Repeat on the other leg.

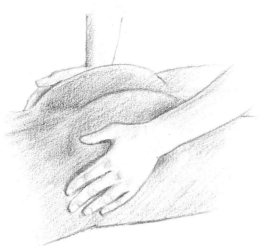

4 Heel-of-hand pressure on buttocks
Facing toward your partner's head, place the heels of both your hands on the hollows at the sides of his buttocks, as shown left. Slowly press your hands in toward each other. Try gently rocking the pelvis from side to side, or use alternating or synchronized circling movements to work into the soft tissue. Go gently if there is any tenderness.

5 Pressing sacrum holes and under iliac crests
Kneeling by your partner's thigh, facing his head, rest your thumbs on either side of the top of his sacrum. Feel for the small hollows, then slowly lean on to your thumbs. Hold, release, then move down the sacrum, pressing the pairs of holes. Now press carefully outward along under the rims of the pelvic bone, as shown right.

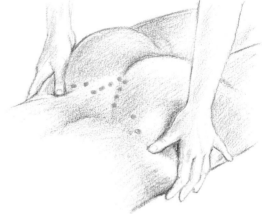

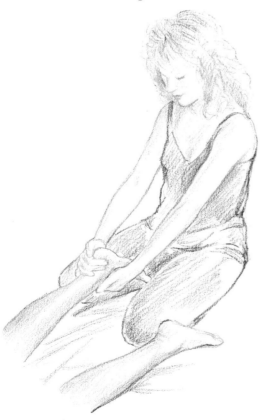

6 Stretching legs
Kneel at your partner's feet and take hold of one foot, one hand cupped around his heel and the other supporting the front of his ankle joint. Now lean back from your pelvis and let your arms go taut like ropes. Let your body take the weight and stretch the leg steadily and firmly. Release, then repeat on the other foot.

Aching hips

The hips act as the body's fulcrum, joining legs with torso. Many people hold tension here, due to lack of exercise, structural imbalance in the legs and suppression of sexuality and anger (both basic drives centred in the hara). This creates stagnation in the pelvis and increasingly limited and painful movement of the hip joints. Pressing in the buttocks around the hip joints and rotating them by moving the legs will increase circulation and mobility and help to relieve discomfort. The whole of the sequence for sciatica (see pp.78-9) will also be useful for warming and loosening the muscles around the hip joint. Try marjoram essence for massaging hips (see p.21).

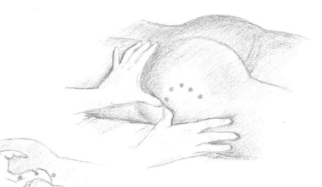

I Pressing with thumbs around joint
Kneeling beside your partner, feel for the hollow just above his hip bone (see diagram). Rest the balls of your thumbs together at this point. Now lean forward from your *hara* and let your body push your thumbs into the hollow. Hold, release, then continue on around the joint in a semicircle. Repeat on other side.

2 Shiatsu rotating hip joint
With your partner on his back, kneel on one knee by his thigh, facing his head. Raise his leg, as shown left, using one hand on his knee and the other on his ankle. Start slowly to rotate the hip joint by describing small circles with his knee. Gradually extend the circles to the point of resistance, then reverse the direction of rotation. Repeat on the other hip.

3 Shiatsu pressing knee to chest
Begin as above, but this time transfer your body weight forward, pressing his knee slowly toward his chest. Stop at the point of resistance and hold for a few seconds. Release gently and repeat on the other leg.

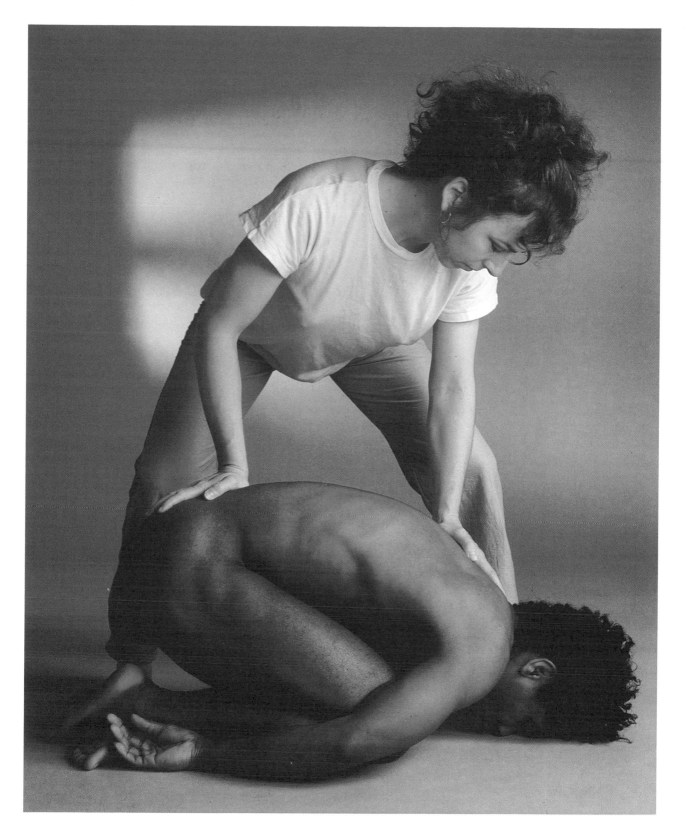

1 Breathing into pain

Lie on your back with your knees up, feet hip-width apart, and your arms and shoulders relaxed. Locate an area of pain or tension in your body, and as you inhale, imagine your breath bringing healing energy and nourishment to this area. As you exhale imagine breathing out the tension or soreness with your breath. Breathe slowly and deeply in this way for several minutes.

Exercises for mid or lower back pain

If we kept our backs healthy and supple with regular exercise and if we were aware of our posture, many back problems would be avoided. Here is a series of exercises to do daily. Never overstrain when exercising and move smoothly and slowly. Do each exercise only for as long as feels comfortable. Breathing properly (i.e. inhaling as you spread out your body and exhaling as you curl in) will aid circulation and help to heal strained muscles. Work up gradually to the half sit-ups and take pain as a warning to go more easily. A pillow under the pelvis may help to ease the lower back.

2 Pelvic lift

Lying as before, with your feet flat on the floor, lift the base of your spine and pelvis slightly by tightening the muscles of your abdomen and squeezing your buttocks together. As you do this, make sure your neck and shoulders remain relaxed. Hold for a count of five and then relax all the muscles and begin again. Repeat.

3 Bringing knees to chest

Lie on your back with your knees up, and hold them with your hands. As you exhale, bring them gradually toward your chest to the point of resistance. You can bounce them very slightly in this position if it feels comfortable. As you inhale, gently lower them again until your feet touch the floor. Repeat.

4 Letting one knee fall out to side
Lie on your back as before, with your knees up and feet apart. As you inhale, let one of your knees flop out to the side. Keep your neck and shoulders relaxed. Lift your leg again as you exhale and on the next inhalation let your other leg flop out to the other side. Repeat.

5 Gentle twist
Start as before and, as you inhale, let both your knees flop to one side so that your pelvis rolls from the hips. Keep your shoulders on the floor as you do this and for extra twist gently roll your head to the opposite side. As you exhale, bring your knees back up to centre again and, on the next inhalation, let your pelvis roll to the other side. Repeat.

6 Partial sit-ups
Lying on your back with your knees slightly bent, gently raise your neck and upper back off the floor as you exhale, stretching your arms forward at the same time. Hold for a count of five and then very slowly uncurl backward so that your back, then your neck, your head, and finally your arms are relaxing again on the floor. Repeat.

LEGS AND FEET

Our legs and feet support us, transport us, and connect us with the ground beneath. They link with our sense of security and stability – or lack of it. Many expressions in our language reflect the legs' connection with security: "to stand on our own two feet"; "to stand our ground"; "to be a person of standing" and "having our feet firmly on the ground". Locking our knees and bracing our legs can give us a false sense of security, but in fact this increases our susceptibility to shock or injury as it makes our joints less flexible. The legs link with the *hara* (our centre of gravity) and the Root *chakra* (our grounding and root situation in life, see p.12). The Root *chakra* is at the base of the spine and it is from here that the nerves emerge to supply the legs and feet, which are indeed our "mobile roots". Our feet are complex structures, each having 26 bones and an arch, which have to support the weight of the whole body above, and act as shock absorbers. Massage brings awareness to our legs and feet, helps to improve our circulation, clears waste and toxins and generally increases our sense of connection with the ground.

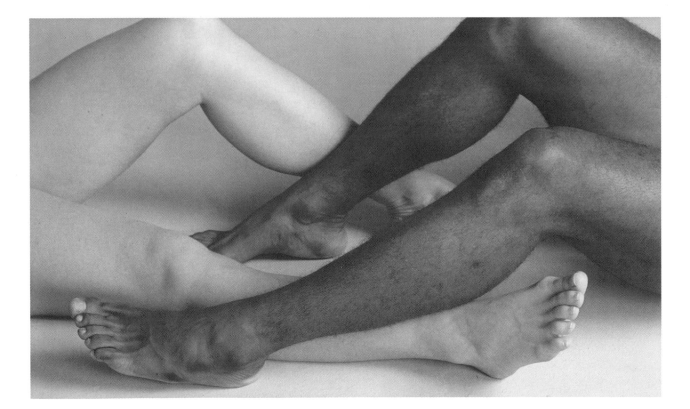

Cramp

Cramp is a painful, sharp and sudden contraction of muscles. It occurs most frequently in the legs or feet, but can happen in other parts of the body as well. Cramp is sometimes caused by salt loss after very excessive sweating, or by poor circulation. It can be violent and come on suddenly in the night. In this sequence we show some alternating kneading and stretching movements for the calf muscle. As well as massaging the leg it is often helpful to get up and walk about in order to stretch the tightening muscles. Marjoram essence may be helpful (see p.21).

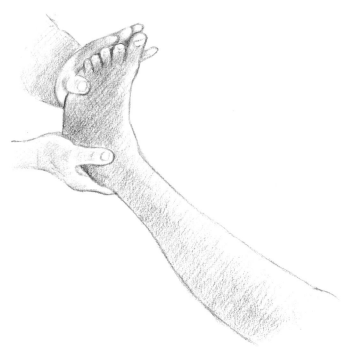

1 Stretching back of leg

Kneel at your partner's foot and, cupping one hand under his heel, lift his leg slowly to stretch the muscles at the back of the leg. To emphasize the stretch you can use your other hand to press his foot back toward his head. Hold the stretch for a few seconds, then release. Then repeat as many times as are necessary.

2 Massaging calf with knee up

With your partner's knee bent, kneel on either side of his foot and begin to work, with both hands, into his calf muscle using slow, rhythmical kneading and wringing strokes. Squeeze, press and lift the muscles, using one hand after the other. You can alternate this muscle massage with stretches of the back of his leg, as shown in Step 1.

3 Kneading the calf

With your partner lying on his front, kneel at his side and begin firmly to knead the calf muscle. Rock your body from your pelvis as you lift, circle, and squeeze with alternate hands. Cover the whole calf area thoroughly.

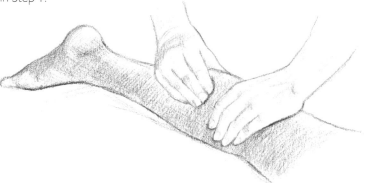

Knee ache, arthritis, sprains and strains

As they are large weight-bearing joints, the knees are subject to powerful forces, making them susceptible to physical stress. This happens particularly if they are usually held braced or locked. The massage sequence shown here will help the healing process after any structural damage from injury has been repaired (see p.90). The strokes will also ease tired, aching knee joints and help arthritic knees (see p.92). The receiver can sit in a chair, if lying on the floor is not comfortable. Try using lavender or rosemary essence (see p.21).

Caution: *If the joint is inflamed or swollen, do not massage it, but work the muscles above and away from the swelling to disperse fluid.*

1 Broad circling of knee joint
Start by cupping your hands under your partner's knee and then begin to describe broad circling and overlapping movements right around the front of his knee with your thumbs. Move rhythmically in alternating circles. As your thumbs work over the front of his knee joint your fingers and palms are sliding under and massaging both the sides and the back of the joint.

2 Deep tissue work
Kneeling between or beside your partner's legs, start to work slowly and sensitively around the knee using both your fingers and thumbs to press into the soft tissue between the bones. You can use small rotating movements, without sliding on the skin, as you press in. Stay present and work right around the knee, keeping within the threshold of pain.

3 Massaging muscles above knee
Rest your hands on either side of your partner's leg, just above his knee, and use your thumbs to make slow, firm sweeping movements, upward and outward, over the muscles above the knee. Pay special attention to this area and then work gradually up the front of the thigh in the same way.

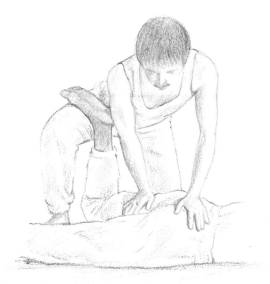

1 Shiatsu palming down back of thigh

With your partner lying on his front, kneel on one knee and support his bent leg on your other knee. Rest one hand on his sacrum and, with your other hand, palm slowly down the back of his thigh. Build up and release each pressure by moving your body weight on to and off your active hand. Repeat on the other leg.

2 Shiatsu kneeling on feet and pressing calves

Carefully kneel on the soles of your partner's feet and place the palms of your hands on his calves. Increase your pressure by slowly moving your body weight on to your knees and hands, and begin to massage his calves. You can also work on your partner's thighs from this position.

Leg ache: Shiatsu

Energy can easily stagnate and toxins can build up in the feet and legs due to lack of exercise and movement. This causes the circulation of blood returning to the heart to become sluggish under the pull of gravity. Many major meridians and nerves run to and from the feet and legs, connecting them to vital organs and glands, and when a buildup of impurities continues the legs ache and the whole of the body is adversely affected. Pressing down on the legs and walking on the receiver's feet activates the movement of energy and encourages the dispersal of toxins.

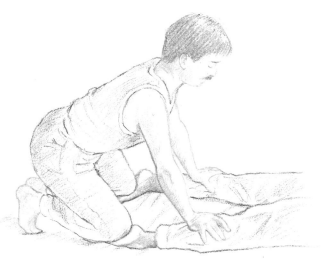

3 Shiatsu treading on feet

For this technique, your partner's feet should lie flat, with the heels falling out to the sides. Using your heels, walk on the soles of his feet. Put pressure only on the insteps and balls of his feet, and take care not to step on his heels. If there is space between his ankles and the floor, insert a rolled towel to fill the gap.

Footache, sprains and strains, arthritis

Foot massage is wonderfully refreshing and relaxing and, because of the hundreds of nerve endings on the sole of the foot that have reflex connections with all parts of the body, it can relax the whole body as well. The sequence here can be used in combination with the foot strokes shown for the whole body (see p.36), and will help in the recovery stage of strains or sprains (see p.90). Try rosemary or bergamot essences (see p.21).

Caution: *Do not massage swollen or inflamed joints. Before treating arthritis see p.92.*

1 Rotating ankle joint
With your partner lying on his front, lift his lower leg. Now clasp the side of the big toe joint and let your inner forearm rest on his heel. Using your forearm like a lever rotate the whole foot in a slow, wide circle, first in one direction and then in the other.

2 Pushing front of foot back
Kneel beside your partner and with one hand press down on his heel and use the other to push the front of his foot back toward his head. Press to the point of resistance, then hold, and release.

3 Pressing down on ball of foot
Kneel up, and with one hand, hold either side of the Achilles tendon, just below your partner's heel. With your other hand, press down on the ball of his foot (not on the toes alone), while pushing the heel up. Lean firmly in to this stretch, but check the limit with your partner.

4 Twisting front of foot to sides
Still kneeling, face down toward your partner's toes. Clasp each side of the front of his foot. Now slowly twist it sideways, first to one side and then the other. Repeat several times.

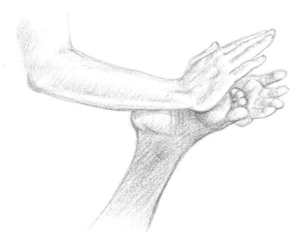

5 Rolling ball of foot between heels of hands

Sandwich the ball of your partner's foot (back and front) between the heels of your hands. Now roll the ball of his foot between them and, with a firm rotating pressure, move from side to side, covering the whole of the area just behind the toes.

6 Stretching toes apart

Hold two adjacent toes between the thumbs and fingers of your hands and slowly pull them apart from each other, stretching the web of skin. Let your partner tell you when the stretch is enough. Stretch all the toes in this way.

7 Pulling toes

Facing up toward your partner's head, hold his foot with one hand. With your other hand, take hold of a toe between your thumb and finger and gently but firmly rotate it a few times. Then stretch it with a steady pull before sliding your fingers to the tip and off. Repeat on every toe.

8 Holding toes in a bunch and shaking leg

Face toward your partner's head and, with one hand, grasp his toes in a bunch between the heel of your hand and the flats of your fingers (avoid "clawing" in under the toes). With your other hand, take hold of the big toe and joint and then with both hands, lift the leg slightly and shake it a little, thereby stretching all the toes at once. Repeat from Step 1 on the other foot.

Sprains and strains

A strain is an injury to muscle fibres or ligaments that have been forcibly stretched beyond their proper length. This can result in some local pain and perhaps swelling. A sprain is more severe and is caused by a violent wrench or twist, causing tearing of the muscle fibres or the ligaments of a joint, resulting in pain, swelling and bruising. The most common areas to be affected are wrists, ankles and backs. These are both common injuries that can be helped by massage in the recovery stages, but you will need to follow the process outlined below. Having ascertained from a doctor that no bones are broken, the best initial treatment for sprains and strains is an ice pack or a cold-water compress if no ice is available. Then you should apply a bandage and support the joint, elevating it if possible. Rest for between 24 and 48 hours, or until tenderness has subsided. Remedial massage treatment can then begin.

Don't work directly on swollen areas, but start with gentle gliding strokes that push up toward the heart, above the injury. In the case of a sprained ankle, for example, work first from knee to thigh, and then from ankle to knee, to help disperse the fluid (see below). As the injury heals you can begin to work all around the area with careful kneading and friction strokes. Finally, where possible, you can work with passive movements to help restore mobility. Always keep within the threshold of pain. You could use a mixture of lavender and rosemary essences (see p.21).

Draining above swelling in sprained ankle

With your partner lying down, his knee supported with a cushion, begin to stroke slowly upward, first on the thigh from knee to top of leg. After several minutes do the same on the lower leg, working above the ankle and up toward the knee. Use alternating hand movements, gently squeezing and pushing in the direction of the heart to aid the dispersal of fluid from the joint along the blood and lymph vessels.

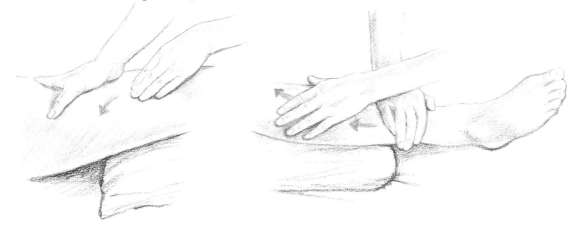

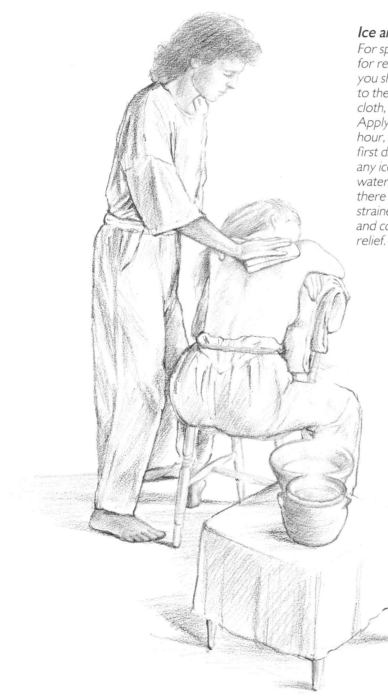

Ice and water compresses

For sprains and strains ice is useful for reducing internal bleeding, but you should never apply ice directly to the skin. Always wrap it in a cloth, or use a bag of frozen peas. Apply ice for five minutes in every hour, for several hours, during the first day or two. If you do not have any ice, a cloth wrung out in cold water is also effective. Where there is persistent aching from strained muscles, alternating hot and cold compresses can bring relief.

Applying hot and cold compresses
You need two bowls, one containing iced water and the other very hot (not boiling) water, and two cotton cloths or small towels. It is useful to start with the hot compress, so wring out one cloth in the hot water, then fold it to shape and apply it to the area of pain for three minutes. Next wring out the cold cloth and apply it for one minute. Continue alternating these compresses for between ten and fifteen minutes.

Arthritis

There are many different kinds of arthritis, all of them involving the joints. The most common are rheumatoid arthritis and osteoarthritis. Rheumatoid arthritis is a generalized disease that can start in childhood, usually in the small bones of the hands or feet. Joints become very painful, swollen and inflamed, and the condition can spread throughout the body. Osteoarthritis is a disease of later life, linked with wear and tear and mechanical deterioration of joints, bones and discs. It is often found first in the lower neck and lower back, and can occur in joints where there have been previous injuries. Massage can help to reduce pain in both these ailments. However, if a joint is swollen or inflamed do not work on it. You may give it hand healing by just resting your hands lightly on the painful area for several minutes while remaining centred. Then work with light gliding strokes above the swelling, in the direction of the heart. Where there is no swelling you can use whatever strokes feel good to your partner, from the section of the book that deals with that part of the body.

Before doing passive movements on arthritic joints check with a doctor to see if this is alright and then always go very sensitively and keep within the pain threshold. Never force movements beyond their range. General soothing, slow stroking and gentle kneading and thumb circling around the affected areas can be comforting and relaxing. Rosemary and lavender essences dissolved in oil will also help to alleviate pain (see p.21).

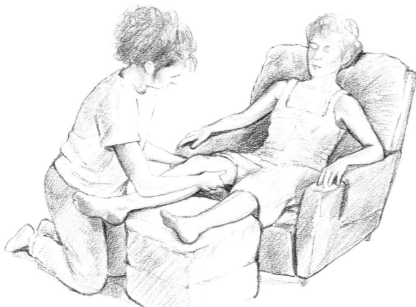

Supporting the limb
As people with arthritis may feel too stiff to climb on to a table or get down on to the floor you can improvise in a variety of ways with chairs of different kinds, and stools or footstools to support the legs. Watch your own posture and avoid bending too much. Sit on the floor or on a stool or chair as you work.

When massage should not be used

There are certain conditions which should not be treated by massage or Shiatsu and these are listed below. It is very important to take note of these contraindications. However, the fact that a person is suffering from any of these ailments does not mean that he or she should be totally deprived of any healing touch. Touch is reassuring, calming and comforting and can help to mobilize the body's own healing processes. So very gentle touching or light stroking on unaffected areas of the body can be soothing and help to ease pain. For any serious problem, though, never massage without first obtaining a doctor's consent. The warning "Don't massage" means don't use any deep strokes on or near the affected areas.

Hand healing
Hand healing is done by first centring (see p.19) and then very gently letting your hands come to rest on a part, or two parts, of the body and holding them lightly there for some minutes. Meanwhile you remain present and aware and visualize your hands as channels for healing energy.

Contraindications
Localized infections or inflammation
Don't: massage where there is an infection or inflammation, as you may spread it.
You may: do very light hand healing through clothes or dressings. With a doctor's consent do gentle stroking massage on parts of the body that are not sites of infection.

Swelling
Don't: massage on swollen areas.
You may: do light hand healing and work above swelling with upward strokes to disperse fluid.

Skin eruptions (i.e. acne, eczema, heat rash)
Don't: massage over skin eruptions.
You may: do light hand healing through clothes and massage on parts that are clear, draining upward to drain wastes from tissue.

Bruising
Don't: massage on bruises.
You may: work upward above the bruise and stroke around it to disperse it.

Varicose veins
Don't: massage on varicose veins, and don't push up from below toward them.
You may: do hand healing, apply cold-water compresses (see p.91), elevate the leg and do gentle gliding strokes above the varicose veins, up toward the heart. If a doctor agrees you can also work with very light, slow upward strokes on either side of the veins, not directly on them. This can relieve the aching caused by swollen varicose veins.

Fever
Don't: massage a person with a fever.
You may: do hand healing. The skin is often hypersensitive during a fever. Stroking or holding may give comfort.

Thrombosis or phlebitis
Don't: massage a person with these conditions, which mean that blood clots are present and massage could dislodge them.
You may: do light hand healing or do very gentle massage of hands, feet or face if a doctor agrees.

Broken bones
Don't: massage if a bone is broken or suspected to be broken. Seek medical help.
You may: give hand healing and comforting touch to other parts of the body for reassurance. In later healing stages consult a doctor, then massage as for sprains and strains.

Tumours
Don't: massage where there are tumours.
You may: do hand healing. If a doctor agrees do gentle stroking of areas such as face, feet, hands and shoulders. Cancer patients can get great comfort from caring touch.

Pregnancy
Don't: use Shiatsu pressure around ankles or massage with any heavy, deep or percussion strokes on lower back or abdominal areas.
You may: with the consent of a doctor, give gentle massage throughout pregnancy, using light and gentle strokes but be particularly careful in the first three months.

Publisher's acknowledgements

Gaia would like to extend special thanks to the following: Sara Thomas, Jane Downer, Chris Jarmey, Sheilagh Noble, Fausto Dorelli, Lesley Gilbert, Peter Sperryn, Sara Mathews, all the photographic models, and the staff at Marlin Graphics Ltd and F. E. Burman.

Author's acknowledgements

First of all I want to thank Chris Sturgess-Lief, who encouraged me to write the book when it was still only an idea. I also would like to thank Jane Downer for her contribution on Shiatsu and her invaluable help and support (and wonderful Shiatsu treatments). Thanks also to Chris Jarmey for his advice. I want to thank Lucy Lidell for her work on the book, and all her support and clarity. Many thanks to Joanna Godfrey Wood for all her hard work, co-operation and patience in editing, also to Susan McKeever, and to Lynn Hector for her design and patience. Thanks to Fausto Dorelli for his beautiful photographs and to Sheilagh Noble for her sensitive drawings. Thanks, too, to Peter Sperryn as my medical advisor, and to Mary-Jane Anderton and Anita Sullivan. Gratitude also to those who modelled for the photographs and drawings: Jane Downer, Terry Williams, Karen Drury, Patti Money-Coutts, Jerry Gloag, Otter Baker, Michael Tirrell, David Kayla-Joseph and friend Mike, Danny Paradise and Margareeta Saari. Finally, special thanks to Bob Moore for his healing and inspiration.

Recommended reading

Brooks, Charles, *Sensory Awareness*, Viking Press, 1974

Downing, George, *The Massage Book*, Wildwood House, 1973

Lidell, Lucinda, *The Book of Massage*, Ebury Press, 1984

Masunaga, Shizuto, *Zen Shiatsu*, Japan Publications, 1977

Montague, Ashley, *Touching*, Harper and Row, 1971

Ohashi, Wataru, *Do-it-yourself Shiatsu*, Unwin Paperbacks, 1976

Tanner, John, *Beating Back Pain*, Dorling Kindersley, 1987

Von Durkheim, Eraf Karlfried, *Hara: the Vital Centre of Man*, Unwin Paperbacks, 1977

Sources of quotes on p.7

Gunter, Bernard, *Massage*, Academy Editions, 1973

Liss, Jerome, *In the Wake of Reich*, Coventure Ltd, 1976

Brooks, Charles, *Sensory Awareness*, Viking Press, 1974

Useful addresses
Sara Thomas
15A Bridge Avenue
London W6 9JA

Jane Downer
92 Chesson Rd
London W14 9QU

Chris Jarmey
(Shiatsu School of Natural Therapy)
Churchfield Cottage
East Kennet
Nr Marlborough
Wiltshire SN8 4EY
tel. 0672 86459

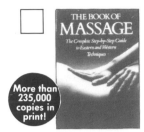
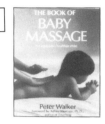
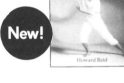
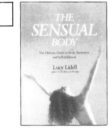
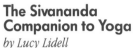

THE
EVERYTHING
WEDDING
BOOK

JUST MARRIED

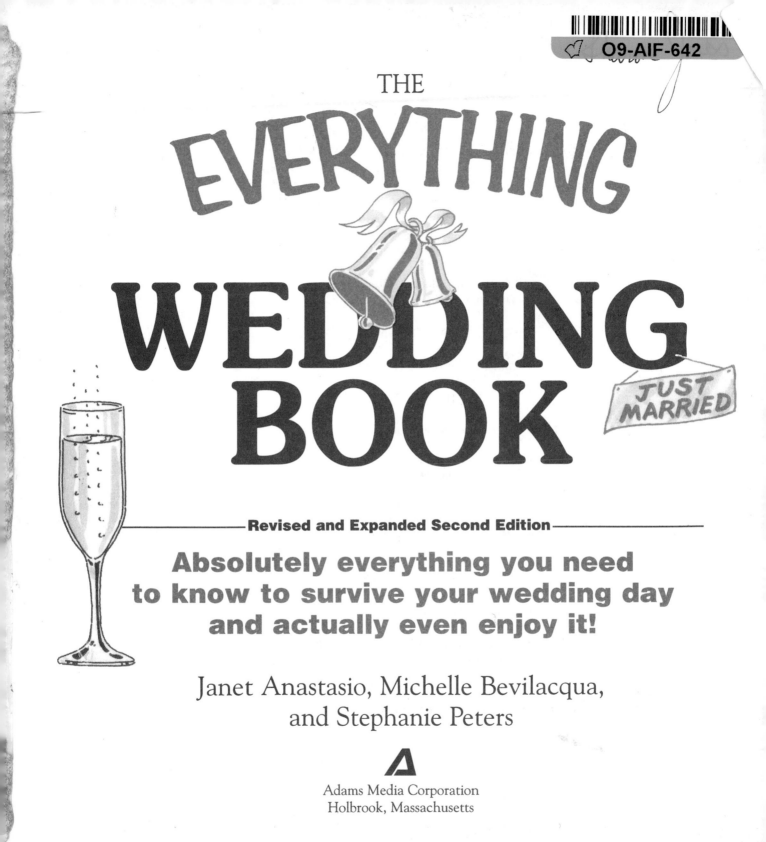

—Revised and Expanded Second Edition—

Absolutely everything you need to know to survive your wedding day and actually even enjoy it!

Janet Anastasio, Michelle Bevilacqua, and Stephanie Peters

Adams Media Corporation
Holbrook, Massachusetts

An Everything® Series Book.
Everything® is a registered trademark of Adams Media Corporation.

Published by Adams Media Corporation
260 Center Street, Holbrook, MA 02343

ISBN: 1-58062-190-2

Printed in the United States of America.

J I H G F E D C B

Library of Congress Cataloging-in-Publication Data
Anastasio, Janet.
The everything wedding book / Janet Anastasio, Michelle Bevilacqua,
and Stephanie Peters.—2nd ed.
p.   cm.
Includes index.
ISBN 1-58062-190-2
1. Wedding etiquette. I. Bevilacqua, Michelle. II Peters, Stephanie True.
III. Title. IV. Everything series.
BJ2051.A53   2000
395.2'2—dc21   99-053197

Illustrations by Barry Littmann and Kathie Kelleher.

*This book is available at quantity discounts for bulk purchases.
For information, call 1-800-872-5627.*

Visit our home page at http://www.adamsmedia.com

CONTENTS

Chapter 8 ♥ What It All Means: A Brief History of Wedding Rituals

Part Two ♥ The Wedding Ceremony

Chapter 9 ♥ I Do, I Do: The Ceremony

Chapter 10 ♥ Making It Legal: The Marriage License

Chapter 11 ♥ The Name Game

Chapter 12 ♥ Places Please: The Wedding Rehearsal and Rehearsal Dinner

Part Three ♥ The Reception and Beyond

Chapter 18 ♥ Love in Bloom: Your Wedding Flowers

Chapter 19 ♥ Let Them Eat Cake: Wedding Cakes

Chapter 20 ♥ Transportation: Getting There Is Half the Fun

Chapter 21 ♥ By Invitation Only: Stationery and Invitations

Chapter 22 ♥ Your Wedding Day: A Possible Scenario

Chapter 23 ♥ Into the Sunset: Your Honeymoon

Chapter 24 ♥ His Home, Her Home— Your Home! Moving into Your First Home Together

Part Four ♥ Worksheets

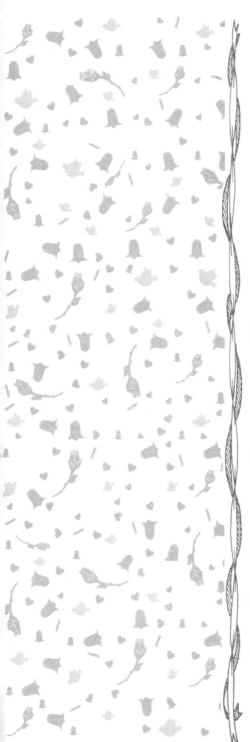

Introduction

Congratulations! You've decided to get married. Once the shock begins to wear off, you're probably going to have a lot of questions about the whole wedding process—not to mention a lot to do. That's where this book comes in.

This book recognizes that planning a wedding can be an overwhelming task. With all the worry and tension that goes into trying to plan the biggest event of your life, tempers and moods are bound to go awry now and then. Relax. These feelings come with the territory and are quickly forgotten once your wedding day comes. You will see that all your work and worry weren't for nothing.

In order to get you to that big day in one piece, we've broken down the wedding planning process into its basic components. If all you want to know is where to have your wedding, what to wear, who should take your pictures, and how to resolve all the other practical issues, there's plenty of that kind of stuff in here.

But this book also explains how to alleviate a lot of the pressure and many of the hassles by using some simple planning. It offers suggestions on how to deal with problems that may arise from difficult family situations, such as serious illness or divorce. And it gives you the lowdown on how to set up exotic weddings, too, if your budget has room for it.

On top of this advice we've included worksheets, planning calendars, budget planners, charts, and checklists in the back of the book so you can keep all the essential information in one easy-to-find-and-use place. That means you can take just one book with you to the many appointments you'll have over the next few months. Dates, names, and addresses will be right at your fingertips—preserved for trips down memory lane once the big day is over.

In short, you should find everything you need in *The Everything Wedding Book*. Keep this book handy and you'll have everything covered!

Part One:

Getting Started

Chapter 1

Your Engagement,
Choosing a Date,
Laying a Plan

Whether he "popped the question" as a complete surprise or the two of you came to a mutual decision after a series of businesslike discussions, you and your fiancé have now decided to get married. So, now what? How do you get from point A (getting engaged) to point B (your wedding day)? Well, that's what this book is here for: to take you by the hand, so to speak, and lead you step by step through that nerve-wracking, frustrating, and hectic process known as planning a wedding!

Protocol

Once you've made the big decision, you'll probably want to tell everyone you know—and even people you don't. But wait! As hard as it may be in all the excitement, calm down, collect yourself, and think about who should be told first. There is a certain protocol that should be followed, and you don't want to offend anyone. (Unfortunately, bowing to protocol is something you're going to have to get used to. Unless you truly feel comfortable throwing courtesy and tradition to the wind, it's usually as big a part of planning and having a wedding as your budget, your gown, and your guest list.)

Announce your engagement in person to both sets of parents. If either set lives too far away for you to do so, call them to pass on the good news. If possible, try to arrange a visit soon so that everyone can start getting acquainted (if they haven't already). Discuss the possibility of getting all the future in-laws together before the wedding.

If your or your fiancé's parents are divorced and/or remarried, think long and hard about which parent to inform first. You know your family better than anyone else does. Do what you feel most comfortable with.

If either you or your groom has children from a previous marriage, make sure they are told of the impending new marriage right away; don't let them hear it from someone else! A parent's new marriage can be a delicate and stressful event for children. Give them all the reassurance they need, try to sense and quell their fears, and make them as much a part of the wedding as the situation allows.

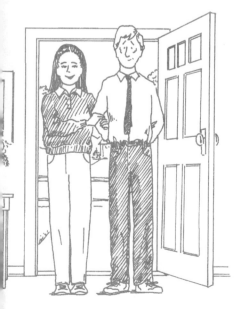

If Your Ex Carries an Ax

Speaking of former marriages, you should also inform your own former spouse (if you have one) of your new marriage plans. The same goes for your fiancé. Don't send the word through someone else, and definitely avoid passing the word via a child. If things are still tense between the two of you, send a note. Issues of alimony and child support may come up; try to resolve them calmly and rationally. You don't want any old problems resurfacing as you start your new life.

Of course, if you feel your former spouse is the type to try to disrupt your wedding, you will want to keep all wedding details quiet. Ultimately, it would be best if he or she did not know of the impending nuptials; you can drop the bomb later. If the problematic former spouse lives out of state, hiding a wedding is a great deal easier, but if he or she resides in the same city, it's important to keep the festivities as private as possible. Make sure family and mutual friends don't spill the beans, and refrain from newspaper and other public announcements.

If you don't have custody of your children but wish them to attend the wedding without the knowledge of your former spouse, get ready for some fancy footwork. Schedule the nuptials for one of your times of scheduled visitation. Though you may feel pangs of guilt, don't tell your children about the wedding in advance; it might put them in a tough position with their custodial parent. (You may have to deal with problems arising from this situation later, but make sure it's understood by all parties that the children had no prior knowledge of your wedding.) Obviously, it will be hard to make the children part of the ceremony under these circumstances, but at least you will have them there.

The issue of a former spouse can be a source of great difficulty for a couple planning to get married. The best course to take is to be open and honest with your fiancé and both of your families; together, you should be able to decide what's best for all.

If either you or your groom were married before to a person who is now deceased, news of the remarriage may be painful to the late spouse's parents. Depending on how close you are to them, you may choose to tell them about your marriage in person or with a tactful note. Whatever the mode, make sure it's you who tells them; don't let them hear it through the grapevine.

"Mom"? "Dad"? How about "Hey You"?

At some point in your engagement, the question of what to call your fiancé's parents is bound to come up. This is one of those issues that shouldn't be that difficult, but always manages to cause some awkwardness or tension between your families.

Your future in-laws might say something directly either to you or to your fiancé. Usually engaged couples continue to call in-laws whatever they did before their engagement.

If the inlaws suggest something you're not comfortable with—"Mom" and "Dad," for instance—explain that you don't feel right calling anyone but your parents "Mom" and "Dad." Suggest you call them whatever your fiancé calls your parents. Regarding stepparents, the easiest solution is to call them whatever your fiancé does.

Start Spreading the News

After all the delicate family matters have been taken care of, it's time to start yelling the news from the rooftops. Tell your friends. Tell your coworkers. Tell the paperboy. Tell the grocery clerk. Tell until you don't want to tell anymore, or until someone sticks a sock in your mouth, whichever comes first.

One easy and time-tested way to spread the word of your impending nuptials is via a newspaper announcement. This announcement is usually made by the parents of the bride; typically, it gives general information about her and the groom, their schooling, careers, and so on. Many couples include an official engagement photo along with the announcement, or a photo of the bride alone. (For more information on engagement photos, see the chapter on photography and videotape services.)

The announcement information is usually sent to the lifestyle or society editor, but you might want to call the paper's offices just to make sure. You should also inquire about any fees you may be charged; this is a common practice these days, arising from the abundance of marriage notices many papers receive.

If the groom's family lives in another city or state, be sure to send them a copy of the announcement form and photo. That way they can arrange for an announcement in their local paper as well.

If you're planning a very long engagement (one year or more), you may want to wait a while before sending an announcement to the newspaper, as they are usually printed no earlier than a year before the wedding. Make sure to tell the newspaper when you want your announcement printed.

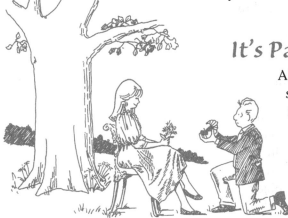

It's Party Time!

Although it is customary for the family of the bride to host some sort of an engagement party, it's perfectly acceptable for the family of the groom (or anyone else) to host such an affair—or do without one altogether if you prefer. Most engagement parties are very informal, with invites made via phone or a handwritten note. The party is usually held either at the host's home or in a restaurant.

The only hint of formality at an engagement party is the toast made by the father of the bride to the couple. This is usually followed by a responding toast from the groom. Anyone else wishing to offer a toast may then do so. When all the toasting is finished, it's on to the celebrating, which is, of course, only a minor version of the big celebration to come: your wedding.

Pick a Date, Any Date

When people learn of your engagement, the first thing you're likely to hear after "Congratulations!" is "When's the date?" Until you set a date, you will have no good answer to this question, and what's worse, you will be unable to go ahead with any of your other planning. Knowing the date is absolutely crucial. Without it, you have no accurate idea of when you will need the ceremony and reception sites; how long you have to find a dress; when you will need a photographer, a caterer, a florist, or any of the other professionals whose time you will be paying for; or even what colors and what types of flowers would look best in that season. A great deal is riding on the date you choose, so unless you don't really care about who, what, when, where, and how your wedding takes place, give the options some careful consideration and then select a date you can stick to.

In Choosing a Date, Ask Yourself...

What season do you prefer? Do you want a country garden wedding in the spring? A seaport wedding in the summer? A celebration at a refurbished farmhouse in the fall? Does the season matter to you at all? If not, is there a time of year that your family or the groom's family finds particularly meaningful? Once you get an idea of the time of year you want, you can start working on the details.

How much time do you have to plan the wedding? Does the availability of a ceremony and reception site coincide with your desired date? Are there conflicts that exist for you, your family, or attendants (such as another wedding, a vacation, a graduation, or a pregnancy/birth)? It's doubtful your matron of honor would enjoy standing beside you in her eighth month in a dress that could double for a tent. By the same token, your parents are unlikely to

Here Is an Example of a Standard Announcement:

Mr. and Mrs. George T. Barker of Boston, Massachusetts, announce the engagement of their daughter, Melissa Ann, to Jeffrey Martin, son of Mr. and Mrs. Wayne B. Martin of Cambridge, Massachusetts.

The bride can also announce the wedding herself:

Miss Melissa Ann Barker has announced her engagement to Jeffrey Martin.

Thank you, Thank you, Thank you...

Show your appreciation and thoughtfulness by sending a thank-you note and a small gift (flowers, a bottle of wine, fancy teas or a coffee sampler, for example) to the hosts of parties given in honor of you and your fiancé. Make sure you also send a prompt thank-you note to anyone who gives you an engagement gift.

appreciate having to choose between attending your wedding and your brother's high school graduation.

Are there military commitments to consider? If either you or your fiancé is in the military, you must work out an appropriate time to take leave. The same is to be considered if there is a close relative or special friend in the military who wishes to be there for your big day.

How many other couples will be getting married around the same time? The peak season for weddings is between April and October, so there may be a lot of competition for everything from flowers to frosting. You may want to consider having your wedding in the off season.

The most popular months for weddings are August, June, and September. December is also popular, most likely because of the festive air and beautiful decorations of the Christmas season. Weddings are usually held on a Saturday, Friday, or Sunday, 11:00 A.M., 2:00 P.M., or 4:00 P.M.

Happy Holidays?

Should you have your wedding on a holiday weekend, such as Memorial Day, Labor Day, or Columbus Day? There are pros and cons to this idea. On the plus side, people may appreciate a wedding on a long weekend; it gives them an extra day to recuperate from the festivities, or to travel if they are coming from another city or state. For you and your fiancé, taking your honeymoon during a holiday week may give you an extra day away (or allow you to save a vacation day for a later time).

But what if your guests have some long weekend vacation plans of their own? This is where problems may arise. Some people, for instance, may not be able to attend a wedding scheduled for the Friday after Thanksgiving because of obligations to visit family who live out of town. On the other hand, your own out-of-town relatives might appreciate the convenience of a single trip combining both the holiday and the wedding.

A wedding during the Christmas season can be a beautiful and spiritual experience, but it can also be very hectic for you, your attendants, and your guests. You will need to plan for a wedding and get your shopping, wrapping, cooking, and similar projects done in time for the holiday, and that can be quite a chore.

If you and/or your spouse is Jewish, there are certain religious restrictions placed on dates you should be aware of. Weddings are not permitted on the Sabbath (Friday evening to Saturday one half hour after sundown) or the major holidays (Rosh Hashanah, Yom Kippur, Passover, Shavuot, and Sukkot). If you have friends who are Jewish you may want to schedule around these holidays so they aren't faced with a tough decision—their religious observance or your wedding.

Party On!

Once the question of "when" is settled, begin thinking about whom you want in your wedding party. It's customary to ask those people as soon as you announce your engagement. That way everyone involved can get an idea of the duties and obligations involved as soon as possible.

Once the initial surprise and excitement of the engagement has subsided, it is time to settle down, put your nose to the grindstone, and, like a field general, start mapping out a battle plan for your wedding. Make no mistake about it, planning your wedding will be a battle: a battle to get everything as coordinated, beautiful, on time, and generally perfect as your most important day should be. It's often a challenge, but take heart; if you go about it the right way, you will get it all done. Occasionally, you may feel it's all too big for you to handle. When that happens, stop, take a breath, and remember that once you start your walk down the aisle, it will all be worth it.

If, however, you really don't feel up to the challenge, don't despair. There are professionals who can help...

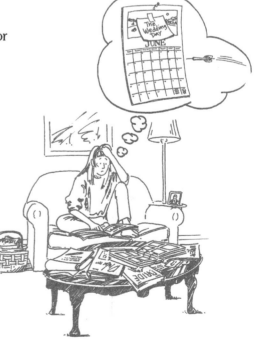

Wedding Consultants

Professional wedding planners may not have quite the same recognition as professional athletes and entertainers, but to many harried brides, they are truly superstars. Otherwise known as wedding consultants, these walking wedding encyclopedias will have the answers to all your questions, or will at least know where to find answers. You'll pay for the expertise, of course—but if your schedule is a hectic one, you may come to the conclusion that it's worth it.

Since weddings are their business, consultants are experienced in just about all areas of wedding planning. They may have knowledge, ideas, and contacts you might not otherwise be able to take advantage of. Not everyone needs or wants a consultant, however, and you shouldn't feel you have to hire one just because someone else does. Some brides enjoy planning their own wedding and have plenty of time to do so; for them the process is as important and exciting as the result. Others, who have at their disposal the past experience of their mother, aunts, sisters, friends, cousins, and so on, ask why they should pay for the advice when they can get it for free.

But there are brides out there who don't have anyone to help them, or don't have the time or energy required to plan the wedding they want. It can be especially hard for women with fast-paced careers to balance the demands of their job and their wedding. If you fall into this category, you may find that a consultant can relieve a great deal of the pressure you face.

Which kind should you choose?

There are two types of wedding consultants: independent and store-affiliated. Independent consultants can help you with all phases of the wedding and may even act as the master or mistress of ceremonies at the reception. A consultant like this can sit down with you and plan your wedding from A to Z, act as the go-between for you and the florist, baker, caterer, DJ/band, and photographer, and do just about everything for you except show up in a white dress on your wedding day.

If you decide to go this route, make sure you're honest about your budget from the beginning. Because of her extended contacts and experience, your consultant should be able to help you stick to your budget, and still include most of the things you really want.

Store-affiliated consultants are those people employed by the bridal salons, reception sites, and other businesses that cater to weddings. Their knowledge may not be as broad as the independent's, but they will be able to help you with any questions you have in their area of expertise.

Stealing the show?

Remember that having a wedding consultant does not mean you have to stand in a corner while someone else makes all the decisions. Your consultant will have as big or small a role in the wed-

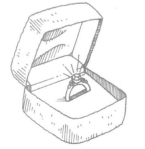

ding as you wish. Don't be afraid to communicate your desires and to double-check that the consultant understands them. If you tell her you'd like the reception band to specialize in harmonies, you may not be thrilled to find out later that she'd booked a barbershop quartet.

Before you hire a consultant, take the time to find out what kind of person you will be working with. As far as store-affiliated consultants go, you get whoever is employed by the store and available at the time you come in. You have no real choice—other than to shop somewhere else. With an independent consultant, on the other hand, you will want to select someone who listens to your needs and ideas, and who you feel is capable of handling the job. Ask friends, family, and coworkers for referrals. If they all come up empty, consult the local phone book and ask people in the industry, such as florists, photographers, and bridal shops.

You will want to avoid someone who seems likely to disregard your wishes and run away with the show. You should also keep an eye out for overall compatibility. Look for someone who seems likely to work well with you and who specializes in the areas you require assistance in. Don't forget to check references either; she may seem wonderful, but she could also be using your money to book herself a cruise around the world instead of a reception site for your wedding.

Costs

The cost of a wedding consultant will vary, depending upon the type and extent of service you require. Some will bill for 10 to 20 percent of the total cost of the wedding, while others will charge a flat fee. Store-affiliated consultants, on the other hand, are usually at your service at no extra charge, provided you are already doing business with their shop. (Is anything ever really free?)

If you think you might want to work with an independent consultant but doubt that you can afford one, don't be afraid to ask around. Some consultants receive commissions from the companies they refer business to, a practice that allows them to offer their services at a lower rate than they otherwise would. And although it may not feel quite as luxurious as working with a private consultant, this book can do much the same job when it comes to providing help in planning your wedding—and at a much cheaper rate!

Tick Tick Tick . . .

You may think you have all the time in the world, but beware: the last thing you want is to suddenly discover that it's three months before your wedding and you don't have a dress yet. Make up a schedule and stick to it. Though your tendency may be to procrastinate in the early months, don't! If it can be done months before the wedding, do it months before the wedding. Don't worry, you won't be bored later; there will be plenty to do as the wedding draws near. Wouldn't you rather be free to deal with those things, instead of being bogged down by tasks that could have been done months ago? Get yourself motivated and go at it with gusto.

Sticking to your schedule is the best and only way to make things go smoothly.

Plan to secure the key items in your wedding (ceremony site, reception site, caterer, photographer, flowers, gown, rings, music) as far in advance as possible. Starting early gives you the breathing room to take your time and make unrushed choices.

Get the terms of EVERY service or sales agreement in writing!

The Diplomacy of Planning

Planning a wedding can be a hectic and stressful experience. Quite often tempers will flair, particularly when nerves act up; we end up wanting to choke our parents, our fiancé, our friends, and anyone else who gets in the way. What you don't need in this already explosive atmosphere is any unexpected sticks of dynamite, issues such as family feuding, friends fighting, and relationship politics in general.

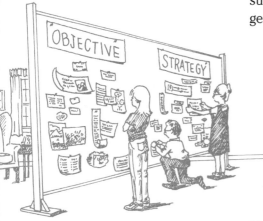

The In-laws and the Outlaws

The bride's family is traditionally in charge of the majority of the wedding details. This can sometimes make the groom's family feel left out, or as if they are being ordered around without consideration. If you're concerned there may be some competition between families, take some steps toward achieving a warm, cooperative environment.

If possible, get the families acquainted a bit before the formal engagement is announced. This way, everyone can relate to each

What to Ask a Consultant

Below is a list of questions that should help you find the right independent consultant for you.

- ♥ How long has the consultant been in business? (Many years in business means lots of experience and contacts. It also means that a consultant is probably reputable, as he or she hasn't been run out of town by dissatisfied customers.)
- ♥ Is the consultant full-time or part-time?
- ♥ Can you get references from former customers?
- ♥ Is the consultant a full-service planner, or does his or her expertise lie only in certain areas?
- ♥ If the consultant isn't a full-service planner, what services does he or she handle?
- ♥ What organizations is the consultant affiliated with?
- ♥ Is the consultant scheduled to work with any other weddings that are on the same day as yours? (You don't want your consultant to be too busy with someone else to meet your needs.)
- ♥ How much (or how little) of the consultant's time will be devoted to your wedding?
- ♥ What is the cost? How is it computed? (Hourly? By percentage? A flat fee?)
- ♥ If the consultant works on a percentage basis, how is the final cost determined?
- ♥ Exactly what does the quoted fee include (or omit)?

Words to the Wise

Whatever you choose and whatever the situation, when you plan a wedding, plan to be honest about relationships, familial or between friends, that may be a source of discomfort. As hard (and embarrassing) as it may be, speak openly and honestly and confront such problems in advance, so that when the wedding day comes, you and your groom need only be concerned with having the time of your lives.

other on a relaxed level, instead of feeling, "I have to like this person because I'm going to be related to her soon." Nor will there be the awkwardness of, "Here, be an instant family!"

With luck, the families will get along and some rapport can develop between the parents. That way, when it comes time to make plans, everybody is already familiar, even friendly, and knows what to expect from one another.

Keep the lines of communication open for all the wedding details, and consult with both families on all major decisions. Have the mother in charge consult with the other mother, to make the latter feel included. "Show up here wearing this!" is definitely the wrong approach.

The groom's family may offer to take on other responsibilities in addition to the rehearsal dinner, or perhaps offer financial assistance. If the bride's family decides to accept, make sure everyone behaves graciously; it wouldn't be wise for the bride's parents to take money from the groom's parents and then refuse to let them make suggestions. If the bride's family declines the money (for whatever reason), they should be gracious and friendly. Make sure they let the groom's family know that even if their money is not needed, their suggestions and input are welcome.

Other ways to make the groom's family an active part of the wedding: include them in the ceremony, perhaps by doing a reading or lighting a candle; have the groom's father walk the groom's mother down the aisle as part of the procession; put both sets of parents' names on the invitation (and anything else you can think of).

For your part, be patient and, most of all, diplomatic; you want to step into the biggest day of your life with your best foot forward.

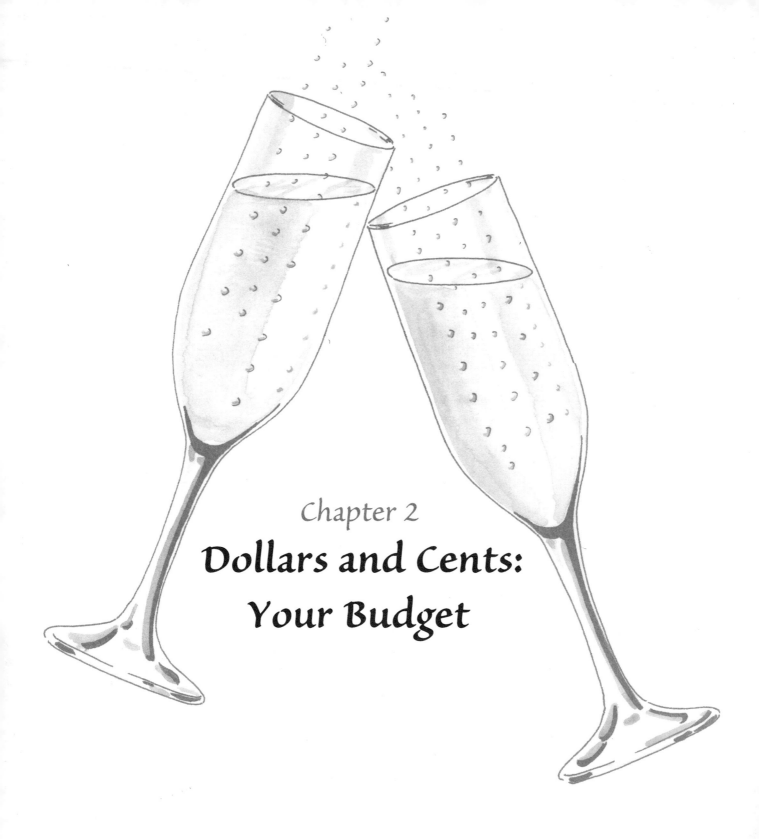

Chapter 2

Dollars and Cents:
Your Budget

For Love or Money

You say money is no object when it comes to your wedding? You say you're one of the very few (and very lucky) people who have an unlimited supply of funds just waiting to be spent on the wedding of a lifetime? Great! Skip this chapter. Go all out and make your wedding an extravaganza filled with all you've ever dreamed of.

If you're like most people these days, though, you'll need to set up a budget. If money is especially tight, it's best to prioritize so that your wedding can have the things that are most important to you. But how to begin?

First, decide on the type of wedding you want. Your job will be to try to construct a budget based on that, using the sources available. Perhaps you and your fiancé don't even want a "big" formal (or semiformal) wedding. You may both shy away from frills and thrills, preferring to avoid much of the headaches and expense by holding a small, simple affair. If this is how you want to go, there are plenty of options: a backyard wedding, a wedding in a home, a civil ceremony—it's up to the two of you. Budgeting such a wedding should be a fairly simple affair.

You may decide, though, that you want as much of the grand, traditional wedding that your budget will allow—in which case planning expenses becomes particularly important. You'll want to make every dollar go as far as it possibly can.

After you decide on the type of wedding you'd like to have, you'll need to figure out exactly how you're going to afford it. The amounts you allocate yourself will help you determine the number of guests you can invite, the location of your reception, the food you will serve, the number of photographs you will have taken, the flowers on display, and many other elements of the celebration.

There are two ways of going about setting a budget. One is to determine what amount of money all of the parties involved—bride, groom, bride's parents, groom's parents can and/or will contribute. Perhaps your parents have anticipated your eventual nuptials and have set aside a lump sum for this use. If you're lucky, this sum plus anything you plan to add will equal the amount you eventually spend.

However, you may find you're more comfortable—and will get a better response—if you can discuss the wedding you want with a realistic picture of what it could cost in hand. If so, you and your fiancé should come up with approximate dollar amounts for each item in your wedding budget before you approach your parents.

If you choose this second option, you'll need to do your homework. The worksheet provided at the end of this book gives you line items found in a typical wedding budget. But how to start filling it in? If you have friends who recently got married, don't be shy about asking them how much they paid for what. Most newly-weds are happy to pass on the wisdom they gained from going through the wedding planning experience themselves. Though your figures may differ from theirs in the end—you may want to spend more on photography than they did, or decide to have a DJ instead of a band—at least you'll have a preliminary figure to plug into the worksheet.

Once you've consulted your friends, pick up the phone. Call a variety of reception sites and caterers and ask for their wedding menus to get an idea of how much per person charges can run. Be sure to ask for any additional fees you may be charged (rental fees, set-up fees, gratuity, corkage, or cake-cutting fees). Do the same with photographers, limousine services, videographers, and any other service you might want. Once you have the paperwork in hand, you can insert cost ranges into the budget to give you a "cheapest to costliest" scenario, or find the average price of each item for an overall approximate picture. Then it's off to the parents to ask the big money question . . .

It is customary for the bride's family to bear the majority of the wedding expenses . . . but circumstances can dictate other arrangements. These days it is not uncommon for the bride and groom to bear the brunt of the wedding expenses themselves. While the idea of paying for your own wedding may take you aback (especially if you've started finding out how much things can cost!), keep in mind that your opinions might have more weight if you are the one writing the check. Of course, the same holds true if you do accept contributions from your parents; if you're spending their money, you'll want to carefully consider all their suggestions.

Words to the Wise

Whether your wedding is a small, informal affair or the gala social event of the season, you'll want to take advantage of the cost-cutting suggestions included throughout each section. (If you're looking to save on flowers, consult the chapter dedicated to flowers, and so on.)

Using a Budget

Work up a budget and stick to it. Decide what the truly important items are and try your very best to fit them in—but realize when it's time to sacrifice for the sake of your pocketbook (and your future finances). Remember that what makes your wedding most special and memorable is joining your life with the one you love, and doing it with the blessing of family and friends.

Sticking to a budget can save you a lot of time and aggravation. You won't take that trip to the city in rush-hour traffic to look at the grand ballroom of a luxury hotel "just to see" because you already know its cost is beyond your means.

There are many compromises you can make that will have

(continued)

Who Pays for What?

The bride and her family:
The groom's wedding ring and gift
Invitations, reception cards, and announcements
Bride's wedding gown and accessories
Fee for ceremony location
Flowers for ceremony and reception (including flowers for attendants)
Housing for bridesmaids
Gifts for bridesmaids
Photography
Music for ceremony and reception
Rented transportation, such as limousines
All reception costs (location rental, food, decorations, etc.)

The groom and his family:
The bride's wedding and engagement rings
Gift for the bride
Housing for ushers
Marriage license
Officiant's fee
Bride's bouquet
Bride's going-away corsage (optional)
Mothers' and grandmothers' corsages
Boutonnieres for groom's wedding party
Rehearsal dinner
Honeymoon

The maid/matron of honor and bridesmaids:
Dress and accessories
Gift for the couple
Shower gift
Contributing to bridal shower
Transportation to and from the wedding

The best man and ushers:
Clothing rental (tuxedo, suit)
Gift for the couple
Contributing to the cost of the bachelor party
Transportation to and from the wedding

Remember, these guidelines are not set in stone. No one will faint or put out a warrant for your arrest if your family, instead of the groom's, hosts the rehearsal dinner, or if the groom pays for the photographs. If circumstances require doing things differently, don't let these guidelines stop you.

Cash, Check, or Charge?

You will have to start tapping into your wedding funds the minute you begin hiring people and places for your wedding because most will require a deposit of some sort. There are three ways to handle payments: cash, check, or charge. It is doubtful that most places will accept cash payments; besides, will you really feel comfortable carrying around a wad of hundred-dollar bills, or happy not having some way, other than this book and your memory, of tracking how much you paid for what, and when? That leaves checks and credit cards.

If your parents have set aside a lump sum for your wedding, you can do one of three things. Ask for the sum to be deposited into your or your fiancé's checking account so you can write checks without the worry of them bouncing. Or have your parents send the checks directly to the person or place being hired (keep in mind, however, that if someone else's check gets there first, they may beat you to the band or reception site you wanted). Finally, you may decide to set up a separate checking account just for the wedding money.

This last option might prove the easiest all around. You know that the money you take from the account was set aside for the wedding only, that you're not accidentally tapping into your own savings. You have the option of adding to the account, should extra money come your way. And finally, you'll have your cancelled checks as proof positive that your deposits and payments were cashed—just in case a question ever comes up.

Using a credit card can also be a handy way of keeping track of your deposits and payments, but be careful to remember how much you've charged each month so you're not surprised when your statement arrives—and be sure to pay off each bill as it comes in so your credit rating doesn't suffer. Remember, weddings can cost thousands of dollars; you don't want to begin your life together with that kind of credit card debt hanging over your head!

Using a Budget

(continued from previous page)

little or no effect on you or your guests' enjoyment of the day. You may opt to get your invitations done by an offset printer instead of having them engraved, have a DJ instead of a band, or hold a buffet instead of a sitdown dinner. The goal is to prioritize so you can spend money on what is most important to you, on the things you are most likely to carry with you from that day into the future. Try to keep things in perspective. Your wedding will be the time of your life because you'll be joined with the one you love, surrounded by friends and family; whether you serve chicken instead of steak is really not all that important.

Tipping Guidelines

Even the most budget-conscious brides and grooms often overlook one very substantial expense—tips! Depending on the size of your reception and your reception location, tipping can easily add from a few hundred to a few thousand dollars to your costs. As a result, whom to tip and how much to tip can often be perplexing dilemmas. Although tipping is, for the most part, expected, it is never required—it's simply an extra reward for extraordinary service. Exactly how much or whom you tip is completely at your discretion. The following are simply guidelines, not rules:

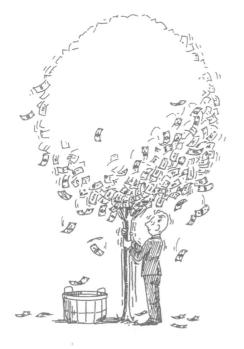

- ♥ Caterers and reception site managers usually have gratuities of 15–20 percent included in their contracts. These are usually paid in advance by the host of the reception. If the caterer or manager has been exceptionally helpful, you may wish to give him or her an additional tip, usually $1–$2 per guest.
- ♥ Waitstaff usually receive 15–20 percent of the food bill. Caterers sometimes include this gratuity in their contract. But if the tip is not included, give the tip to the head waiter or maitre d' during the reception.
- ♥ Bartenders should be tipped 15–20 percent of the total bar bill. If their gratuity is already included in the catering contract, an additional tip of 10 percent is common. It should be paid by the host during the reception. Don't allow the bartender to accept tips from guests; ask him to put up a small sign that says, "No tipping, please."
- ♥ Restroom, coat check, or parking attendants should be pre-paid by the host, usually $1–$2 per guest or car. Ask the staff not to accept tips from guests.
- ♥ Limousine drivers usually receive 15–20 percent of the bill. Additional tips are at the host's discretion.
- ♥ Musicians or DJs may be tipped if their performance is exceptional. Tips usually run about $25 per band member. DJs are tipped about 15–20 percent of their fee.
- ♥ Florists, photographers, and bakers are not usually tipped; you simply pay a flat fee for their services.
- ♥ An officiant is never tipped; he or she receives a flat fee for performing the service. A religious officiant may ask for a small donation, around $20, for his or her house of worship, but a civil officiant is not allowed to accept tips.

Chapter 3

Ringing in a New Life: Your Wedding Rings

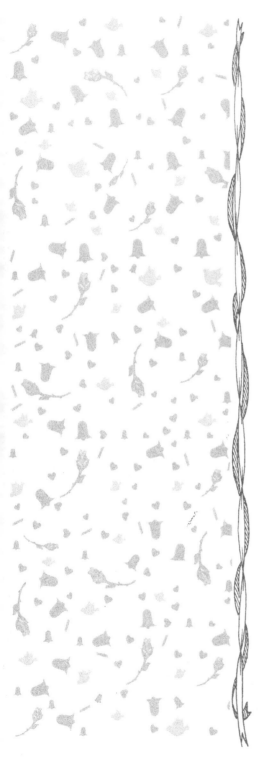

Odds are that, by the time you look at this, you are already able to read by the glare of your diamond engagement ring. That may be a bit of an exaggeration, but it is true that most brides-to-be these days have their engagement ring before they publicly announce their betrothal—and start looking through books like this to help them plan. Even if you're part of this majority, you might want to read the section on diamonds just in case you or your fiancé plan to purchase diamond wedding bands.

Before you and your fiancé start to consider purchasing rings from a jewelry store, ask your friends and family to recommend a reputable jeweler. If no one has any suggestions, the next best thing is to pick a store that appeals to you, appears to stock jewelry in your price range, and is a member of the American Gem Society. Members of the AGS must meet high standards of quality and reputability, so when you choose one of these stores, you know you'll be getting the best—and you won't be getting taken.

Some Tips of the Trade

Beware of a jeweler who displays rings under a light (particularly a blue one). Sometimes this special lighting serves to make the ring appear much more brilliant (not to mention buyable) than it is in reality. Ask to see the ring—and all its potential flaws—in plain daylight.

Make the final sale contingent upon your taking the ring to an appraiser of your choice to verify value and price. Some jewelers will try to dupe you into buying a ring for much more than it's worth by having their appraiser (or one they recommend) "confirm" the ring's inflated value.

As a general rule, spend no more than three weeks' salary, or about 6 percent of your annual income, on each ring. Yes, you want good-quality rings that will stand the test of time, but by the same token, you don't want to be paying for them when your twenty-fifth wedding anniversary rolls around. These are rough guidelines, of course; if you have more to spend, by all means, go ahead. Conversely, if 6 percent seems a bit steep, go with a price range that is more appropriate for you.

Before handing over cash, get a purchase agreement that includes stipulations for sizing and return. Does the store offer a money-back guarantee if the ring is returned within the designated time frame? Any sizing, tightening, or cleaning required during the first six months of ownership should be free.

Your purchase agreement should describe the ring in full for insurance purposes. Rings can be insured under your homeowner's policy.

Engagement Rings

If you're already wearing an engagement ring, feel free to skip this section—or read it just for the fun of it. But if you don't have one yet (and plan on getting one), subtly slip this chapter under your fiancé's nose. There just may be some stuff here that will interest him.

If your fiancé is very traditional, he'll want to shop for the ring on his own and surprise you with it later. Perhaps he'll take you window shopping to get a general idea of what you'd like, but make the final purchase himself. On the other hand, maybe you'll do the whole nine yards together, right down to walking out of the jeweler's store with the ring on your finger. Maybe you'll even help pay.

Some would-be grooms feel that their future bride's input is essential. An engagement ring is an important, expensive purchase; if you're going to be wearing something on your finger for the rest of your life, you might as well have some say in what it's going to look like.

Diamonds

A diamond ring is the most popular kind of engagement ring. That diamond on the ring finger of your left hand is immediately recognized by potential suitors as a sign that you're no longer in the game.

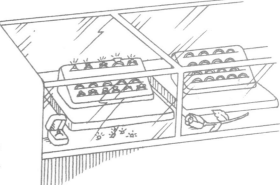

There are four guidelines to go by when judging the quality of a diamond: clarity, cut, color, and carat, also known as the "Four C's." The diamond you or your fiancé purchases should pass the test in each of these categories.

Clarity

The clarity of a diamond is measured by the number of its flaws or imperfections (either interior or exterior). Clarity, broadly

Round

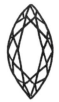

Marquise

Pear

Oval

Square

speaking, is the most important factor in determining the beauty of a given stone: a stone with low clarity, for example, will have a number of imperfections when viewed under a gemologist's magnifying glass.

Cut

The cut of a diamond is the stone's physical configuration, the result of the process whereby the rough gem is shaped. The diamonds you will be shown by a jeweler have had many cuts made on the surface of the stone to shape them and to emphasize their brilliance. The most common shape is the "round" (or "brilliant") cut, which incorporates a flat, circular disc shape at the top of the gem, a modest, tapering edge around that disc descending to the gem's broadest point, and a sharper-angled taper to a point at the bottom. (Other common options include pear-shaped, oval, and marquise cuts.)

Color

The color of the diamond is also a major factor in determining its value. Stones that are colorless are considered to be perfect. The object, then, is to find a stone that is as close to colorless as possible—unless, of course, your personal preference dictates otherwise. (Many people prefer to wear stones with a slight discoloration, even though these stones are not—financially, at any rate—worth as much as higher-quality diamonds.)

Carat

The diamond's carat weight refers to the actual size of the stone. (Unlike the carat weight of gold, the carat weight of a diamond is simply a physical measure of the weight of the stone—not a measure of quality or purity.) Bear in mind that carat weight alone can be misleading. A three-quarter-carat-weight, colorless, flawless diamond will almost certainly be appraised higher than a two-carat-weight stone with several flaws and a murky, yellowish tint.

The Ring

After the stone is selected, it's time to think about the ring you're going to attach it to. Most people choose to go with a yellow gold ring, although white gold and silver are options. How do you judge the value of a gold band? Generally by carat weight and appearance. As mentioned above, the term *carat* does tell you something about purity when it's applied to gold. The carat system designates how many parts out of 24 are pure gold in a given piece of jewelry. (Since gold is such a soft metal, it is sometimes blended with another, stronger metal.) Therefore, a wedding band that is "18-carat gold" is three-quarters pure. While it may be tempting to choose "pure" gold, gold strengthened with another metal is much more durable. This is why jewelry made of 18-carat gold is generally more wear-resistant than that made of 24-carat gold.

The way the diamond (or any other stone) is placed on the band is known as the setting. Some rings are set high, meaning that more of the stone is exposed, away from the band; others are set low. Before you decide on a setting, consider the everyday treatment your ring will get. If you work with your hands, or are often in an environment where you're likely to knock your ring finger against something and scratch or dislodge the stone—architects, engineers, schoolteachers, nurses, and hairdressers beware—you might want to have your ring set low.

Diamonds Aren't a Girl's Only Best Friend

Don't feel that you're restricted to diamonds for your engagement ring. Perhaps you'd prefer to wear a ring featuring your birthstone, or a stone you've always loved. What about a ring that features some small cluster diamonds around a precious stone of another kind? You may also choose to design your own ring, and have it specially made just for you. Remember, whatever you decide, go with a reputable jeweler.

Bands on the Run

Not too long ago it was common for men to skip wearing wedding bands altogether. Today, more and more husbands are wearing them. If your groom plans to wear a band, the two of you should plan on visiting jewelry stores together. Some couples wear matching bands; other couples prefer that the bride pick the band that suits

Words to the Wise

The size of your hands and fingers will affect the way the ring looks on you. Women with larger fingers are better able to wear larger rings, which may look gaudy on petite hands.

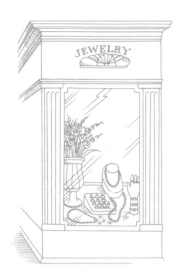

her, and the groom does the same. Sometimes the bride buys her band as part of a matched set with her engagement ring; in any event, the band you purchase should complement your engagement ring. (Often, women who don't have an engagement ring prefer to purchase a diamond wedding band rather than a plain one.)

Many couples choose to have the inside of their bands engraved, usually with the date of the wedding and their future spouse's name or initials. While etiquette dictates that you pay for the groom's band and he pay for yours, the two of you should feel free to work out whatever arrangement you see fit.

Order your wedding bands three to six months before the wedding. This will give you plenty of time to make sure the rings are fitted properly.

Care and Cleaning

You've spent all that time and money on the perfect rings; you certainly don't want to lose them down the drain or allow food crumbs or paint chips to become imbedded in the setting. Below is a list of ring "Dos" and "Don'ts" to help you keep them clean, safe, and out of the septic tank.

Don't . . .

♥ . . . put rings on the edge of the sink when you're washing your hands or doing dishes; it's far too easy for them to fall down the drain. Given the large number of preventable ring "drownings" that occur, your best bet is to keep rings safely on fingers, not only around sinks, but also when you're near swimming pools, toilets, or other dangerous bodies of water. Another hazard: rings can be soiled by chemical soaps and cleaners which often linger in these vicinities.

♥ . . . expose your rings to harsh chemical soaps or cleansers, as staining may result. (Other hazards include food, paint, and good old dirt.)

♥ . . . wear your rings when doing laundry or heavy cleaning. Not only do you not want the rings soiled by the detergents, but it's doubtful your diamond would look the same after going through the rinse cycle.

♥ …wear your rings if you're going to be doing any heavy work that requires using your hands a lot, such as yard work. You may chip your diamond or knock the setting loose.

Do . . .

♥ …have your rings checked once a year to make sure the settings are sturdy and to give them a good cleaning.

♥ …store a diamond ring in its own box or box compartment. (Diamonds will scratch less durable stones.)

♥ …keep rings in a safe (and memorable) place when you remove them.

Should You Reuse Rings?

If either you or your fiancé has been married before, don't use the rings from that marriage in your new one. Wearing the rings that were part of a marriage to someone else is insensitive and in very poor taste.

What do you do with those old rings? Some choose to sell them to make a complete break with the past, but there are other options. Women may have their engagement ring reset and worn as regular jewelry. If there are children from the previous marriage, you may decide to put the rings aside for them.

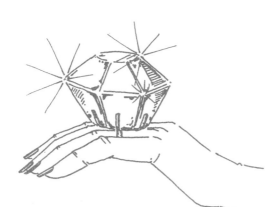

Birthstones By Month

January: Garnet

February: Amethyst

March: Aquamarine

April: Diamond

May: Emerald

June: Pearl

July: Ruby

August: Peridot

September: Sapphire

October: Opal

November: Topaz

December: Turquoise

Chapter 4

The Few, the Proud, the Soon-to-Be-Broke: Your Wedding Party

Having the right group of people in your wedding party can provide much comfort and laughter during an occasionally trying time. Surround yourself with close friends and family members you can depend on and you may just find that those pre-wedding parties, fittings, and rehearsals are going more smoothly than you expected—and are even fun!

With good planning and a little luck, you won't have to worry about the best man losing the rings, or a bridesmaid complaining that she doesn't like the color of her dress. You need your attendants to help you out of such minor disasters, not into them! By choosing the right people in the first place and doing a little work beforehand to prepare, you can be sure that you're the nervous wreck who's being propped up on the big day, not someone else.

How Many People—And Who?

Your wedding party can be as big or small as you like. Formal weddings usually have a larger number of attendants than informal ones, but you can feel free to bend tradition here if you think it's appropriate. Think about which close friends and family members you and your groom would really like to have in the wedding. Brides often feel obligated to have certain people in their wedding even if they're not that close. Don't bow to your mother's pressure to have your cousin as a bridesmaid if you really don't like her. (However, if not asking them promises to cause family strife, you may want to consider including them in some other way.)

Once you have a list in mind, write it all down. If you're lucky, the number of ushers will equal the number of bridesmaids; if not, you may have to do a little cutting and juggling. The general guideline is one usher for every fifty guests. One concern is that all the bridesmaids have a partner to walk them down the aisle, and to dance with them during scheduled dances at the reception. But having a couple of extra ushers is no crime: they can walk with each other down the aisle, and they probably won't shed a tear over not dancing.

As soon as you figure out who you want in your wedding party, get out there and ask them. Sometimes, due to monetary problems or other conflicts, one of your first choices may have to decline. You want to make sure you have enough time to dig up a replacement. Even if you're

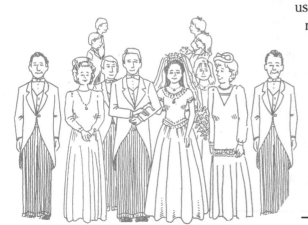

absolutely sure everyone you want will say yes, don't wait until the last minute to ask them. Being part of a wedding is a big and often expensive responsibility; you want to give everyone ample time to plan and save. Six months is the absolute minimum amount of notice you need to give everyone involved.

If your closest friend lives far away

The maid of honor has considerable responsibility before the wedding, but you shouldn't let distance stop you from having your best friend beside you on your special day. Keep in mind that an out-of-town maid of honor won't be there to help you with as much pre-wedding planning as would someone who lives locally.

Maid or matron?

The word "maid" suggests single women, but there's nothing wrong with having married attendants. They're still called bridesmaids, but a married maid of honor is called a matron of honor. Many designers now offer maternity-style bridesmaid dresses. Bear in mind that if your matron of honor will be eight and a half months pregnant at the time of your wedding, you may need a standby.

Meet my best friend, Bill

What if your best friend is a guy? There's no reason why he shouldn't be included in your wedding party. Just don't make him wear a dress, dance with an usher, or do any of the traditionally "feminine" duties, such as helping you get into your wedding gown or arranging your train and veil. If he's taking the place of your maid of honor, he's called the honor attendant; if not, he's simply another attendant. He stands on your side, and in the processional and recessional he can walk in before the rest of the bride's attendants, or, if there are more bridesmaids than ushers, escort one of the bridesmaids. Also, it's perfectly acceptable for your fiancé to have a female usher. She's still called an usher, but she shouldn't escort female guests to their seats.

Above all else, try to select attendants who are comfortable working with people, who don't get flustered easily, and who have known you or your groom for a while. This is no time for surprises.

If you're up front about what you expect all attendants to do, you shouldn't run into any complications. But if you do have an attendant who doesn't seem to "get it," give her the benefit of the doubt. After

Housing Your Attendants

If any of your attendants are coming from a distance to be in your wedding, try to arrange for them to stay with another friend or family member. If alternate housing is not available, pay for rooms at a nearby hotel. But if your attendants would rather stay at a hotel than with your Aunt Martha, they should pay for the hotel themselves. Don't offer to put the bridesmaids up with you; things will be crazy enough without worrying about being hospitable to houseguests.

all, maybe your maid of honor thought your mom would want to address wedding invitations for you. Perhaps you could copy this list of attendants' duties and give it to all your attendants so as not to single anyone out. If this doesn't work, try talking to her. Maybe she has other things going on in her life that are preventing her from helping you out. But unless her behavior is extreme, you're going to have to just grin and bear it.

Kids' Stuff

If you or your fiancé has younger relatives, you might want to let them play a part in your ceremony. This is especially true if one of you has a child from a previous marriage. Junior bridesmaids are usually between ten and fourteen; flower girls are younger. Little boys, usually under ten, can be ringbearers. Other little boys and girls, called trainbearers, can walk behind the bride, carrying her train. Try to avoid having children under five in your wedding; their behavior can be pretty unpredictable. And if you just have too many nieces/nephews from which to choose, you might want to forget about having kids in the ceremony altogether. Choosing one child over another could cause strife.

Flower girl

The flower girl is the last person down the aisle before the bride. Traditionally, she sprinkles fresh flower petals for the bride to walk on, but many brides have been known to slip on the petals, so you may want to think twice about this. As an alternative, you could have her toss paper petals, or carry a pretty basket of fresh flowers.

Ringbearer

The ringbearer precedes the flower girl in the procession. He carries the rings, which are displayed on a satin pillow and tied with a ribbon. For those of you who are worried about the ringbearer losing or eating your rings, don't worry; the rings he carries are fake (and to be doubly safe, perhaps sewn or otherwise secured to the pillow). The best man and/or maid of honor have the real ones.

What Do They Do?

Maid/matron of honor

- Helps the bride address envelopes, record wedding gifts, shop, and other important pre-wedding tasks
- Arranges a bridal shower (with bridesmaids)
- Helps the bride dress for the ceremony
- Pays for her own wedding attire
- Arranges the bride's train and veil at the altar
- Holds the groom's ring until the appropriate point in the ceremony
- Holds the bride's bouquet while she exchanges rings with the groom
- Signs the wedding certificate (with the best man) as a witness of the wedding
- Stands in the receiving line (optional)
- Helps the bride change clothes
- Takes charge of the bridal gown after the wedding
- Assists the bride in any additional planning

Bridesmaids

- Pay for their own wedding attire
- Help organize and run the bridal shower
- Keep a gift record at the shower (usually one bridesmaid only)
- Assist the maid of honor and the bride with pre-wedding shopping or other tasks
- Help the bride dress for the ceremony (with maid of honor)
- Stand in the receiving line (optional)
- Provide guests with the rice or birdseed to throw at the married couple (if ceremony site allows)

Best man

- Organizes the bachelor party/dinner (optional)
- Rents (or purchases) his own formalwear
- Drives groom to the ceremony
- Holds the bride's ring until the appropriate point in the ceremony
- Gives payment check to the officiant either just before or just after the ceremony (the money is customarily provided by the groom and his family)
- Gives payment check to other service providers, such as chauffeurs and reception coordinators (if the families wish him to)
- Returns the groom's attire (if rented)

Ushers

- Rent (or purchase) their own formalwear
- Arrive at the wedding location early to assist with set-up
- See to important finishing touches, such as lighting candles, tying bows on reserved rows of seating, and other tasks as required
- Escort guests to their seats
- Meet, welcome, and seat pre-assigned guests of honor (such as grandparents)
- Roll out aisle runner immediately before processional
- Oversee transfer of all gifts to a secure location after reception
- Help decorate the newlyweds' car

Page or trainbearer

The only duty of the page/trainbearer is to carry the bride's train and help to arrange it neatly. Strictly speaking, this job is only necessary if the bride has a very long train, but you may wish to have one or two even if your train is short. (One more way to include cute kids in the wedding.) Although most people assume that pages are always boys, there's nothing wrong with them being girls, too.

And Don't Forget ...

The father of the bride

On the surface, the father's duty is to accompany his daughter to the church, walk her down the aisle, and "give her away." In reality, his more important (and unspoken) responsibilities are usually (a) to be depressed that his daughter has grown up and no longer considers him the most important man in her life, and (b) to wonder how he's going to pay for all this. He may even try to figure out how to prevent this "giving away" nonsense.

The mother of the bride

Though you may not realize it, the mother of the bride is considered part of the wedding party. And why not; after all, your father gets his moment in the sun, why not the woman who endured hours of labor to give you life! At the onset of the ceremony, the mother is the last person seated before the processional begins. But, like your attendants, she has plenty to do before the wedding, both officially and unofficially.

Official duties
- Helps the bride in choosing her gown and accessories, and assembling a trousseau
- Helps the bride select bridesmaids' attire
- Coordinates her own attire with that of the mother of the groom
- Works with the bride and the groom's family to assemble a guest list and seating plan
- Helps address and mail invitations
- Helps the attendants coordinate the bridal shower

Words to the Wise

It bears repeating: if you have doubts about the dependability of any of the friends and family on your list of potential members of the wedding party, think twice before you ask them. It could be an awful strain on the relationship if you had to take back your offer because someone turned out to be more of a headache than a help. And it would be a big strain on you to end up having to worry about whether everything's going to come off smoothly if you opt to hold on to the person.

* Assists the bride in any of the hundreds of things she may need help with before the ceremony
* Occupies a place of honor at the ceremony
* Stands at the beginning of the receiving line
* May act as hostess of the reception
* Occupies a seat of honor at the parents' table

Unofficial duties

* Listens to the bride complain that she cannot find the "right" gown
* Argues with the bride dutifully any time she needs someone to argue with, and otherwise helps the bride to vent frustration
* Provides invaluable emotional support
* Persuades the father of the bride not to declare bankruptcy and skip town before the wedding

The groom's parents

These people have the easiest job of all. They sit at the parents' table during the reception, have their picture taken, and think about how they don't have to pay for all this.

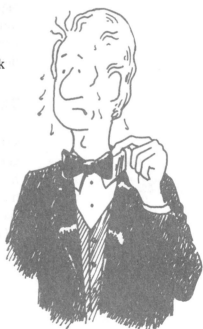

Finding a Place for Everyone

If there are any special family members or friends that you couldn't fit into the wedding party but would still like to be part of the ceremony, don't despair; there are ways to fit them in. You might have them do a Scripture reading, light candles, or hand out ceremony programs. Is a close friend musically talented? Perhaps she could sing a song or play an instrument. Be creative! Between you, your groom, and the officiant, you should have no trouble finding ways to include everyone.

Attire

Now you've got your wedding party. Everyone should have a good idea of what they're supposed to be doing and where they're supposed to do it. All that's left to decide is what they're going to be wearing when they do it.

Deciding whether the party should dress formally or casually is the easy part; the type of wedding you're planning will tell you that. Finding something everybody likes and looks great in, however, is a whole new can of worms. (Warning: you may end up concluding it would be easier to dress the worms.)

First, decide on your wedding colors. These should be colors you really like a lot because you'll be seeing them on your bridesmaids, your flowers, your wedding favors, your decorations, and even your cake. If you have a couple of favorites that go well together, go with them. If your favorites happen to clash, though, you might consider picking only one—a purple and orange wedding would just not be pretty.

In a quandary as to what colors to pick? There are some guidelines that can help you decide. If your wedding will be in one of the warmer months, cool pastel shades like ice blue and pale pink work very well. In cooler months, forest green, midnight blue, burgundy, or other warm tones can give the wedding a cozy feel. However, you shouldn't be afraid to choose bridesmaids' dresses in your favorite color just because someone told you it wasn't right for the season. Just be sure the dresses are of a fabric and style appropriate for the time of year. Don't dress your bridesmaids in velvet if you're getting married in July, and don't have them wear short sleeves in March.

Start looking for your bridesmaids' dresses as soon as you finalize the wedding party. The women need to begin the process early because their dresses have to be made and altered. The men can afford to wait a while because, as usual, finding the right attire for them is much easier; a few tucks here and there to some rented tuxedos and they'll be ready to go.

The bridal party

When searching for bridesmaids' gowns, check the formal dress section of a quality department store in your area before you go to a bridal salon. You may find appropriate dresses your attendants can wear again in the future—and at a cheaper price than salon dresses.

Whether you buy from a department store or a bridal salon, avoid outfits that look great on one or two people but lousy on everyone else. Try to find something everyone finds acceptable. It's not fair to make your bridesmaids wear a style that is wrong for them just because you like it. Even if something is unflattering on only one bridesmaid, it's wise to forget that style and find something else; you don't want anyone to feel awkward or unattractive. These are special people in your life; don't make them wear pink and red polka dot dresses with yellow fringe. Remember, they are paying good money for dresses they may never wear again; help them to feel beautiful and comfortable that one day.

Traditionally, the members of the bridal party wear the same style dress, but you shouldn't be afraid of a little variety. Consider having everyone wear the same style dress, but each in a different color, creating a rainbow effect. If you really want to make your bridesmaids happy, allow each one to pick out whatever dress looks best on her (as long as it meets your basic color and style guide-lines). This approach works especially well in a black-and-white wedding, with each woman wearing a different-style black-and-white gown. Another option is to dress the bridesmaids uniformly, but have the maid of honor wear a dress of a different style or of a slightly different shade from the rest.

Attendants do not have to troop to the bridal shop as a group for fittings. Once dresses have been ordered, they can go for alterations at their own convenience; just be sure to give them a dead-line for getting it all done. (For details concerning time frames, see the calendar worksheet in the back of the book.)

Out-of-town bridesmaids

If one of your bridesmaids lives far away and can't make it to town for the fittings, ask your salon about alternate arrangements. If you can, send her a photo of the dress you have in mind, and make sure it's something she will feel comfortable wearing. Then ask her for her measurements so that you can order her dress along with the others. Once the dress comes in, send it to her so she can have alterations done at a bridal salon in her city. Don't ask your bridesmaid to order a dress at her own bridal salon. All of the dresses should be ordered together so that they come from the same dye lot; otherwise, the shades of color may vary.

The same rule applies to shoes: if all of your attendant's shoes have to be dyed the same color, it is best to have them dyed together, to ensure an exact color match.

Words to the Wise

If you send a gown to an out-of-town bridesmaid, she may have trouble finding a salon willing to do the necessary alterations. Unfortunately, it is common practice for bridal salons to refuse to work on dresses not purchased in their shop. The only way to combat this nasty practice is for your bridesmaid to start looking around for options as soon as possible. If she's lucky, she'll find a bridal salon that is an exception to the alterations rule; if she's not, she should look into hiring a seamstress.

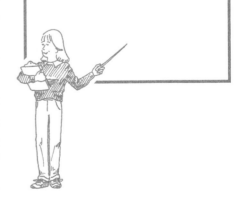

Made to Order

If you just can't find a ready-made dress everyone agrees on, you might consider turning to dress patterns and finding someone to custom-make the bridesmaids dresses. If you're lucky, you have a friend who's handy with needle and thread and has time on her hands to make and alter as many dresses as you need. If not, you'll have to turn to a seamstress. The upside about custom-made dresses is that you get to choose just the material and style you want; the downside is it's time-consuming, could be costly if you have to hire a seamstress—and the results are by no means certain.

The little women

A junior bridesmaid can wear the same dress as the other brides-maids, or a different style that is appropriate to her age. In a black-and-white wedding, she should not wear solid black; a white dress with a black pattern or trimming is perfectly acceptable.

Flower girls wear either long or short dresses that match or complement the other dresses. If you have a hard time finding something appropriate, don't fret; a white dress trimmed with lace or fabric that matches the other dresses is a lovely option.

The mothers

The mother of the bride usually has first choice when it comes to picking out a style and color for her gown. She then consults with the mother of the groom, who (you hope) picks out a dress color and style that complements, rather than copies, the bride's mother's dress. It's best if the mothers' dresses don't clash with the color scheme or style of the wedding. If your bridal party is in elegant long gowns, it's doubtful you'd appreciate your mother showing up in a beaded flapper dress.

The men

As indicated earlier, the choices for men's attire are usually so simple that they're liable to drive any woman crazy. All the groomsmen dress the same, in a style and color that complements the groom's outfit. Most likely, the men will be wearing some form of tuxedo or suit, depending on the formality of the wedding. To brighten up a plain tuxedo, have the ushers wear cummerbunds and bow ties that match the bridesmaids' dresses.

For a formal wedding, the fathers of the bride and groom should wear the same style and color as the attendants. Otherwise, they can wear nice suits.

Most men rent their formalwear. Your best bet is to have your men go at least a month before the wedding to reserve their attire. In the busy wedding months between April and October formalwear may be hard to find; if your wedding falls during this time, make sure the guys look around and reserve things extra early.

Any male attendant who lives out of town should go to a reputable tuxedo shop in his area to be measured. Have him send the measurements to you so you can reserve his attire with the rest of the group's.

Be sure to have him include shoe size; as hard on the feet as they may be, matching rented shoes that go with the tuxes will make your wedding party—and pictures of them—look much sharper.

Remember to ask your formalwear shop about exact prices, including alterations. Also inquire about their return policy and the time of return.

The little guys

Ringbearers and male pages can dress exactly as the other men in the party, or they can wear dress shorts or knickers to make them stand out—and look especially adorable.

Gifts for the Wedding Party

It's customary to show your gratitude to the wedding party by giving each member a little gift. Let them know you appreciate all the time, money, and aggravation they've spent helping to make your wedding day something you'll all enjoy.

After being on the receiving end of so much giving over the course of your engagement, you may be a little rusty on how to do it yourself, so here are some suggestions to help jog your memory.

What to give the bridesmaids
Possible gifts include:
- ♥ Jewelry (possibly something they can wear for the wedding, such as earrings or a bracelet)
- ♥ Datebook
- ♥ Stationery
- ♥ Monogrammed handkerchiefs
- ♥ Perfume
- ♥ Silk scarf
- ♥ Jewelry box
- ♥ Monogrammed purse mirrors
- ♥ Gift certificate (to a bed and bath shop, for instance)
- ♥ Something related to a favorite hobby of the bridesmaid

It is most common to give all of the bridesmaids the same gift, but if you want you can individualize a bit by including a monogram, or giving each woman the same gift in a different color. (The same is true of the men's gifts.)

One Size Doesn't Fit All

There are salons out there that will tell a woman she should order a size much bigger than she would normally take, just so they can charge a fortune for alterations. If your friend is 4'11" and weighs ninety pounds, don't let the salon convince her she needs a size sixteen dress with additional length; and don't give your business to that salon.

You may have a bridesmaid who insists she's going to lose fifteen pounds before your wedding. Just in case things don't work out, coax her into a dress that suits her present body, not the one she envisions; she can always have the dress altered down a size later, but making a too-small dress bigger is a much greater challenge.

Tea for two, three, or more

Because bridesmaids usually wind up doing the lion's share of pre-wedding work compared to groomsmen, you may want to do a little extra to show your appreciation. Custom once called for the bride to take her attendants out for tea. Since not many people go out for tea anymore, many brides treat their bridesmaids to lunch or dinner several days before the wedding. If you're getting married in the late afternoon or evening and are feeling exceptionally calm, you can take your brides-maids out for a nice brunch the morning of the wedding.

The groomsmen
Possible gifts include:

♥ Money clip
♥ Datebook
♥ Cologne
♥ Silk tie
♥ Travel or shaving kit
♥ Gift certificate (to a sporting goods store, for instance)
♥ Something related to a favorite hobby of the groomsman

You know your friends and family better than anyone else, so with a little thought you should be able to find something for everyone. Don't forget to get a little something for the children in the wedding party (it's doubtful that a boy under fourteen would appreciate a shaving kit).

The parents

Often forgotten in this whole gift-giving frenzy are the parents of you and your groom. Perhaps they are providing most of the funds for the wedding, perhaps they are just lending moral support. In any case, it's nice to remember the people who brought you here on your wedding day.

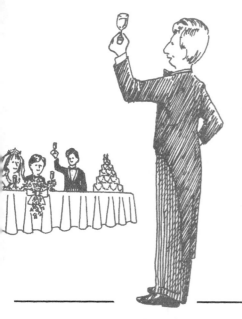

Possible gifts include:

♥ A special wedding photo
♥ A weekend getaway (to relieve all that wedding stress)
♥ A gift certificate (for dinner, clothes, or hobby items)

Chapter 5

The Guest List (and Other Nail Biters)

Hammering out your guest list can be a smooth, effortlessly enjoyable process.... NOT. NOT unless you have a completely tension-free family life, an endless supply of wedding funds, unlimited reception space, and a magician who'll whip up a seating plan that pleases everyone. If you're NOT one of the lucky .0001 percent of the population who fit into this category, read on...

There will probably be a few rough spots along the way. The best strategy for addressing these problems is to hit them head on; don't try to ignore them or push them aside until the last minute. You'll be surprised how much easier things can get when you are resolved not to let anything beat you.

Below you will find a few scenarios to be aware of, and some suggestions and strategies you can add to your Tough Issue Arsenal.

Guessing the Guest List

If money is no issue, you should be able to invite as many people as you want to your wedding, provided that your reception site will hold them all. (People have been known to rent out airplane hangers for large gatherings.) But if, like most of us, you're on a budget, you'll have to do a little more fancy dancing. Start out by listing everyone you'd ideally like to have: perhaps the total number is not beyond your reach. (It's not that you're not as popular as you thought; you're just more selective than you give yourself credit for.) If you do end up having to cut people, don't throw everyone's name into a fishbowl and ax anyone whose name is picked out. Instead, set up boundaries for your list and stick to them. In most cases the guest list is divided evenly between the two families, regardless of who is paying for what. Established couples often split the list three ways: the bride's parents, the groom's parents, and the couple. Each invites one-third of the guests.

Some Boundaries to Consider

No children

That you're not inviting children is usually implied to parents by the fact that their children's names do not appear anywhere on the invitation. Just to be safe, however, make sure your mother (and anyone else who might be questioned) is aware of your policy. What is the cut-off point between children and young adults? It's up to you to pick an age. (Eighteen or sixteen are common cut-offs.)

If you do decide to have a no-children policy, stick to it—no matter what. You can't make an exception for your favorite cousin, who happens to be fourteen, because it's a sure bet other parents will ask, "What's she doing here if mine couldn't come?" If there are children who are very special to you, consider making them part of the wedding; that way they'll be present for your big day, and you won't be offending anyone else.

Another option: excluding children from the meal, but telling parents to feel free to have them come by later to enjoy the fun.

No coworkers

If you were counting on talking to people at the wedding to help strengthen business ties, this may not be the best option. But if you do need to cut somewhere, and you feel comfortable excluding work acquaintances, this may be the way to go.

No thirds, fourths, or twice-removeds

If you have a large immediate family and many friends, you may want to exclude distant relatives from the guest list. Again, be consistent. As long as your third cousins don't have to hear that your second cousins twice removed have been invited, they should understand your need to cut costs.

Ceremony, but no reception

If you both feel it's important to have a large guest list, you may want to consider inviting more distant relatives and less intimate friends to the ceremony only. To do this, you'll need to order separate reception cards that correspond with the invitations to the ceremony. For the guests who will be invited to the ceremony only, simply omit this card. (While this option may help cut costs, it could also leave the ceremony-only people feeling more slighted than if they hadn't been invited at all. After all, the party is the big attraction, no matter how touching or beautiful your ceremony is.)

Words to the Wise

If you do set up boundaries for your guest list, remember to apply them across the board. Making exceptions for certain people is a good way to offend others and create more headaches for yourself.

"And guest" or not "and guest"?

You will probably want to allow any "attached" guests to bring their significant others. It is also nice, but not necessary, to give unattached guests the opportunity to bring someone. This is especially appropriate for people who may not know many others at the wedding, as it will help them feel more comfortable.

If you can't afford to invite single guests with a date, they will almost certainly understand. Remember, however, that engaged guests should be allowed to bring their fiancés, no matter what.

Married guests are almost always invited with their spouse. One exception to this rule: if you are very friendly with some of your coworkers and would like to invite them, you can include them as a group without their spouses.

Always give your attendants the option to bring a date, even if they're not involved with anyone at the time. These people have worked hard (and taken on a hefty financial burden) to be part of your wedding; give them the courtesy of sharing the day with someone special to them.

Return invitations?

If a distant relative or acquaintance invited you to his or her wedding, this does not obligate you to return the favor. These people will understand if you make them aware that you're cutting costs and having a small affair. If people approach you and assume they're being invited when they're not, be honest with them—and quick. Don't go home and stew for weeks about how to break it to them. Waiting only makes things more awkward, and it also causes people to wonder whether something happened over that time to make you change your mind. The best approach is to be honest right then and there; tell them you'd love to have them, but you're having a small wedding and it is impossible to have everyone. It may be a little awkward, but it beats dashing expectations later.

Last-minute invites

Because it's realistic to anticipate some regrets (on average, about 20 to 25 percent of invited guests will be unable to attend), you and your fiancé may decide to send a second mailing of invitations to people on a "wish list." If so, your first mailing should be

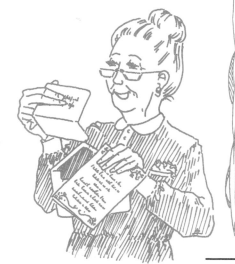

sent ten to twelve weeks before the wedding date; the second should be sent no later than five weeks prior.

Remember, you may have to adopt certain policies out of necessity, financial or otherwise. If it were up to you, you'd make everybody happy, but you can't, so try to do the best thing for everyone. There are bound to be some tempting exceptions that come up to challenge any policy, but it's much better in the long run to be consistent.

The Other Nail-Biting Issues

Divorced parents

If a divorce between your parents or your groom's parents was amicable, be thankful. You won't have to plan around family tensions. If, however, the relationship between the ex-spouses is best compared to the situation in Northern Ireland or Beirut, you'd better map out a battle plan of your own to deal with it.

Do as much as you can before the wedding to prevent any "scenes" at the wedding. This is your big day; you don't want anything to happen that will upset or embarrass you.

Speak with the parents openly and honestly; request their cooperation and their best behavior. With luck, they will be able to put aside their grievances for one day for your sake, but it's best to take precautions. Remind them of how much this day means to you. Divorced parents often think they're big enough to handle the situation but find that when the moment arrives emotion and tension gets the best of them.

To be safe, don't schedule events that require divorced parents to interact. Seat them at separate tables, each with his or her own family and friends. If necessary, have their tables situated as far away from each other as you can without offending one of them. (Your mother may be upset if her table is by the door while your father's is next to the head table.)

Stepparents, stepchildren, steptension

In the same vein, if either one or both parents have remarried, consider yourself lucky if all the "exes" and "steps" get along. If there are tensions, some planning is in order. If your natural mother and your stepmother are on the verge of ripping the earrings out of

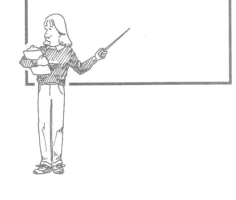

Words to the Wise

When deciding upon a policy that affects the wedding, it is vital for you, your groom, and your families to agree on everything—and communicate key decisions. Compromise and understanding are also essential. Imagine the tension at future family gatherings if you'd set a policy of "no coworkers," only to have the groom's parents discover that the bride's father invited half of his office.

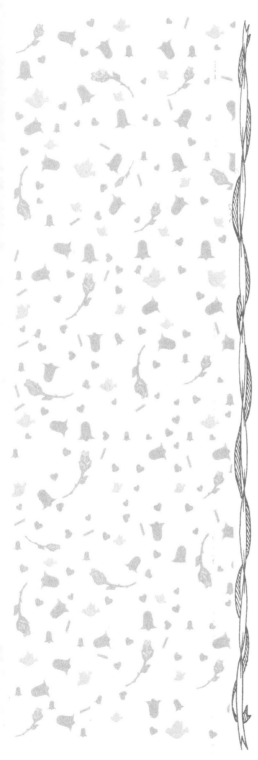

one another's ears whenever they catch sight of each other, consider asking your stepmother to step aside on the wedding day. This may be hard for you if you're at all close with her, but she should understand the delicacy of the situation and want to help you. Celebrate your wedding with her at another time, at a small party or a nice dinner. Of course, if yours is a "like mother, like daughter" situation, and you can't stand the sight of her either, this will be an easy choice to make.

If either you or your groom always seems to be on the verge of fisticuffs with a stepparent, then it is definitely wise to ask them not to attend the wedding. Talk the matter over with your natural parent to find out the most tactful way to handle this.

In some cases, a stepparent will be an integral part of planning or financing the wedding. If your mother has remarried to a man you have grown close to, you may want him to hold a place of honor at the wedding. Just make sure you allow your natural parents their moment in the sun, too.

The "ex" factor

No surprise here: one's ex-spouse and ex–in-laws are usually left off the guest list. Even if things are very amicable, the presence of your ex-spouse might be upsetting to your new groom (and vice versa). Former mates and family members are generally an unpleasant reminder of the past. Remember, this is a day dedicated to your future. In all but the most special cases where everyone feels comfortable, inviting an ex-husband, ex-wife, or ex–in-law is a bad idea.

Death/illness

If there is a death in the immediate family, postpone your wedding until everyone has had a chance to mourn. Reschedule for a later time, when you're sure that everyone will be able to celebrate happily.

A family member who is very ill during your engagement may request that you not postpone if they pass on. If this should happen, try to honor his or her wishes, as hard as this may be. You might have a special prayer said during the ceremony, or share a moment of silence or a special reception toast dedicated to the person's memory.

If a close loved one is terminally ill, you may want to schedule your wedding for as soon as possible, so that person can see and enjoy it, and you can be comforted by his or her presence. Alternatively, you might plan the wedding far enough in advance so that if the person has passed on, the mourning period will be finished and family and friends will be ready to move on.

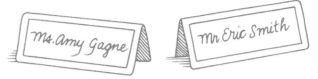

Here's Looking Up Your Old (Ad)Dress

Once you've finalized your guest list, be sure you have all the pertinent information correct: names correctly spelled, proper titles (doctors, religious and military personnel, etc.), and the right addresses. You might also wish to list phone numbers; they can come in handy if you need to call a late RSVPer, or if any family members or friends want to contact guests to invite them to showers or other parties in your honor.

If you're not 100 percent sure you've got the information right, don't hesitate to ask someone who would know, or ask the person in question. There may be a moment of embarrassment (you're inviting this person to your wedding but you don't know where she lives?), but it's better than learning you've misspelled a name on invitations and place cards, and given it out wrong to whoever needed it.

Out-of-Town Shouldn't Mean Out-of-Mind

Since your out-of-town guests will be traveling some distance to be with you on the big day, you should try to make things as pleasant and convenient for them as possible. Start by helping them find a place to hang their hats over the course of their stay, whether with family members, friends, or local hotels. Generally, guests pay for their own lodging (unless either the bride's or groom's family can offer to pick up the tab), but it is customary for you to make reservations for them, or at least provide enough information so that they can do it themselves.

Some hotels will offer a lower rate for a group of rooms. Grouping your out-of-town guests in one hotel has several advantages: the group rates will lighten the burden to their pockets; they can mingle with the other guests during the downtime between wedding events; and they can carpool to and from the festivities.

Though grouping everyone at the same hotel is preferable, some guests may not be able to afford the hotels you choose. Others may have another hotel that's a favorite—or may simply want their privacy. Don't assume anything about your guests' financial situation; include a note with their invitation that lists several lodging options. Detail the prices and any special features of each place, and inform your guests about where you are trying to coordinate group rates. After that, the ball is in their court.

Once you find out where your guests will be staying, you might go the extra mile and arrange to have a small gift awaiting them in their rooms (if your finances permit). A bottle of wine or a fruit basket would be a welcome sight to weary travelers, especially if they've just spent several hours on a plane seated between a screaming baby and a neurotic businessman, for example.

Another way to make your out-of-town guests feel welcome is to invite them to the rehearsal dinner, and to any other wedding events that are going on while they're in town. Inviting them makes them feel like the trip was worth it, that they really are missed, and it certainly beats staring at the four walls of a hotel room, or sitting in your aunt's living room watching TV while she's off whooping it up at the rehearsal dinner.

Don't forget to enclose detailed maps to all the events for those unfamiliar with the area. You don't want guests to have traveled across country for your wedding only to miss it because they got lost a few miles from the ceremony site. As a further precaution, consider putting a trustworthy friend or relative in charge of herding up the out-of-town group and transporting them from place to place. This person would also be in charge of airport pick-ups and drop-offs.

If out-of-town guests bring children with them who are not invited to the wedding, talk about finding a baby-sitter well in advance. (Some churches have baby-sitters on hand.) Children can

The Bride's Book

Want to have a keepsake book that you will cherish as the years go by? Consider making a Bride's Book. Purchase a nicely bound notebook, alphabet tabs, and dividers. Head each section and large divider with the desired category, then enter the names and addresses in a column down the left half of the page. Rule columns down the remaining width of the page for these notations: Reception only or Reception and Dinner (R or R/D), Accept or Regret (A/R), Gift, Thank-you Note (N). Make separate sections for your announcement list and your supplier list.

If you prefer a smaller notebook, use the facing right-hand page for the notations next to each name. You can even go for a looseleaf set-up; rule a page once, photocopy it as many times as you need pages, and go on from there. You can use different-color paper for each category in the looseleaf, and you will also be able to photocopy the filled-out pages to give your mother-in-law a set of names and addresses (so that she can help check the responses).

As you write, think about each family. If they have children over eighteen who will be invited, you need a separate card for each young person. Invitations are never sent "and Family."

If some of the single people will be invited to bring a friend, note that on the card, so that you count that card for two guests when you make your head count later on.

In your Bride's Book you may want to keep a copy of your menu, with notes about the food. When you plan your next big party you'll recall that the baked Alaska was delicious or that the Chinese tidbits were a disaster.

A Typical Page in a Bride's Book:

BRIDE'S FAMILY	R/D	A/R	Gift	Note Sent
GREEN, Mr. and Mrs. Charles 201 West Chestnut Street Chicago, IL 60610 (R—Uncle Charles, Aunt Sarah) 312–864–8084	D	A	Cut Glass Bowl	11/17/99

be invited to the rehearsal dinner even if they're not going to the ceremony.

Trying to accommodate everyone's needs may sound like a headache, but remember, with planning, willingness to compromise, and a little luck, the moments of tension will all evaporate once your wedding day arrives. Then the only "hitch" will be the one that happens when you and your groom are joined for life.

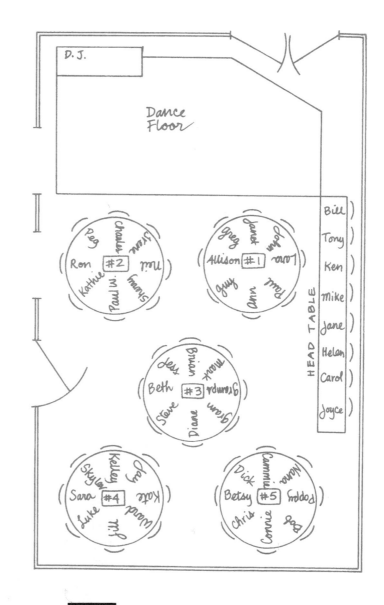

Chapter 6

Party Time: Bridal Showers (and Other Wedding Parties)

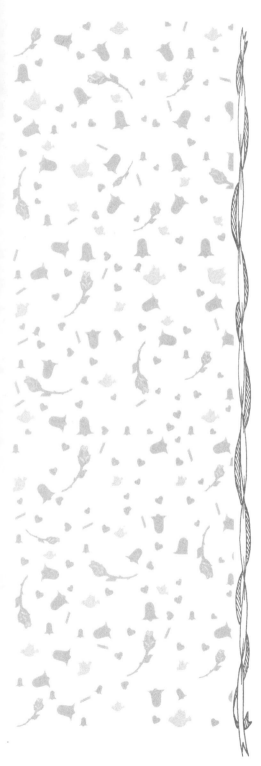

Most of us know that a bridal shower is not where the members of the bridal party stand in the tub and take turns soaping up under the shower head. So why is this party named after a hygiene ritual? Legend has it that the bridal shower originated in Holland, where a disapproving father once refused to provide his daughter with the dowry necessary for her to marry a less-than-wealthy miller. Back then, a woman could not marry without a dowry, so her friends, pitying her situation, "showered" her with gifts in order to provide one for her.

These days, you don't need presents from your friends and family to get married, but shower gifts do go a long way toward helping you and your fiancé set up your household and your future life together.

In the past, etiquette dictated that a bridal shower could only be sponsored by your friends; today, as with many things related to weddings, that has changed. Family, friends, coworkers, and anyone else who feels so inclined may throw a shower for you. The most common sponsors are your bridal party, in combination with your mother and other close family members—but who's to say what other generous (and ambitious) people might come down the pike.

The typical shower is held either at a small function hall or in someone's home, depending on the size of the guest list. The guests are women only, but your fiancé usually comes along for the ride, so he can spend the time looking awkward as you open box after box, especially the ones with lingerie inside.

By the way, it was customary in the past to keep the specifics of the shower—time, date, location, and so on—a secret from the bride until the last possible moment. These days, however, it is more and more common for the bride (who may have a busy work schedule) to take an active part in planning the festivities.

Invites and Vittles

Showers are generally informal. You may wish to send invitations (you can buy them ready-made in any stationery store) but it's perfectly acceptable to make phone calls if your guest list is small enough. It is customary to provide guests with refreshment (remember, they will have to sit for two exhausting hours "oohing" and "ahing" while you open present after present). The menu can be as simple or as complicated as the hosts want it to be; there are no fancy etiquette rules to follow here. Of course, if the guest list (and the budget) is big enough, your hosts may wish to hire a caterer to lower the hassle factor.

Shower menu suggestions

For a breakfast shower:

Bagels	Fresh fruit
Croissants	Omelettes
Muffins	Belgian waffles
Doughnuts	French toast
Danish	Pancakes
Coffee cake	Bacon
Juices	Sausage
Mimosas	Ham

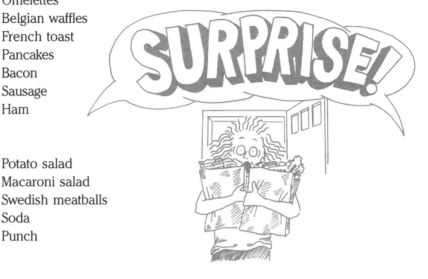

For an afternoon shower:

Cold-cut platters	Potato salad
Tuna salad with rolls	Macaroni salad
Seafood salad with rolls	Swedish meatballs
Pasta salad	Soda
Garden salad	Punch

Appetizers:

Calzone (rolled pizza)	Beef teriyaki strips
Fried chicken wings	Shrimp cocktail
Stuffed mushrooms	Scallops
Crab cakes	Chicken fingers
Zucchini appetizers	Vegetable platter with dip
Meatballs	

Desserts:

Brownies	Raspberry squares
Pistachio surprise bars	Lemon squares
Frosted pumpkin bars	Congo bars
Dutch apple cake	Strawberries dipped in chocolate

Another featured dessert can be a shower cake. Shower cakes are not like wedding cakes, which are usually crafted by a skilled baker and can cost a small fortune. If your hosts choose, they can order a shower cake from a bakery, but they can also bake one

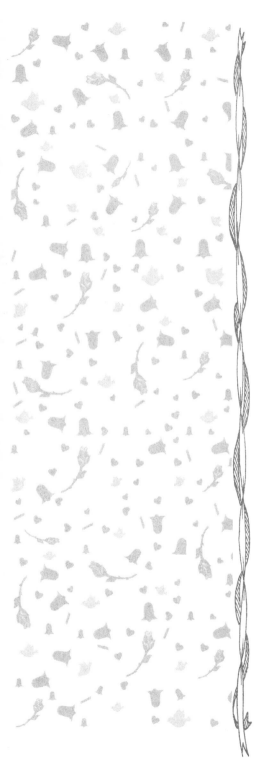

themselves. Shower cakes can be simple or elaborate, depending upon how ambitious and creative the hosts are feeling. The cake can be shaped like a heart, a basket, a gift-wrapped package, an umbrella, or anything else that seems appropriate.

The Gift Recorder

The most important thing to remember for any shower is to assign someone the task of keeping track of your gifts. If you are able to bring this book with you and use the recorder in the back pages, great. If not (the shower was a surprise so you didn't have the book with you), any kind of notebook will do. Put someone you trust in charge of recording what each gift is, and most importantly, who sent it. Pick someone who can keep things organized even when things get hectic, so that you can write out your thank-you notes properly after the shower.

Shower Games

Nothing kinky here. These are just a way to liven things up a bit for your guests. Even the most engaging party games can encounter some initial resistance from a party-pooper or two. If you offer prizes for the winners of these games, though, even the biggest cynics may be encouraged to play. (Some ideas for prizes appear later in this chapter.)

"Guess the Goodies"

Fill a large decorative jar with white or colored candied almonds. Ask the guests to figure out how many almonds are in the jar. They can take as long as they want to hazard a guess; at the end of the shower, they hand in their answers on a slip of paper. The person who comes closest to the number without going over wins the jar and the almonds. (You can substitute chocolate kisses, M&M's, jelly beans, or anything else you can think of.)

"Mish-Mash Marriage"

Scramble the letters in words associated with love and marriage: kiss (siks), love (voel), garter (tergar), and so on. Set a time limit for the guests to figure out the scrambles; the one who completes the most gets a prize.

"Mystery Spices"

Find ten jars filled with different spices. Place masking tape over the labels; spread the jars out on a table and let the guests try to guess what's in each jar. They may shake, examine, and even open and sniff the jars—but they may not read the labels! Set a time limit for this game, otherwise your guests may excuse themselves to run to the supermarket and check out the spice smells there. In the end, the spices can go either to the person who correctly guesses the identity of the most jars, or to the bride, to start her spice rack. (Of course, you'd probably prefer the latter.)

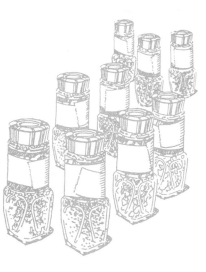

"Bride's Chatter"

Assign someone to keep a record of the bride's comments while she's opening her gifts. After she's through, read the comments back to the group. Taken out of context, the remarks are sometimes hilarious.

"Famous Couple Trivia"

Trivia is all the rage these days, so why not develop some trivia questions with a love theme for your shower?

Sample questions:

- ♥ What famous singing TV couple of the '70s had their own show? (Hint: "I've Got You, Babe.")
  (Sonny and Cher)
- ♥ What was Roy Rogers's wife's name? (Hint: It wasn't Trigger.)
  (Dale Evans)
- ♥ Who were Lucy and Ricky Ricardo's best friends?
  (Fred and Ethel Mertz)

The only limitation is your own imagination. Set a time limit for answers, and give a prize to the winner.

"Memory Game"

After the bride-to-be has opened all of her gifts, she is asked to leave the room for a few minutes. (It's a good idea to explain the purpose of the game in advance, lest the bride think the guests are planning to run off with her gifts.) Once she's left the room, pass out pencils and paper to the guests and ask them to answer questions about the guest of honor: What is she wearing? What color are her shoes? Does she have nail polish on? Is she wearing earrings? What is her middle name? Add any other questions you can think of. The person with the most correct answers wins.

"Right Date Door Prize"

Ask all of the guests for the date of their wedding anniversary (or birthday, for single guests). Whoever has a date that comes closest to the wedding date wins a prize.

"Bride's Bingo"

This game can be bought at most stationery and card stores. Bride's Bingo is the same concept as regular bingo, only words associated with weddings replace those boring numbers.

"Pin It on the Groom"

This certainly sounds like it has some potential, doesn't it? If your live groom is not willing to volunteer his services (which is 100 percent likely), draw the silhouette of a man on a large piece of paper. Attach a photo of the groom's face to the top. Blindfold the guests, spin them, and have them try to pin a flower on his lapel. Of course, this is a variation on Pin the Tail on the Donkey.

"Magnetic Personality"

Magnetized word kits are available at most bookstores. Simply spread the selections out on a big cookie sheet, then pass the sheet around with instructions for guests to create meaningful words of wisdom for the bride. The resulting sentences, poems, and one-liners can be hilarious and touching. A word of caution for less-worldly guests, though: sometimes the "words of wisdom" can be a bit shameless.

"Don Pardo, please tell them what they've won."

It's a good idea to give game prizes to the winning guests. But what kind of prizes? New cars? Small appliances? An all-expense-paid tropical vacation for two? Perhaps. But your hosts might also consider these suggestions:

Shopping list pads	Fancy recipe cards
Note cards or stationery	Fancy soaps
Coffee/tea mugs	Hand lotion
Candy	Cocktail napkins
Bubble bath/bath oils	Unusual pens and pencils
Funny, decorative magnets	Mixed nuts
Coasters	

To guard against the possibility of a riot, astute hosts will have more than one prize on hand for each game, just in case there's a tie. If there are no ties, the remaining prizes may be raffled off. Have the guests pick numbers between 1 and 100. The guess closest to the number selected by the hosts wins.

Theme Showers

At a theme shower, guests are told to bring a gift that fits in with a set theme, such as a kitchen shower, a linen shower, a lingerie/personal shower, a recreation shower, a money tree shower (in which guests attach envelopes containing bills and checks to a small tree, later presented to the bride and groom), a honeymoon shower, and so on.

Some theme showers dictate the guest list and the menu. In a Jack and Jill shower, for instance, the women bring their husbands or significant others, presumably kicking and screaming in protest, along to the shower. Another example is the barbecue shower, which is usually co-ed, and is typically held in someone's backyard.

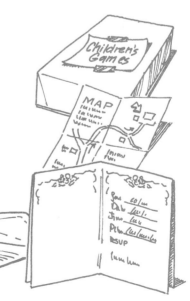

It's in the Mail

With today's booming mail-order business, one way your hostess can be sure your friends will shower you with gifts you really would like is to

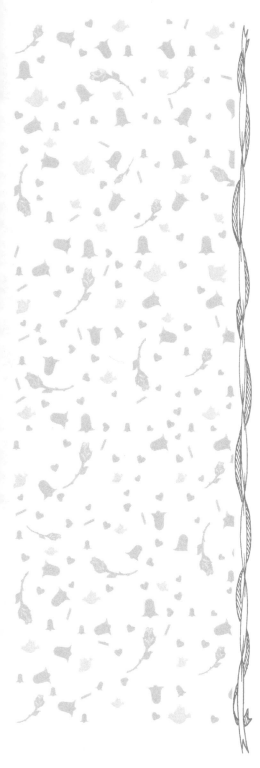

have a "catalog shower." In the invitation, guests are asked to bring their favorite catalogs so that the bride and groom can order from them. Men friends, as well as women, are invited.

Using catalogs saves everyone, including the happy couple, any number of shopping trips and can even eliminate using a bridal registry, if that's distasteful to you. You can agree on a price limit—for instance, fifty dollars per gift. Of course, this need not stop a group of your friends or relatives from joining together to give you something more costly. You can add to the pool of catalogs any that you particularly favor, providing for guests who do not bring one and ensuring that certain types of gifts such as tools, camping supplies, and garden equipment will not be overlooked.

The bride and groom are given markers which they use to circle items they would like to receive as gifts. After everyone has had a pleasant time eating and "window-shopping," the hostess collects the catalogs and makes up a master list for the guests to use as a shopping guide. Think of the time, energy, and shoe leather saved by using the phone and the almighty credit card to complete an order and have the gifts delivered. And the bride does not have to wear a hat made of the ribbon bows from all the gifts she's unwrapped!

Just so the bride and groom go home with some gifts under their arms, the centerpiece can be a set of decorated baskets—one containing handy kitchen utensils, another garden tools, and a third bath accessories—with cards naming them as the first installment of the gift shower.

Multiple Showers

Often, different groups sponsor separate showers for the bride-to-be. Perhaps her college friends will have a small one, her coworkers another, and the groom's family yet another. In such cases, it's best if those in charge can coordinate with each other. That way, each shower has a different theme, and there are likely to be fewer repeat gifts. After talking the ideas over, the college friends might decide to throw a lingerie/personal shower, the coworkers a domestic/pantry shower, and so on.

But don't get too excited. In most cases every group of people you know will not be throwing you a separate shower.

Other Pre-wedding Parties

The bridal shower is just one of several festive occasions that may occur over the course of your engagement. This means, of course, that you should be prepared to party your brains out during your engagement—and sit home with nothing to do after you're married.

The bachelor party

You've heard all about this. The woman popping out of the cake; much eating, drinking, and making merry (with emphasis on the latter two). In the past, this party was held the night before the wedding, but too many hung-over grooms and weaving green ushers have led more and more rational adults to schedule this high-culture event about a week before the wedding. Tradition dictates that the groom is to signal the end of the party with a toast to his bride, but it is quite possible that by the end of the night, he doesn't even remember her name, in which case the end of the party is signaled by the collapse of the groom onto the nearest flat surface.

The bachelorette party

Why should the guys have all the fun? These days the bride-to-be is getting her night on the town, too; and the proceedings are bound to be a little livelier than the shower.

Attendants' party

An attendants' party gives you the chance to turn the tables—to honor the people who've been honoring you. Usually this party is scheduled to take place about a week or two before the wedding, to give all the harried planners a chance to relax and pretend to forget about the impending fuss. In a happy (for them) reversal of fortune, your guests are freed from the burden of bringing you gifts. If you and your groom wish, you may now give your attendants the gifts you've bought for them (another common time is during the rehearsal dinner). The guest list does not have to be limited to the attendants; family and close friends would probably also enjoy the breather. To keep the

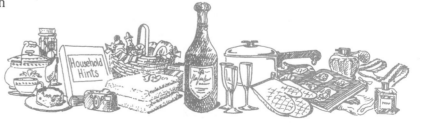

atmosphere relaxed, consider having a barbecue, a park picnic, or a day at the beach (weather permitting, of course).

Post-wedding Party

If your "wish list" guest list includes extended family and distant friends who live far away but near one another, you might want to consider traveling to them for an informal party after the wedding instead of inviting them to the wedding. They will still be able to celebrate your marriage with you, but will be spared the expense of travel; you'll have found an easy way to trim your guest list. You and the host (usually a close friend or relative) should agree on the date well in advance so she can have time to plan and send out invitations, and you and your spouse can make your travel arrangements. Be sure to send wedding announcements to each person on the post-wedding party guest list before the invitations are mailed; otherwise, the invitation—and the fact of your marriage—may come as a surprise.

Another time to consider a post-wedding party is if your parents' guest lists are too large for your budget (remember, though, that parents should always be allowed some guests at the wedding). Ask them nicely if they would mind not inviting all twenty couples, some of whom you don't even know, and instead consider hosting a post-wedding party.

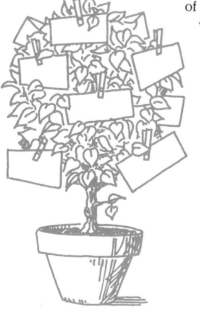

Barbecues, pool parties, buffet luncheons, and cocktail parties are all good choices for this type of party. Be aware that many people may feel obligated to bring gifts. If you are uncomfortable with this, be sure the invitations state "no gifts, please."

Chapter 7

It Is Better to Give . . . The Gift Registry

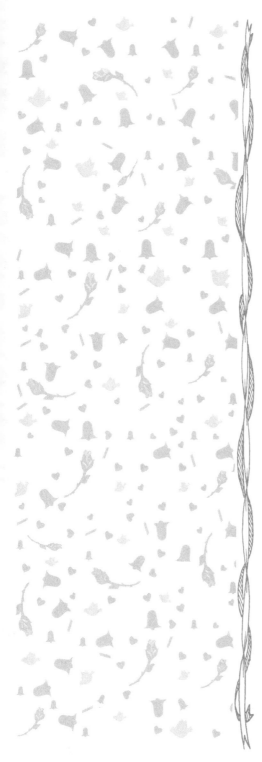

News flash: one of the perks of getting married is that people shower you with gifts. The idea behind all this gift-giving is to help the new couple in setting up their home and starting their life together. You pay these generous friends and family members back by showing them a wonderful time at your wedding—and by having a long, happy marriage.

The gifts probably will start arriving soon after you announce your engagement and will continue in a steady stream until the wedding. Etiquette dictates that people have up to a year after the wedding to send a gift, so you may be getting scattered presents long after the honeymoon. The gift organizer in the back of this book allows you to keep a record of what you receive, from whom, and when. Organizing things this way will be a great help when you sit down to write those thank-you notes.

The Gift Registry

Though some of your friends and family have probably already decided on the perfect gift for you, there are no doubt others who would appreciate a few hints. That's where the gift registry comes in. Gift registry is a free service provided by most department, jewelry, gift, and specialty stores. Couples go in and "register" for a list of gifts they would like to receive. When friends and family go into the store, they give the registry attendant your name, and he or she provides them with the list. As each item is bought, it is removed from the list, helping to prevent duplication.

You and your fiancé should put some careful thought into what store or stores you will register with. Make sure the store has a variety of quality items, in the colors and styles you want. (In other words, don't pick a place because you love their bath towels but despise everything else.) You might consider registering with a few specialty shops, but have some pity on your guests—you don't want to send them traipsing all over the world. It's best to register with one high-quality department store that is sure to have almost everything you need. Another advantage of these stores is that your registry can often be sent to their branches in other cities and states—a key point for out-of-town guests.

If such a department store is just out of the question, you may want to consider registering with a store that provides efficient catalog order service. Once guests know the name of the store you've chosen, they simply call to receive the catalog and a copy of your registry. They can at least see a picture of what they're getting you, and have the added convenience of only having to pick up the phone to buy your gift. The gift can be mailed to them, or directly to you. Hopefully, the sender will remember to ask the store to include a card stating whom the gift is from, or will send a follow-up card once they're sure the gift has arrived. Otherwise, you may be wondering for months who sent you the lovely glassware you wanted.

Before registering with a store, ask about the policy on returns and exchanges—you don't want to be stuck with duplicate or damaged gifts. Find out if the store will take responsibility if you receive gifts intended for another couple, and vice versa. Though it may seem far-fetched, people with names much more exotic than Smith or Jones do share their names with someone else out there; if they've both got bridal registries at the same store, there can be a mix-up. To prevent this, the store should use your groom's name or the wedding date as an additional point of reference when asking friends and family which couple they want to buy for.

Take your time and browse through the store. Items to be on the lookout for include a formal dinnerware (china) pattern, a silverware pattern, glasses, pots and pans, linens, appliances, and anything else you can think of. When you decide on the styles, patterns, and colors you want, add that item to the list. Try to achieve some balance in your final list; mix in everyday kitchen items with fine dishware. And even though you may feel awkward, don't be afraid to ask for a few "big money" items like a television or a VCR; you may be helping out friends or family looking to chip in for just such a gift.

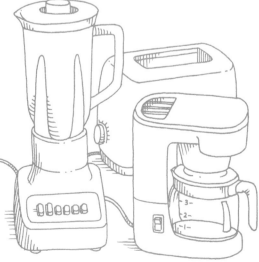

A carefully assembled gift registry can help put you on the road to a beautiful, functioning, and well-stocked home. It will also help ensure that you don't get Art Deco when you wanted Victorian, that you aren't sitting, overwhelmed, in front of a pile that contains five juicers, three blenders, a neon beer sign, and a lava lamp; and that, at least at the outset of your marriage, something actually matches something else at the dinner table.

Returning/Exchanging Gifts

What if (God forbid!) someone does send you that lava lamp—with a matching fringe lampshade? Your first instinct would probably be to immediately throw it out, burn it, or exchange it for something else. But it's not as simple as that. The people who bought you that gift did so with the best of intentions, spending a good deal of their time, energy, and money on you. Imagine how hurt they'd be if they visited your house a week after the wedding, expecting the lamp to hold a place of honor, only to find that you'd exchanged it for some napkin rings.

The best thing you can do to avoid this awkward situation is to wait until about a month after the wedding to exchange any unwanted or duplicate gifts. It is customary for you to display all of your gifts somewhere in your home in the days before the wedding; anyone visiting at that time is likely to look for their gift and even ask your opinion of it. After the wedding, when everything is put away in its proper place, guests are less likely to make an issue out of their gifts (you hope!). This is also a good policy regarding gifts you receive at the reception. If your aunt actually gives you a painting of Elvis on black velvet, you may want to consider keeping it around so that she can see it when she comes to visit you. After the first visit, odds are you'll be exchanging it for something else or "storing" it in the basement.

Another advantage to waiting is that you will have a better idea of the things you still need after all the presents are in. Exchanging the lamp for a toaster only to receive another toaster two weeks later will end up adding to your frustration (and your time in the returns line).

If you do return an unwanted gift, don't let the giver know about it. Send a prompt thank-you note expressing your gratitude for the thoughtfulness expressed in the gift. Hopefully you won't get caught in this web of deceit, but if you do, explain the gift's return as tactfully and sensitively as you can.

Damaged Gifts

If you receive a damaged gift, try to track down the retailer who sold the item; ask whether it was insured. If it was, tell the person who gave you the gift so she can get her money back and perhaps buy something else. Uninsured gifts that are damaged should be quietly exchanged for the same item; there's no need to upset or worry the sender.

Gifts at the Reception

Gifts can get lost or damaged at the reception. Tell everyone who might be asked to pass the word that you'd prefer things be sent directly to your home. Any gifts that are brought to the reception should be put together on an out-of-the-way table or in a closet. Wait until you get home before opening anything; the chances of losing or breaking something at the reception are greater if the gifts are opened. Ask that someone be in charge of watching the gifts and making sure they find their way home.

Thank-You Notes

As soon as you receive a gift you should send out a thank-you note. As hard as it will be given the many notes you'll be writing, try to be warm and personal. Always mention the gift, and, if possible, how you and your fiancé will be using it—this small touch will prevent people from feeling you just sent them a form letter. When sending notes for gifts you received before the wedding, sign your maiden name.

Here are some examples of good thank-you letters.

Dear Ann and Billy,

Thank you so much for the beautiful painting. We plan to hang it over the living-room fireplace for everyone to see. The colors really brighten up the room.

Fondly,
Ann

Dear Aunt Mary:

Thank you for the lovely wine glasses; they really round out our bar set. Jim and I are looking forward to your next visit, when you can have a drink with us.

Warmest regards,
Ann

Gift Display

In some parts of the country it is popular to have a gift display at the reception site. Gifts are set out on a table, often arranged in groups (appliances together, dishes together, and so on) and garnished with flowers or greenery. Gift displays are extra work: someone has to be in charge of transporting the gifts back and forth and setting up the display.

If you do decide to have a gift display, arrange for some security to watch the table and prevent the gifts from being stolen or damaged.

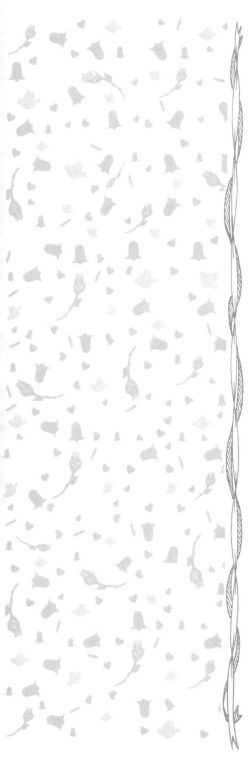

When You'd Prefer Cash

Perhaps you and your fiancé would prefer gifts of cash to put toward buying a house, a car, or another big-ticket item. If this is the case, do not express this wish on your invitations. Ask someone responsible and tactful, such as your parents, to spread the word around. This approach keeps things low-key... and helps to let people know what the money will be used for, so they don't think their generosity will be keeping you supplied with cigarettes and beer.

Register for your dream house? Yes!

A new kind of cash gift is springing up that may be worth looking into. Your friendly HUD (Department of Housing and Urban Development) and a few mortgage lenders have moved into modern times by recognizing the desire of every young couple to own their own home, a goal that so many find difficult to achieve. (The home ownership rate for people under 35 is 58.8 percent as against a national average of 65.4 percent.)

HUD has announced a bridal registry initiative in which an engaged couple can open an interest-bearing savings account at any one of thirty FHA-approved lenders around the country. Your family or friends can contribute toward a down payment.

The etiquette ladies may shudder, but this is becoming an acceptable way to ask for a money gift. One bank, at least, offers cards explaining the program which you can mail out with your invitations. Tacky? Maybe, but better than receiving unwanted crystal stemware or silver that needs polishing. In some participating mortgage institutions, if you decide not to buy a house, the cash belongs to you. Get the straight information by calling 1-800-CALLFHA.

Thank-you notes for gifts of cash

Dear Ed,

Thank you so much for your generous gift. Mark and I have narrowed it down to two houses and are having a hard time deciding between the two. When we do, we hope you'll be one of the first dinner guests.

Cordially,

Ann

"No Gifts, Please"

Though there are not very many of them out there these days, some couples actually do not want or need wedding gifts. This sometimes happens when the couple is older and more established. (Other couples are simply well-off to begin with and don't like to see money wasted.) If you and your groom are part of this lucky group, you can let your guests know with a simple statement on the invitation: "No gifts, please."

In Case of Cancellation

If the wedding is cancelled, you must return all gifts, even ones that were personalized or monogrammed. Return the gift with a small note explaining the cancellation (there's no need to give messy details). If the wedding is postponed, you can keep the gifts, but even if the wedding is delayed, do not delay your thank-you notes.

It's Lovely . . . But Who Sent It?

Occasionally the card that comes with a gift is lost (or just not included in the first place). If this happens to you, put your keen detective skills to work. Most of the time the senders do not realize there is no identifying card (if they did, they would probably contact you) and are waiting anxiously to hear from you.

If the gift arrived in the mail, check for the return address. No luck? Check to see whether the gift was purchased from the store where you are registered. If it is, there should be a record of who bought it.

If the gift was brought to the reception, your job will be a little harder. Go through your guest list; try to figure out which people hadn't yet sent a gift by that point. With any luck, there will be only a handful of people who went to the reception who were late in giving gifts. Perhaps you can narrow it down from there. Or perhaps the gift itself will be a clue about its sender: if your great-aunt has always sent demitasse spoons as wedding gifts, and you got a set with no name, you've probably found your culprit.

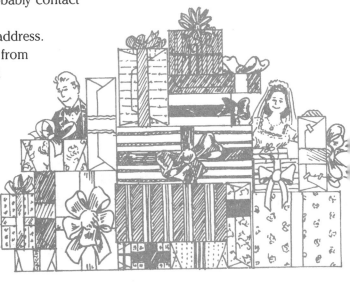

Sample Registry

The categories listed below are those traditionally registered for; for specific items in each category, see the checklist at the back of the book.

Formal dinnerware	Luggage
Casual dinnerware	Home electronics
Formal flatware/silverware	Ready-to-assemble furniture
Casual flatware	Formal table linens
Glassware	Casual table linens
Bar and glassware	Master bedroom
Hollowware	Guest bedroom
Gifts/home decor items	Master bath
Small electric appliances	Guest bath
Cutlery	Grooming aids for the bride
Bakeware	Grooming aids for the groom
Kitchen basics	Intimates for the bride
Cookware	

Tableware

Tableware is broken into four categories, depending upon whether you eat on it, eat with it, drink from it, or serve things from it: dinnerware/"everydayware," silverware/flatware, glassware, and hollowware.

Your best bet is to pick the style, pattern, and color of your dinnerware first. Choose the rest of your tableware with an eye to matching or complementing the dinnerware.

Dinnerware

Dinnerware usually refers to fine china, although some couples also request a set of "everyday" dishes. Most couples already have dishes and utensils, but sometimes this "set" is a mishmashed collection of blue-tinted glasses, dull knives, and three different kinds of hand-me-down plates. Obviously, the china is the more expensive, and if you were forced to choose, you'd probably select the china as the gift and pick up the everydayware yourselves. Only you know how much room is on your registry and what your priorities are; if the second set is a priority, make room for it. There are two types

of fine china: porcelain and bone. Porcelain is made from refined clay and minerals that make it nonporous, which means it cannot be stained by food. The main ingredient in bone china is bone ash. This china has an almost translucent glow; if you hold it up to light, you can see through it.

"Everydayware"

"Everydayware" may seem self-explanatory, but there are actually several kinds of everydayware to choose from, so your choice might be more complicated than you'd think.

Stoneware. Like porcelain, stoneware is made from clay, but the clay is grainier and rougher, making it very durable.

Earthenware. Earthenware is also made from clay, but it is less durable than stoneware, and it may be stained by food.

Oven-to-tableware. From the name, you already know you can cook with it. Oven-to-tableware contains a little porcelain and a mixture of other clays. It is usually guaranteed to be safe and untarnished by the oven for a certain number of years.

Plastic. The highest-quality plastic dinnerware is known as Melamine, and is very durable and stain resistant. Not too many couples use plastic these days, but you might consider it as a spare set for picnics, vacations, and camping trips.

Whether you're choosing dinnerware for formal or everyday use, you will want to choose the design of the plate carefully. Some plates are rimmed or shouldered, meaning they have a slight lip around the edge; others are rimless (also called coupe), completely level all around.

When trying to decide how many place settings you should order, think about your lifestyle and the degree of entertaining you do. Perhaps you have a lot of big formal dinner parties; you'll need a good number of formal place settings. But if your style is geared more toward pizza and beer than shrimp cocktail and roasted duck, you'll probably only need a small set to start you off.

The standard formal place setting consists of a dinner plate, a salad/dessert plate, a bread and butter plate, a coffee cup, and a saucer. Everydayware bread and butter plates are replaced by soup bowls.

Should You Return It?

If you know that a family member or friend is the type to ask to see the gift he gave you every time he visits, don't exchange his gift. No matter how much you dislike it, it will be nothing compared to the anguish you'll all feel when he finds out you took it back.

Here's another tip. Remember that with every gift you register for, you must provide the pattern, the quantity, and in some cases, the material and color. Being specific will ensure that no one (least of all you) is confused about what you want.

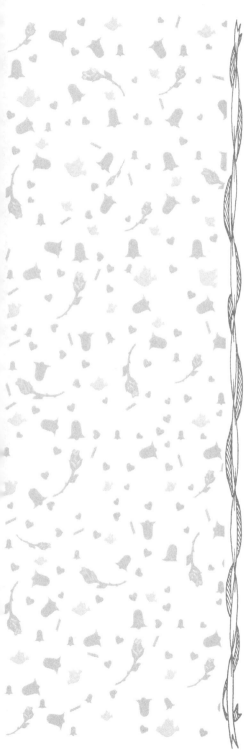

Silverware/flatware

What most of us know as silverware is referred to as flatware in the stores and by those in traditional circles. As you would expect, flatware is just about anything that you eat with short of chopsticks: forks, spoons, knives, and even serving utensils. Since you won't want to place your best china next to stainless steel utensils with plastic handles, you should put some thought into getting some high-quality flatware.

The best flatware you can buy is made of sterling silver. Some families treat their sterling silver as an heirloom and pass it down through the generations. These days, many couples are bypassing the highest-quality silver and opting for something that is both elegant and less expensive.

There is no denying the elegance and style of sterling silver—but don't hide it away in a cupboard, and use it only on special occasions. Regular use of your silver will help to bring out a special glow (called a patina) in the silver that is caused by small scratches. Since you can use it every day, and it tends, with good care, to get better with use and age, you may consider forgetting the middle-of-the-road stuff and going with sterling silver as your standard flatware.

Glassware

Glassware is absolutely anything you drink out of or pour a drink from: beer glasses, wine glasses, cocktail glasses, champagne glasses, pilsner glasses, brandy snifters, water goblets, wine decanters, you name it. Your glassware can be as elegant as crystal, right down to everyday juice glasses. The main divisions for glassware are based on how it's made and how it's decorated.

Glassware can be hand-blown or machine-made. Pieces of hand-blown glass are so fine and delicate that they are considered works of art. If you and your fiancé live life like it's a roller derby, you might want to take a pass on the artwork and go for something a little sturdier.

After it is made, glass can be decorated and styled in many ways:
Full-lead crystal is the highest quality glassware you can buy. The glass must meet standards for its lead content (24 percent in the U.S.). Although you might wonder how lead could make such a difference (after all, they used to make pencils out of it!), it does

provide an amazing sparkle—and also makes the crystal softer, which aids in the creation of delicate designs.

Lead crystal contains less lead; it is usually used to make goblets, pitchers, and bowls. Its products are considered to be very high quality.

Pressed glass. Molds are used to create raised patterns on the glass.

Etched glass. Designs here are made using wax and acid.

Cut glass is decorated by hand using a stone wheel, or a machine that performs the same function.

Lime glass is made from combinations of lime and soda. This is the inexpensive, "everyday" glassware.

If you want a really different look, consider colored glass, milk glass (opaque), or cased glass, which looks two-toned.

Hollowware

Hollowware is serving bowls and dishes, such as soup tureens, vegetable dishes, salt and pepper shakers, creamers, sugar bowls, and so on. The choices of style and composition are very broad here: sterling silver, pewter, glass, wood, silverplate—the list goes on and on. Obviously, you'll be looking for what best complements your tableware scheme.

Linens

Linen items are not restricted to the kitchen. Yes, you should consider napkins (not the kind you use once and throw away), tablecloths, and place mats—but don't forget towels, face cloths, sheets, and pillow cases.

Cookware

Most better-quality cookware (pots and pans) comes in several different forms, depending upon what an item is made of. Before you sign up for anything, find out about the different options: Which one is most durable? Most likely not to fade or scratch? Best at conducting heat?

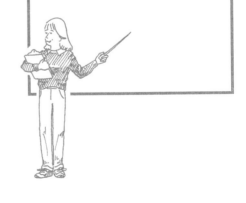

Words to the Wise

Beware of a deal on fine china that seems too good to be true. Often, discontinued patterns are drastically marked down, which is fine for the moment—but down the road if you want to replace a broken piece or add a new one to the set, it's bad news.

Although there are some outlet stores that specialize in discontinued patterns, there is no guarantee that you will be able to find yours there.

Your options for cookware:

Aluminum is the most popular variety on the market. It spreads heat quickly and evenly, and is the lightest cookware you'll find. (It's pretty easy to clean, too!)

Porcelain enamel conducts and spreads heat like metal, but it also has a surface that's extremely easy to clean. Porcelain enamel won't stain or scratch, and you certainly won't find little shavings from the pan's bottom in your food.

Stainless steel, alas, is not a very good conductor of heat. It is durable, though, and it will not dent, scratch, stain, corrode, or tarnish. Sometimes stainless steel can be combined with copper or aluminum, which takes care of the heat-conducting problem.

Glass and pyroceramic cookware has an all-in-one quality that is ideal for someone with a hectic schedule (or a disdain for washing a lot of dishes). In it, you can prepare a meal in advance, freeze it for a later date, cook it in the oven, and serve from it on the table. It's also nonstick and easy to clean. Its downfall: it won't behave the same way as metal if you drop it on the floor.

Copper. People have been cooking with copper longer than with any other metal. It is the best conductor of heat you can find, and it helps to keep food warm if it has to sit around a while. Make sure any copper cookware you buy is bonded with stainless steel, silver, or another surface, as it is dangerous for food to come in direct contact with copper. Mashed russet potatoes would turn into rusted russet potatoes in a straight copper pan, because copper will stain food. (Copper is not for those who don't like expending a little elbow grease; it has to be polished periodically to maintain its shine.)

Microwaveable cookware has a name that speaks for itself. Unless you plan to cook every single meal you'll ever eat in the microwave, microwave dishes should be considered a supplement to your other cookware. Get a few "nukeable" items, though—there's nothing quite as depressing as thinking you can cook that casserole in 10 minutes instead of 45, only to discover you don't have a safe dish.

Before you list cookware on your registry, consult with the salesperson on the pluses and minuses of each make. Get recommendations from friends and family, preferably those with the same cooking habits. Remember to ask if the cookware comes with a nonstick surface; this feature can save you quite a bit of cleaning time—and add years to the life of your S.O.S. pads.

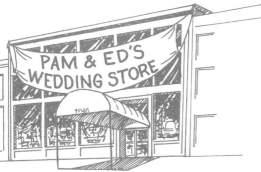

Chapter 8

What It All Means: A Brief History of Wedding Rituals

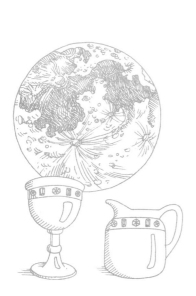

ave you ever wondered why a bride wears a veil? Why people throw rice at the newlyweds? Why it's called a honeymoon when neither you nor your fiancé is named Honey? These traditions (and many others) have been a part of weddings for centuries. It's a pretty good bet you'll see some of them at yours, and for many weddings to come. So read on to get the inside scoop on how they came about.

The Honeymoon

In ancient times, Teuton couples would marry beneath a full moon, then drink honey wine for thirty days after; hence the name. (Too bad today's honeymoons rarely last for thirty days!)

Throwing Rice

The tradition of throwing rice began in the Orient. Rice (which symbolizes fertility) was thrown at the couple in the hope that this would bring a marriage yielding many children.

The Bridal Shower

As noted elsewhere in this book, this custom is believed to have started in Holland, where legend has it that a disapproving father would not provide his daughter with a dowry so that she might marry a less-than-wealthy miller. Her friends provided her with the then-essential dowry by "showering" her with gifts.

The Ring Finger

The third finger on the left hand is considered the ring finger. All engagement and wedding rings are worn there because centuries ago that finger was believed to be connected by a vein directly to the heart.

The Wedding Cake

Wedding cakes originated in ancient Rome, where a loaf of wheat bread was broken over the bride's head to symbolize hope for a fertile and fulfilling life. The guests ate the crumbs, believed to be good luck. The custom found its way to England in the Middle Ages. Guests brought small cakes to a wedding; the cakes were put in a pile, which the bride and groom later stood over and kissed. Apparently, someone came up with the idea of piling all the cakes together and frosting them, creating an early ancestor of the multi-tiered wedding cakes of today.

Diamond Engagement Ring

In medieval Italy, precious stones were seen as part of the groom's payment for the bride. The groom would give a gift of such stones, which symbolized his intent to marry.

The Wedding Ring

The idea of the wedding ring itself dates back to ancient times, when a caveman-husband would wrap circles of braided grass around his bride's wrists and ankles, believing it would keep her spirit from leaving her body. The bands evolved into leather, carved stone, metal, and later silver and gold. (Luckily, you only have to wear them on your finger nowadays—and the groom usually reciprocates.)

Trousseau

When French brides went to their new home with their new husband, they brought their clothes and other meager possessions with them in a small bundle. The French word for this bundle was "trousseau." When the standard dowry became more than what you could carry in a small bundle, the name was no longer adequate, but it stuck just the same. Today, the gifts a bride-to-be receives at her wedding shower could be considered a modern-day version of the trousseau.

Words to the Wise

Find out if your family and friends are planning to throw rice at you. If they are, suggest they throw birdseed instead; it has the same theatrical effect, and it is not deadly to the nearby birds, as rice is. (Their digestive systems simply can't handle rice; any they eat will kill them.)

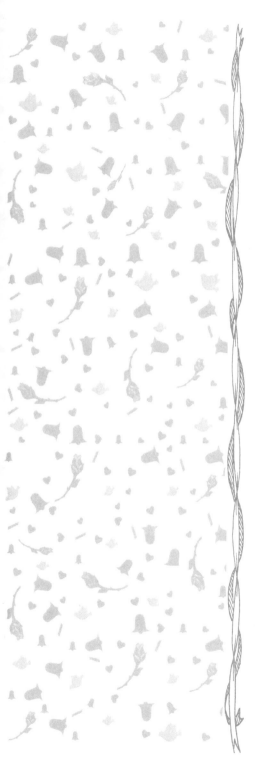

"Something Old, Something New, Something Borrowed, Something Blue"

The odds are pretty strong that you'll be wearing all of the above on your wedding day. But do you know why? The old is to stand for a bride's ties to her past; the new represents her hope for the future; the borrowed means friendship; and the blue is for faithfulness. These things are only significant symbolically, but try to get a bride to the altar without them.

Carrying the Bride Across the Threshold

Yet another wedding custom originated in Italy—Rome, to be exact. The bride had to be carried across the threshold because she was (or pretended to be) reluctant to enter the bridal chamber. In those days, it was considered ladylike to be hesitant at this point—or at least look hesitant. (Another legend has it that the bride was carried over the threshold to protect her from any evil spirits lingering there.)

The Best Man and Ushers

Speaking of reluctance, the potential groom used to take a group of his friends with him while in pursuit of the bride—you guessed it—to help him capture her. Often as not, young brides were "kidnapped" from a protective family which typically included a few big brothers. Sometimes there would even be a battle between competing suitors. If a potential groom wanted to show that he meant business, he took along the "best men" for the job of helping him fight for his love. Aren't you glad you live in the 20th century?

The Maid of Honor and Bridesmaids

These were the women who helped the bride get away from her overprotective family and other suitors so that she could be captured by the groom she wanted. When such quaint methods of getting the bride and groom together faded in popularity, the honor roles survived.

Giving the Bride Away

This custom is closely related to the throwing of the shoe, but probably not as painful. Back when a daughter was considered her father's possession, some formal transfer was necessary during the wedding ritual. Today, the custom symbolizes the parents' acceptance of the bride's passage from child to adult, and a sign of their blessing of her marriage to her chosen groom.

The Veil

Veils were originally meant to symbolize the virgin bride's innocence and modesty. These days, our society considers the veil a purely romantic custom. But in parts of the Middle East and Asia, the veil is still used to hide the bride's face completely. The first lace veil is said to have been worn by a woman named Nelly Curtis, George Washington's adopted daughter, who married one of his aides. Apparently, the first time the aide ever saw her she was behind a lace curtain. He was mesmerized by her beauty. Nelly, the story goes, made herself a lace veil for the ceremony in an effort to duplicate the effect.

Tossing the Garter and Bouquet

This dignified custom began in the 1300s in France, where guests used to chase the bride and tear off her garter because they believed it was good luck. To save herself, her leg, and her dress, the bride began removing it voluntarily and tossing it into the eager crowd. Later, the bouquet was added to this toss. The lucky recipient of the bouquet is now believed to be the next woman in the group to get married. The man who catches the garter is supposed to be the next groom.

Wedding Customs from Other Cultures
Africa

Though many women might not consider the sentiment well-wishing, the common greeting to a new bride in some tribes is,

"May thou bear twelve children with him." Some African ceremonies include the binding of the couples' wrists with plaited grass.

Belgium

The bride takes a family handkerchief with her name newly embroidered on it with her to the wedding. After the ceremony, it is framed and displayed in the family house until another daughter gets married; then she carries it and adds her name.

Bermuda

The new husband and wife plant a tree to symbolize their love and union.

Czech Republic

The bride wears a wreath made of rosemary to symbolize love, loyalty, and wisdom.

China

In the Chinese wedding ceremony, a goblet of honey and a goblet of wine are tied together with a red ribbon. Red is the color of love; the ribbon stands for unity. The bride and groom take a drink to symbolize a union of love. After a wedding dinner that might feature delicacies like bear nose, the guests receive fortune cookies for good luck.

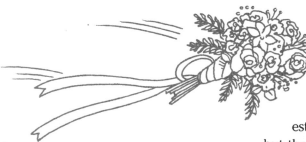

Egypt

For the rowdiest wedding procession you're likely to see, head to Egypt. Belly dancers, men brandishing swords, and people blowing loud horns all accompany the wedding party and guests as they troop from the ceremony to the reception. In an interesting twist, the guests wear traditional Egyptian clothing, but the bride dresses in a Western-style wedding gown.

England

In the English countryside, the bride and her attendants walk to the church on a floor strewn with flower petals, meant to guarantee a smooth and joyous path through life. As the couple enters the church, the bells chime; when they exit as husband and wife, they chime again, only to a different tune. (Bells were once believed to ward off evil spirits.)

Finland

In days gone by, the bride-to-be was crowned with gold during the ceremony. Afterwards, she was blindfolded and surrounded by all of the unmarried female guests. The bride groped around blindly until she picked someone to pass the crown to. The one the bride crowned was believed to be the next to wed (much like the bouquet-catcher).

France

Couples drink a toast from a "coupe de marriage," a two-handled silver cup. The cup is passed down through the family to future couples. For a refreshing change, the guests bring the flowers to the reception, to help the couple celebrate life and their new beginning. (Considering how big your florist's bill can be, you'll probably wish this idea would catch on here.)

Germany

In another tradition that some American women might like to see catch on in the United States, both the bride and groom wear gold bands as a symbol of their engagement. A custom not too many American women are likely to be fond of, however, is the one that encourages the groom to kneel on the hem of the bride's dress during the ceremony, as a sign that he is now her boss. The bride sets him straight by getting up and stepping on his foot.

Greece

During the ceremony, the bride and groom wear crowns made from flowers, signifying their entrance into marriage. The couple takes three sips of wine and walks around the altar three times with the priest, which symbolizes the Trinity. The groom's Godfather (or another honored male family member, known as *koumbaros*) has an important part in the ceremony: he is the one who crowns the couple.

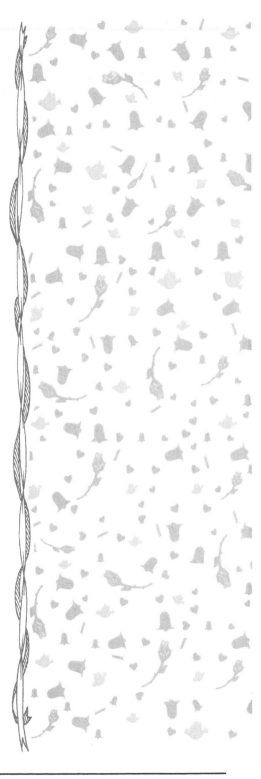

Holland

An awning or canopy of sorts made of evergreen is set up for the couple; they sit under it on thrones during a pre-wedding party given by the families. The evergreens are meant to symbolize everlasting love. As the couple "holds court," the party guests approach them to wish them luck and happiness.

India

The families of both the bride and groom prepare puffed rice for the ceremony as a symbol of fertility and good luck. The groom's brother douses the new husband and wife with flower petals at the ceremony's end. Henna dye is used to paint designs on the couple's hands; the couple usually leaves their handprints on the outside door of their new home for good luck.

Ireland

Many Irish believe there is a lucky day for weddings, one that comes but once a year: New Year's Day. For good luck, a swatch of Irish lace may be sewn into the bride's gown; the couple also receives a horseshoe to put up in their new home. Although they are now popular in America simply as friendship rings, Claddagh rings remain the standard Irish wedding ring. The heart, crown, and hands found on the Claddagh symbolize love, loyalty, and friendship.

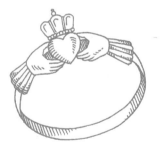

Italy

The lucky villagers are recipients of cakes and other baked goodies passed out by the bride and groom as they wind their way through the streets. For the departing couple, there are no clanging cans on the back of the car; instead, the front grill is decorated with flowers to symbolize the road to a happy marriage.

Japan

Part of the Japanese wedding ceremony requires both the bride and groom to take nine sips of sake. They may be a little tipsy after the nine sips, but they are considered married after the first. During the ceremony, the bride will leave to change clothes three to four times. (And you thought finding one wedding gown was tough!) As usual, the groom has it easy, wearing only one black kimono. Guests at a Japanese wedding are very lucky—not only are they fed and entertained, but the wedding favors they receive from the couple's families sometimes equal up to half the price of the gifts given to the couple.

Lithuania

The parents of the bride and groom give them gifts that stand for the elements of marriage: wine for joy, salt for tears, and bread for work.

Mexico

The couple is joined by a white silk cord wrapped around their shoulders to signify their union in marriage. In some ceremonies, the silk cord is replaced by a large string of rosary beads, wrapped around the couple in the form of a figure eight. After the ceremony, the couple dances in a heart-shaped circle formed by the guests.

Philippines

Here, they also use the white silk cord. Unlike in the United States, the groom's family pays for the wedding; they also give the bride old coins which stand for prosperity. In return, the bride's family gives the new couple a cash dowry.

Poland

For the privilege of dancing with the bride, guests put money into the pockets of an apron she wears over her wedding dress. The money collected from this "Dollar Dance" is supposed to go toward paying for the honeymoon. (Imagine how many dances it would take for a trip to Hawaii.)

Romania

If you have a feeling you may be a hungry bride, Romania is the place to marry; there, guests shower the newlyweds with nuts and candy, meant to symbolize prosperity.

Russia

Oh, to be a guest here. Rather than bring a gift to the wedding, all non–family member guests receive a gift.

Old Shoes

Once these were thrown at the bride by her father; the act symbolized his yielding possession of her to the groom. Shoes used to symbolize ownership and power over a woman.

Spain

The bride embroiders a shirt for the groom, which he wears on their wedding day; she herself wears orange blossoms and a mantilla. In an unusual turn, the bride and groom wear their wedding bands on their right hands.

Sweden

The couple is sure to smell very nice here. The bride carries a bouquet of herbs in hopes that the fragrance will ward off trolls; the groom's attire comes complete with some thyme sewn in. In an era of pumps and high-heels, one Swedish tradition is no longer popular, but in the old days, the bride kept her shoes untied for the entire wedding day. (In case you're wondering, yes, she would even consummate the marriage with her shoes on!) If, in the course of her night's sleep, the shoes should slip off, it was a sign that she would bear children easily. (The idea apparently being that kids will slip out as easily as the shoes slip off.)

Switzerland

Junior bridesmaids begin the wedding procession by throwing colored handkerchiefs to the guests. Those who catch a hanky are supposed to give money to help the couple start out. (Lucky them!)

United States

In the early days of the country, guests did not give appliances or money to the couple—they provided the newlyweds with some stamina-giving sack posset, a drink consisting of hot spiced milk and brew.

Before the Civil War, African-American brides believed that the best days to get married were Tuesdays and Wednesdays because that would ensure a long and happy life with one's husband.

Wales

The bride's attendants receive a gift of myrtle from the bride; the flower's blooming is said to predict another wedding.

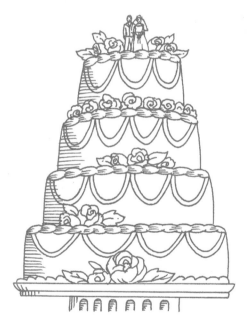

Part Two:

The Wedding Ceremony

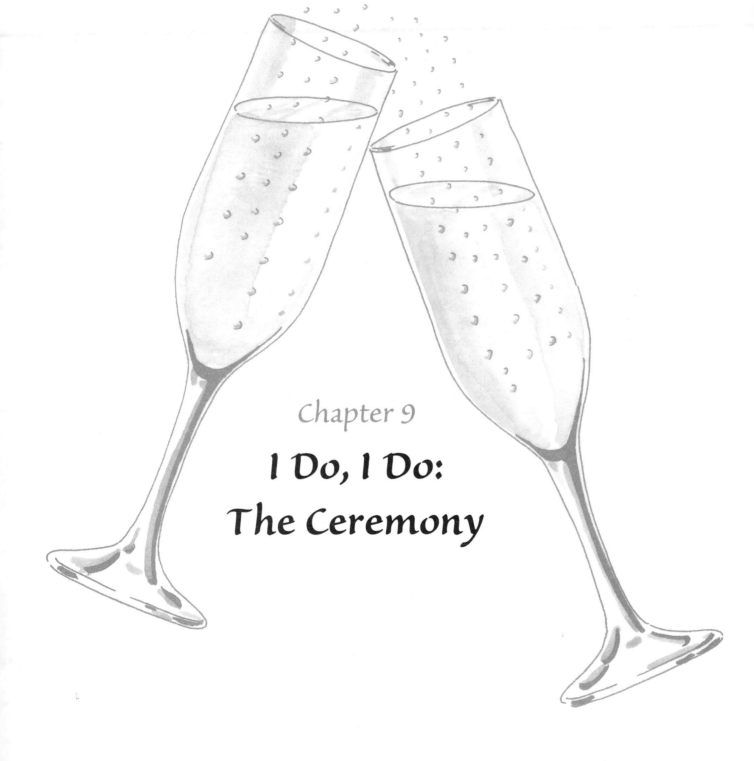

Chapter 9

I Do, I Do:
The Ceremony

The wedding ceremony is that nerve-wracking and frightening experience you have to survive in order to get to the reception. If you find it helpful, you can ease the ordeal by visualizing the terrific party that awaits you once you make it past this part.

The ceremony is what takes you from being an engaged couple to being a married couple. Depending upon your personal convictions, this transformation can be either religiously based or a strictly civil (legal) act. If either of you has any doubts about which of these options is best, you should address them early on. Until you get the groundwork laid for the ceremony, you will probably find it hard to plan much of anything else.

Going to the Chapel?

If you decide on a religious ceremony, consult with your officiant about pre-marriage requirements. Religions differ in their rules and restrictions, as do different branches within the same religion. Your first meeting with the officiant should clear up most of the technical details and give you the opportunity to ask questions. After everything is settled, the way will be clear for you to personalize your ceremony with music, Scripture readings, special prayers, and even your own vows.

Although religions differ too much to make a blanket statement about each one's approach to the marriage rite, the following should give you a general idea about what to expect from some of the major religions' ceremonies.

Roman Catholic Ceremony and Preparations

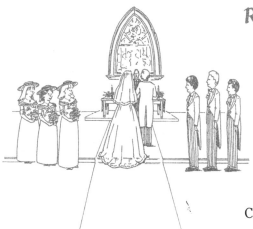

If you're getting married in the Roman Catholic Church, you probably already know that it has some hefty pre-marital requirements. If you've been married before, your challenge is pretty daunting. Technically, it is impossible to remarry in the Catholic Church if your first spouse is still alive. Even a civil divorce will not do the trick; you must receive an annulment. Essentially, an annulment nullifies your previous marriage; once the annulment is granted, the earlier marriage never existed in the eyes of the Church. The annulment procedure is complicated (and intimidating),

Pre-Marital Counseling

Who hasn't heard engaged couples groan at the prospect of spending a series of evenings or even a whole weekend in pre-marital counseling? Before you add your voice to theirs, do one simple thing: ask them what they thought of it. Their answers may surprise you.

Many couples today, no matter how long they've been together, avoid addressing serious issues about their future lives together. They may be certain they already know their partner's position on having children, for example. But if the question has never been asked, then how can they be so sure of the answer?

Pre-marital counseling helps couples open the lines of communication. It gives both partners the chance to let their innermost feelings be known. Even though such counseling is overseen by religious officiants, nothing is taboo: sex, birth control, children, family, intimacy, compatibility, commitment, and other related issues are all brought up for discussion. And while there may be religious overtones at times, many couples find that the officiant is more concerned with getting the partners to speak freely than preaching his or her religion's views on the topic at hand.

So when the time comes for pre-marital counseling, try to keep an open mind. That's what it's all about, after all.

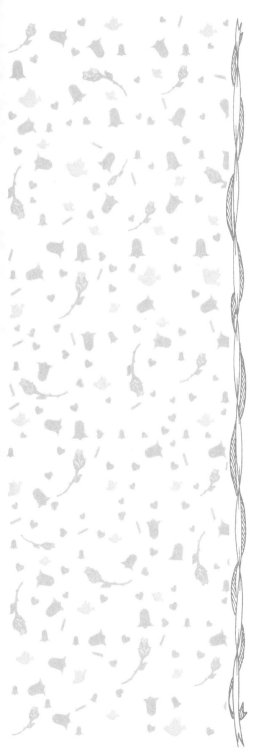

requiring a great deal of paperwork on the part of the person applying; it can cost quite a lot, too. (The Catholic Church has special sliding fees, and makes exceptions for those in difficult financial circumstances.)

It bears repeating: without an annulment, a divorced person cannot marry in the Catholic Church, so if either you or your fiancé will need an annulment, you'd best set the wheels in motion at least a year before you plan to wed—it can take that long. The priest cannot reserve a wedding date within the Church until the annulment has gone through. (Note, though, that a previous marriage that did not take place within the Church does not require an annulment. From the Church's point of view, a civil-ceremony marriage that ends in divorce was never a marriage in the first place.)

If you don't have to worry about any of this, congratulations. You may move to the next step, pre-marital counseling, also known as Pre-Cana ("pre-marriage"). This required counseling is some of the most extensive marriage preparation work you can undertake. What can you expect from Pre-Cana? A lot of talking between you, your groom, and your priest about your religious convictions and important marriage issues; workshops with other engaged couples; and even some compatibility quizzes.

If you need to go through pre-marital counseling, contact the Church soon for their scheduled meetings. Group counseling programs (where many couples meet for a series of evenings or a weekend retreat) are scheduled throughout the year, but space is limited, so sign up right away for the time frame you want.

What about the ceremony itself? Contrary to popular belief, the Catholic ceremony does not go on and on and on. Although you have the option of having a complete Mass (which adds about fifteen minutes to the total time), this is not a requirement. From the moment the organ announces your arrival at the altar to the time you walk back down the aisle with your new husband, approximately half an hour will have elapsed. So what is going on?

♥ Introductory Rites. The ceremony starts with opening music selections; once you reach the altar, the priest greets you and your guests, offers Penitential rites, and says an opening prayer.

♥ Liturgy of the Word. This is when the reading you have chosen will be read, perhaps by special friends or family members. At the completion of the reading, the priest gives a brief homily that focuses on some aspect of marriage.

♥ Rite of Marriage. Here's where you see some action. After the declaration of consent, the rings are blessed and exchanged. What most people don't realize is that the exchange of vows, not the ring exchange, is the act that marks the official moment of marriage.

The Protestant Ceremony and Preparations

The Protestant religion encompasses many different denominations, but the basic elements of the marriage ceremony are the same. Here's a brief overview of what to expect:

♥ The ceremony begins; members of the wedding party walk up the aisle.
♥ The couple welcome their guests.
♥ A Prayer of Blessing is said.
♥ Scripture passages are read.
♥ There is a Giving in Marriage (affirmation by parents).
♥ The congregation gives its response.
♥ Vows and rings are exchanged.
♥ The celebration of the Lord's Supper takes place.
♥ The unity candle is lit.
♥ The Benediction is given.
♥ The Recessional takes place.

Protestant marriages, regardless of denomination, have far fewer requirements and restrictions than Catholic marriages. An informational meeting with the clergy is required, but pre-marital counseling is optional. And there is no need for an annulment if either party has been divorced.

Jewish Ceremonies and Preparations

Judaism, too, has different "divisions" that adhere to different rules; however, in the Orthodox, Conservative, and Reform traditions, certain elements of the wedding ceremony are basically the same.

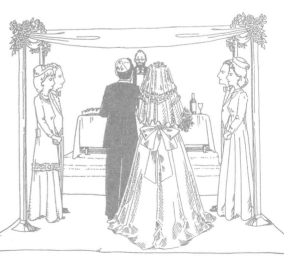

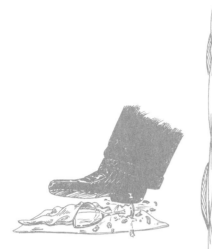

- ♥ The marriage ceremony is conducted under a *huppah*, an ornamented canopy (optional in the Reform ceremony).
- ♥ The Seven Blessings are recited.
- ♥ The bride and groom drink blessed wine; the groom then smashes the glass with his foot. The glass is wrapped in a napkin, presumably to prevent flying shards from landing in someone's eye. The ritual symbolizes the fragility of life.
- ♥ The newly married couple is toasted with the expression "Mazel tov!" ("Good luck!")

Jewish marriages within the Orthodox and Conservative branches have a few stipulations that are rigidly adhered to. Weddings cannot take place on the Sabbath or any time that is considered holy. Both Orthodox and Conservative ceremonies are performed in Hebrew or Aramaic only; neither branch will conduct interfaith ceremonies. Men must wear yarmulkes, and the bride wears her wedding ring on her right hand.

Reform ceremonies differ from Orthodox and Conservative in a few ways. In English-speaking countries, the ceremony is performed in both English and Hebrew. The bride wears her ring on her left hand. As in the Orthodox and Conservative traditions, however, Reform ceremonies cannot take place on the Sabbath or during holy times.

Preparations for ceremonies differ, depending upon the tradition. Check with your rabbi for specific details.

If Yours Is an Interfaith Marriage...

The Catholic Church will sanction a marriage between a Catholic and a non-Catholic providing all of the Church's concerns are met. Contrary to popular belief, it is not necessary for, say, a Jewish person to convert to Catholicism in order to marry in a Catholic ceremony.

In marriages between a Protestant and a Catholic, officiants from both religions may take part in the ceremony if the couple wishes. However, in a Jewish-Christian wedding, even the most liberal clergy rarely will perform a joint ceremony in the temple or church. These ceremonies usually take place at the actual reception site.

A Note on Eastern Orthodox Ceremonies

The Eastern Orthodox (including Greek and Russian Orthodox) wedding ceremony is very similar to the Roman Catholic one, but features some additional rituals that have important symbolic value.

Many rituals in the Eastern Orthodox ceremony are performed three times—to represent the Holy Trinity. Wedding rings are blessed, then exchanged, three times. (Rings are worn on the right hand.) Crowns are placed on the couple's heads and switched back and forth three times. After the Gospel is read, the bride and groom each takes three sips from a cup of wine. The congregation sings "God Grant Them Many Years," and the couple walks hand-in-hand around the ceremonial table three times.

Meeting Your Chaplain

During the meeting with your officiant, be sure to get all the details concerning rules and restrictions, your church's feeling on interfaith marriages, any required commitments to raise children in your religion, and so on. Don't be afraid to ask questions; you want to make sure you and your church are on the same wavelength on these important issues.

Here is a list of questions you may wish to ask the officiant.

♥ Are the dates and times you're interested in available?
♥ What are the requirements for getting married in this church/synagogue?
♥ What are the pre-marital counseling requirements?
♥ Who will perform the ceremony? (You may be close to a particular officiant, only to find that he or she is not available at the time you want.)
♥ Are visiting clergy allowed to take part in the ceremony? If so, who will be responsible for what?
♥ What does the church or synagogue have available with regard to aisle runners, musical instruments, and musical talent? Is the church organ in good working order? What is the policy for bringing in your own organist (or other musicians)? Is there enough room at the site for you to bring in additional singers and players?

Words to the Wise

If you'd like to have a religious ceremony, but are attracted by the idea of having the ceremony on a yacht, in a ballroom, or in some other exotic locale, check with your officiant about the policy on performing an "off-site" ceremony.

♥ Are there any restrictions on decorations? On music?

♥ Will you be allowed into the ceremony site well in advance of the wedding to attend to decorations and set-up?

♥ Is another wedding scheduled for the same day as yours? If so, is there enough time between the two ceremonies to set up decorations and otherwise get things ready?

♥ Are there any restrictions on where the photographer and videographer may stand (or move) during the ceremony?

♥ Can your friends and relatives take part in the ceremony, as, say, readers or singers?

♥ Will you be allowed to hold the receiving line at the site—in the back of the church or synagogue, for instance, or in a courtyard? Is there enough room for this?

♥ What is the cost for the ceremony and the use of church or synagogue personnel and facilities? (This payment is typically referred to as a donation. It does not go to any single individual, but to the church or synagogue as a whole. These days, the suggested amount will range from $100 to $200.) The best man is traditionally responsible for giving the payment to the officiant at the ceremony's conclusion.

♥ How much parking is available?

♥ What arrangements are made for heating during the colder months or ventilation/air conditioning during the warmer months? (There's nothing worse than a bride shivering at the altar or a groom fainting from the heat.)

♥ If yours will be an interfaith marriage, will participation from another officiant be allowed? May other cultural and religious customs be included in the ceremony?

Let's Be Civil!

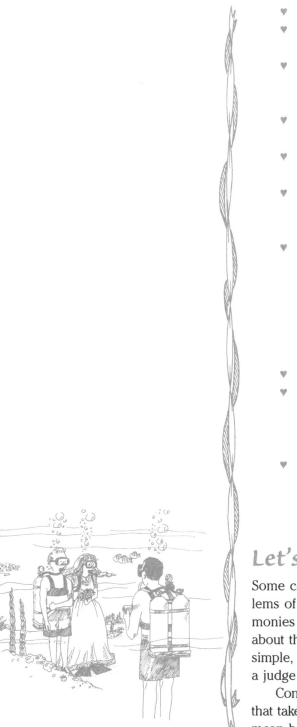

Some couples choose to bypass the tension and potential family problems of an interfaith ceremony by having a civil ceremony. Civil ceremonies may also be the best option for couples who are unsure about their own religious convictions—or who simply prefer a small, simple, and inexpensive ceremony. The officiant in a civil ceremony is a judge or other civic official legally qualified to perform a marriage.

Contrary to the stereotype (a barren scene in a judge's chambers that takes all of twenty seconds), being "civil" does not necessarily mean being boring, quick, or small. If you like, you can have a civil ceremony with all the trimmings of a traditional church wedding. Granted, it won't be in a religious setting, and no religious officials will be present, but you can still summon up a scene of power and drama. After all, your civic official isn't tied to a chair in City Hall. Get him or her out of the office—and into a hotel ballroom or a country club or on a yacht or anywhere else you feel like having your wedding. Civil ceremonies not held at City Hall or the courthouse are usually held at the reception site, which tends to make things more convenient for all involved. It doesn't make much sense to rent a country club for the ceremony, then move everyone to a hotel ballroom for the reception. (See the section on receptions for more location ideas.)

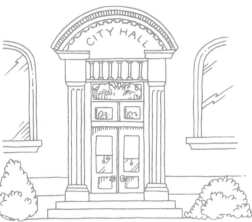

If you prefer to hold your ceremony in the civic official's office, think twice about your wedding attire. You may not feel comfortable coming and going in a full-length white gown. The dress code is a street-length dress or suit for the bride, and a suit for the groom.

Further questions about a civil ceremony, such as who exactly will be performing it, can be resolved with a call to City Hall—or whatever office in your area handles marriage licenses.

Forward, March!

If either you or your fiancé is in the military, you may want to consider having a military wedding. Military weddings are very formal affairs; they can look quite impressive, what with all of those uniformed guests and wedding party members. This type of wedding features what is perhaps the most visually stunning conclusion of them all: the newly married couple walks arm-in-arm from the altar beneath an archway of crossed swords!

A groom serving in the armed forces must wear his dress uniform in the ceremony. As part of his outfit he may wear a sword or saber, but never a boutonniere. If the groom does sport something with a long, sharp blade, the bride stands on his right, presumably to avoid getting blood on that nice white dress. If he doesn't wear a sword, she stands on the left.

A military bride has the choice of wearing her dress uniform or a traditional wedding gown. Other military personnel in the wedding party, male or female, usually wear military garb.

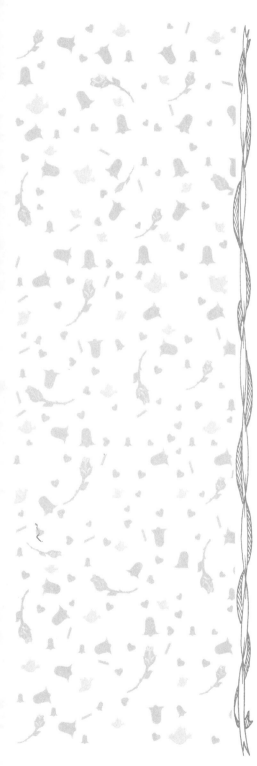

As if doing a seating plan for a regular wedding weren't stressful enough, the seating at a military wedding has to account for high-ranking officers and special officials. These people must be seated in places of honor. The remainder of the military guests should be seated by rank. And if you thought you'd seen enough of swords at the ceremony, you're not through yet; tradition dictates that the bride and groom cut the first piece of their wedding cake with a sword.

With the exception of the attire, some matters of protocol, and the use of weaponry, a military wedding can be as much like a traditional wedding as you wish.

Making the Ceremony Your Ceremony

The readings

Scripture readings at your wedding will, of course, be religious, but you don't have to recycle the same ones you've heard at a dozen other weddings. Your officiant will provide you with a list of recommended readings, most of which focus on some aspect of togetherness and marriage. If you have a favorite passage you'd like to have read, ask your officiant if it would be possible to include it in the ceremony.

The music

Music can add a new dimension to your ceremony, enhancing both its spirit and its meaning. You will have a broad range of choices here as well. Most officiants request that the songs you select be religious, but generally that doesn't mean you're restricted to music you only hear in a church. If you can find commercially released songs that meet the criteria, there should be no problem in their making it onto this "play list." If you have a friend or relative with a good singing voice or talent for playing an instrument, perhaps he or she can be persuaded to sing or play a special song. It would be best if he has experience performing in front of an audience; there's nothing more nerve-wracking than having your soloist come down with stage fright just when he's about to perform.

The rest

How else can you personalize your ceremony? Some couples like to acknowledge their debt to their parents by offering special

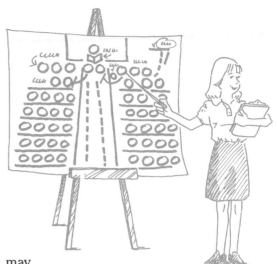

readings or prayers that focus on family themes. Or, as you walk up the aisle, give a single flower from your bouquet to your mother and your groom's mother. Consider including a wine ceremony or a ceremony for the lighting of the unity candle. You might also take your vows by candlelight, and have the church bells ring as you are declared husband and wife. Be sure to consult with your officiant first about restrictions. Be creative!

Writing Your Vows

You may want to formalize your commitment with something unique, something specific to your relationship or situation. You may want your marriage vows to be something truly meaningful to both of you. This is not to say that traditional vows can't be meaningful—but vows you create yourself are more personalized.

Before you break out your pad and pen to write the ultimate love sonnet or go memorizing the words to that special poem, though, let your officiant know about your intentions. Some religions can be strict about what vows must be said, while others are willing to bend a little.

Once you have the officiant's go-ahead, you and your fiancé should consider doing some soul-searching. The following questions and guidelines offer a good start. Each of you should take time to think about your answers and write them down. Doing so will provide you with valuable source material to help you develop the vow you're looking for.

♥ How do you, as a couple, define the following terms: love, trust, marriage, family, commitment, togetherness.

♥ How did the two of you first meet?

♥ What was the first thing you noticed about your partner?

♥ List any shared hobbies or other mutual interests you have.

♥ What was the single most important event in your relationship? (Or, what was the event that you feel says the most about your development as a couple?)

♥ How similar (or different) were your childhoods? Take a moment and try to recount some of the important parallels or differences here.

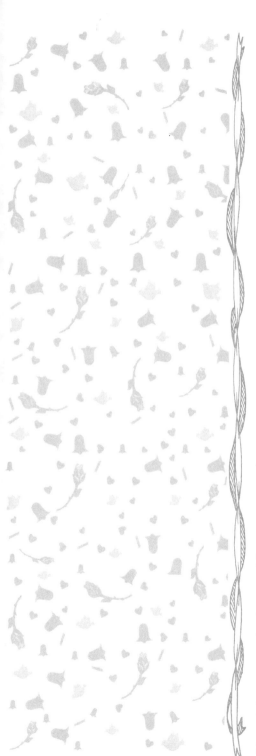

♥ Is there a song, poem, or book that is particularly meaningful in your relationship?

♥ Do you and your partner share a common religious tradition? If you share a common religious tradition, is there a particular Scriptural passage that you as a couple find especially meaningful?

♥ How do you and your partner look at personal growth and change? What aspects of your life together are likely to change over the coming years? How do you anticipate dealing with those changes? How important is mutual respect and tolerance in your relationship? When one of you feels that a particular need is being overlooked, what do you think is the best way to address this problem with the other person?

♥ Do you and your partner have a common vision of what your life as older people will be like? Will it include children and grandchildren? Take this opportunity to put into words the vision you and your partner share of what it will be like to grow old together.

Love letters

Arriving at answers to these questions can give you the foundation upon which to build your vows. But you may find that this material is not enough to get across the full meaning of what you want to say. Don't despair. Chances are someone else has said it already. William Shakespeare, Elizabeth Barrett Browning, John Lennon—you may just need to find the perfect quote, poem, or song lyric to complete the mood.

If you're like most people, you can't quote poetry off the top of your head. Luckily, there are many books of quotations available to point you in the right direction. Checking the index under "love," "marriage," "wedding," "husband," "wife," and other key words, will direct you to appropriate passages. Your librarian or a local bookstore can help you find books of love poems and wedding vows. (Valentine's Day may be the perfect time to find the latest books of love quotations.)

Don't forget the traditional . . .

Just because you've decided to exchange your own vows doesn't mean you can't use the time-honored words of your church or synagogue (again, provided your officiant approves). Many Scriptural passages speak eloquently of the bonds of love and marriage. Consult your religious leader for suggestions and for ways to adapt the passages to fit your ideas.

. . . and the nontraditional

Perhaps you and your partner have already composed the perfect paragraph, with no need to answer questions, consult sourcebooks, or discuss Scripture. It says exactly what both of you want to say—but the question is, Who says it? Instead of playing rock, paper, scissors to decide who has to write a second, lesser vow, consider having both recite the same paragraph. After all, it's how the church has been doing it for years.

Once you have gathered all the poems, quotes, lyrics, and Scriptural passages that appeal to you, put them with the answers to the above questions. Then set about the task of writing a first draft of your unique wedding vows. Let yourself go—there is no right or wrong way to write your vows. But don't be surprised if it takes you a few drafts to develop a vow that is right for you.

Getting the ballpoint rolling

Having trouble getting started? Here are some sample wedding vows:

Example 1: Memory lane

Groom: *The first thing I noticed about Kathy was her radiant smile. We were both auditioning for a show in college, and when I asked her what type of piece she had prepared, she said she planned to make it all up on the spot—and then she smiled at me. Kathy, your warmth and spontaneity have won my heart utterly. From this day forward, I will stand by your side. You are the one I will be true to always. Let us make our lives together. I pledge to you my future. I will share all my tomorrows with you and no other.*

Bride: *The first thing I noticed about John was his unceasing energy. As he waited for the director to call him in, he couldn't seem to sit still, and when I told him my plans for the audition, he stared at me as though I were mad—but mad in an interesting*

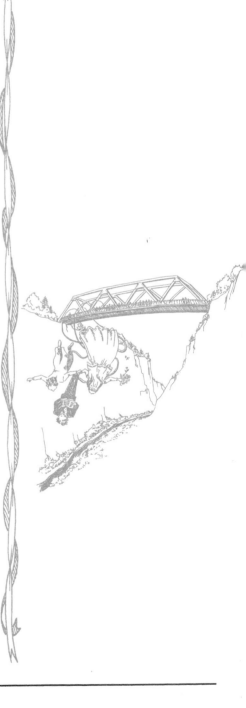

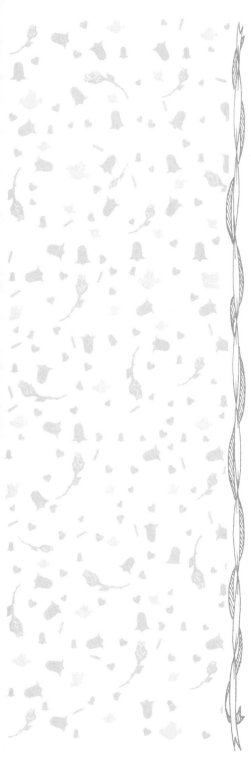

way. What he didn't tell you just now was that I got the lead role in the show and he wound up in the chorus. But John, from that day to this, and for all the days that follow, you will always be my leading man. From this day forward, I will stand by your side. You are the one I will be true to always. Let us make our lives together. I pledge to you my future. I will share all my tomorrows with you and no other.

Example 2: Poem, verse, or song intro

Bride: *Grow old along with me!*
Groom: *The best is yet to be.*
Bride: *The last of life, for which the first was made.*
Groom: *Our times are in His hand*
Who sait, A whole I planned;
Youth shows but half.
Trust God, see all nor be afraid!
Bride: *God bless our love.*
Groom: *God bless our love.*
Bride: *John, in this assembly of friends and family, I take you today as my husband. I do this in the certainty of my soul, and knowing that you are my true life partner. I will love you, honor you, and cherish you for the rest of our days, so long as we shall live.*

Groom: *Kathy, in this assembly of friends and family, I take you today as my wife. I do this in the certainty of my soul, and knowing that you are my true life partner. I will love you, honor you, and cherish you for the rest of our days, so long as we shall live.*

Example 3: Religious intro

Groom: *From the beginning of creation God made them male and female.*
Bride: *This is why a man must leave father and mother . . .*
Groom: *. . . and the two become one body. They are no longer two, therefore, but one body.*
Bride: *So then, what God has united . . .*
Groom: *. . . man must not divide.*
Bride: *John, today, in the gathering of this honored company, we unite in God's love. I pledge myself to you as your wife, and will be faithful to you for all of our days.*

Groom: *Kathy, today, in the gathering of this honored company, we unite in God's love. I pledge myself to you as your husband, and will be faithful to you for all of our days.*

Example 4: Nontraditional vows (both recite same vow)

I come here today, (name), to join my life to yours before this company. In their presence I pledge to be true to you, to respect you, and to grow with you through the years. Time may pass, fortune may smile, trials may come; no matter what we may encounter together, I vow here that this love will be my only love. I will make my home in your heart from this day forward.

Remember, the right way to compose your own wedding vow is your way. The examples you have just seen are offered as general guidelines only. Let your imagination be your guide to developing vows that are meaningful to both you and your partner.

Renewing your vows

Renewing your vows is a wonderful way to tell your partner that what you promised years before still holds true today. Consider reflecting on some of the key events of your lives together—establishing a home together, starting a family, changing careers, fulfilling dreams. Here's a starting point:

Once before I have stood with you before family and friends; once again I take your hand as my partner. (Add details of life together.) (Name), I take you this day and for all days as my (husband/wife).

Second or subsequent marriages

Celebrate finding a new love with special vows that emphasize learning from the past, looking to the future, and committing to a new life of happiness together. Example:

Today we look to the future. (Name), I enter into this marriage with joy and with a firm sense of the importance of sharing our lives as husband and wife. Let us always respect and care for one another from this day forward.

Great Names in Romantic Writing

Anne Bradstreet
Elizabeth Barrett
  Browning
Willa Cather
Emily Dickinson
John Donne
Ralph Waldo Emerson
Ben Jonson
John Keats
Anne Morrow
  Lindbergh
Henry Wadsworth
  Longfellow
John Milton
William Shakespeare
Percy Bysshe Shelley
Virgil

Double Your Pleasure

Let's say a sister, close friend, or relative wants to share your wedding day. You, of course, would tell her to Get Lost. Okay, maybe you're glad to share this day with someone who's special to you. (If it's your sister, certainly your parents will appreciate having to pay for only one wedding instead of two.) Whoever the special person is, the two of you will have memories to share for the rest of your lives.

Before you consent to a double wedding, realistically consider your relationship with the other bride-to-be. If the two of you are likely to be pulling each other's hair out at the altar, or have drastically different opinions on religion, fashion, music, or other issues, you may want to "just say no" rather than risk any embarrassment at the wedding. In other words, you should only agree to a double wedding if the memories you and your potential fellow-bride will share for years to come are likely to be pleasant ones.

If you do decide on a double wedding, there's a great deal of "killing two birds with one stone" to do. Fortunately, most of it saves you money. You send out one invitation for both couples, buy one set of flowers, have one DJ or band. It would be best for everyone's eyes and ears if the level of style and formality between the two wedding parties was the same. Long, flowing purple dresses in one party and orange polka-dotted mini-skirts in another will not make for a pretty picture. Similarly, it's doubtful that your DJ will appreciate alternating heavy-metal tunes for one couple with classical recordings for the other.

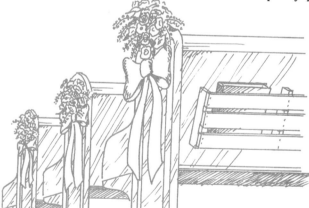

The main piece of protocol to be aware of in a double wedding is that the older of the two brides proceeds down the aisle first with her wedding party, and does other key things first. As you might imagine, two full wedding parties can get rather large, so find a place that can accommodate everyone. Aside from the fact that everything is done twice, the double wedding can be just like any other wedding.

As far as bridal showers and other pre-wedding events go, it's up to you and the others involved to decide whether or not to do things jointly. It's certainly easier on everyone else if the two of you have a joint shower, but if either of you feels the need to retain a sense of individuality, you might tactfully request doing some things separately.

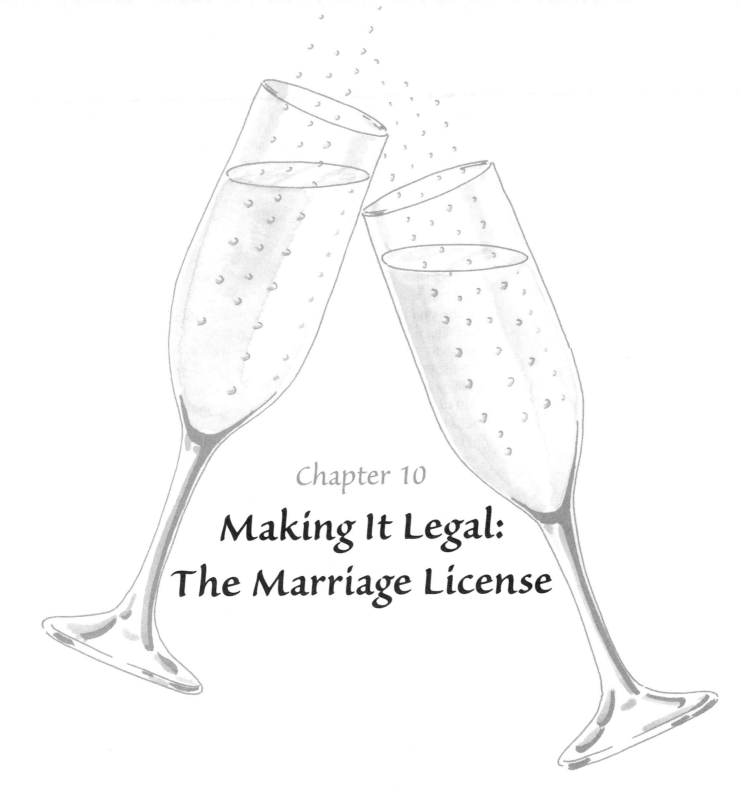

Chapter 10

Making It Legal:
The Marriage License

What do driving, fishing, hunting, boating, selling alcohol, and getting married have in common? Legally, you need a license for every one of them. Admittedly, you're not threatening the public safety by getting married (unless you're planning a particularly festive reception), but that license binds you as a couple in the eyes of the law. As an added bonus, the blood test required to get the license helps you make sure you're not mistakenly marrying your long-lost brother or any other closer-than-they-should-be relations.

Licensed to Kiss

The criteria required to get a marriage license varies from state to state. Contact your local marriage bureau (usually at the City Clerk's office) to find out what requirements you have to meet, what steps you have to take, and how much time is involved. You should start the actual license process one month before your wedding, and earlier if you'll be sending out of state for birth certificates and other records. Some states require a waiting period between application and receipt of the license, but usually it's no more than a week.

Just as you have to be sure to apply for the license in time, you must guard against getting it too early, as marriage licenses do expire. In some states they may be good for 180 days; in others, only twenty.

Thicker Than Water

Yes, the blood test protects you from inadvertently marrying your relatives, but it also protects you, your groom, and any future children from the consequences of a serious disease either of you may have. Depending upon the state in which you are getting married, your blood sample may be screened for venereal diseases, genetic diseases, and AIDS.

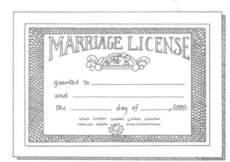

The Rules and Requirements

Regardless of where you get married, you will need to be aware of a number of guidelines common to all states.

- ♥ You and your groom must apply for the license together.
- ♥ You must both have all of the required paperwork (birth certificates, driver's license, proof of age, proof of citizenship).
- ♥ You both need completed blood tests and doctor's certificates from both doctors.
- ♥ You must provide proof of divorce or annulment (in the case of a previous marriage).
- ♥ You must pay a fee. The fee usually ranges from $10.00 to $30.00.

Witnesses for the Institution

Plan on dragging your best man and maid of honor along when it comes time to sign the license. They need to be there as witnesses, to prove that you weren't harassed into the institution of marriage.

The Dotted Line

When the time comes for you to sign the license, you should already have decided on what your married name will be. The license is the first legal document you will sign with your new (or old) name, so make sure it's what you want it to be. (See the section on name changing for more details.)

So, Are You Married Yet?

Having a marriage license doesn't mean you are legally married; it just means you have the state's permission to get married. To be valid and truly binding, the license has to be signed by a religious or civil official. When the ceremony rolls around, you leave the license with your officiant. There is no going off into a back room during the ceremony (à la Charles and Di and other members of the aristocracy) to have a grand signing ceremony. The officiant simply signs the license after the completion of the ceremony and sends it back to the proper state office.

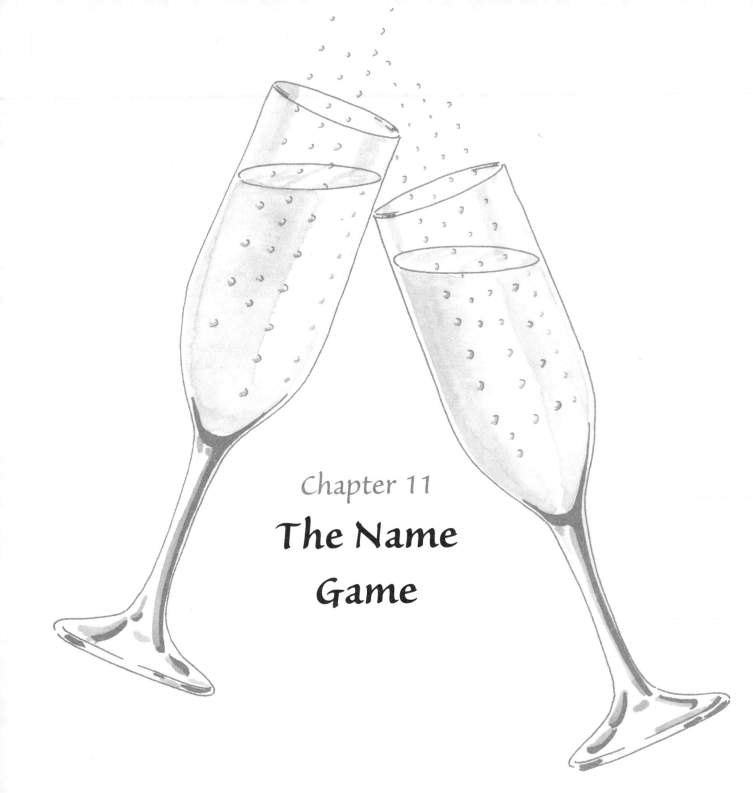

Chapter 11

The Name Game

W hat's in a name? Names can be important. Never as much, perhaps, as when you're deciding whether or not to take your husband's. For years you've probably taken your own surname for granted. But now, faced with its possible loss, you may find yourself more attached to the old girl than you'd realized. This is the name you went through school with, the name you went to work with, the name you made friends with, the name everyone knows you by. How can you let it go? On the other hand, maybe your last name is ten syllables long, or no one ever pronounces or spells it right, and you can't wait to get rid of it.

If taking your husband's name is an easy decision, congratulations. Your life is much simpler than a lot of people's. For many brides, however, the decision is quite difficult. In the past, it was rare for a married woman to keep her own name. Now it's very common; there are even multiple options to accommodate just about any name combination or situation. If you are in a quandary over names, remember that these days the only ones who'll probably care are you, your husband, and perhaps your present and future family. So don't let the "What will people think?" problem worry you at all.

If you'd like to take on your husband's name, but don't want to completely abandon your own, here are a few avenues to explore:

Jennifer Andrews
Jennifer Miller
Jennifer A. Miller
Jennifer Andrews Miller
Jennifer Andrews-Miller
Mrs. Jennifer Miller
Ms. J. A. Miller

First, Last, Middle?

How about using your maiden name as your middle name, and your husband's as your last? In this case Jennifer Andrews marrying Richard Miller becomes Jennifer Andrews Miller.

A Little Dash Will Do

Another popular alternative is to hyphenate the two last names: Jennifer Andrews-Miller. That little dash means that the two separate last names are now joined to make one (like a marriage). You keep your regular middle name, but saying your full name can be a mouthful: Jennifer Marie Andrews-Miller. If both names are fairly short and easy to pronounce, hyphenating is a great option. If, however, Jennifer Martinalletti marries Richard Radovanowsky, she may want to think twice before committing to Jennifer Martinalletti-Radovanowsky. There are few dotted lines in the world that would accommodate that signature.

Your Name, Your Business

Some women choose to take their husband's name legally, but use their maiden name for business. In everyday life and social situations, you'd use your married name, but in the office, you'd use the same name you have always used.(Imagine how grateful your office supply manager will be to learn you won't need new business cards and letterhead, and that the telephone directory can remain the same!)

The Name Remains the Same

Many women choose not to change their name at all. If you decide to keep your maiden name, you should be sensitive to how your in-laws might react. Explain the reason for your decision (for example, that you've already established a career identity with your maiden name) and emphasize that your decision in no way reflects a lack of respect for their family. You may reassure them by saying that you plan to use your husband's name socially and/or that your children will take your husband's name, if that's the case. Ask your spouse to voice his support of your decision.

Until people are aware of your decision to keep your maiden name, there may be times when you are incorrectly referred to with your husband's name. If this should happen, be patient; it's a common assumption. You can either let it pass, or politely correct the person, depending on how important the issue is to you. As a way to avoid this awkwardness, you may wish to take the initiative and introduce yourself to strangers first: "Hi, I'm Jennifer Andrews, Richard Miller's wife."

Some women who keep their maiden name will choose to use their husband's name in conjunction with their children. Rather than calling the school and saying, "This is Jennifer Andrews, Kenny Miller's mom," they opt for the simpler "This is Mrs. Miller, Kenny's

Hers for Him?

Fresh from the "things you'll probably never see in your lifetime" department, the newest idea is for your husband to take your last name. A slightly more likely option is for both you and your husband to have a hyphenated combination of both last names: Jennifer Andrews-Miller, and Richard Andrews-Miller. If you and your fiancé are nearly coming to blows on this subject, consider dropping both of your last names and finding a new one together.

mom." Many mothers also do this for the sake of their young children, who may not understand (or be able to explain to friends) why their mother has a different name than theirs.

One point to consider when keeping your own name concerns taxes. If you file jointly with your husband, but use your own name, the government may ask for proof of your marriage. On the other hand, if you use your husband's name on a government document when the name is not legally yours, you can get into trouble. When dealing with the government and any other tricky legal issues, be sure to clarify your legal name right up front.

And the Winner Is . . .

Whatever your decision on the name issue, make sure you're comfortable with it by the time you sign your marriage license; that's the first official place for your new (or old) name. If your name has changed, there are a lot of people, places, and things out there that will need to be updated with your new identity. Take a look at the worksheet in the back of the book, then start compiling whatever information you need to contact each place in quick order.

Spreading the News

You can inform people of your decision in one fell swoop, or through a series of individual notices. Newspaper announcements reach the most people the fastest; for a more personal touch, you can send out At-home cards (see the chapter on stationery) that include your name choice. As for the wording of these announcements, you can be very subtle: "The bride will keep her name." Or to really make sure everyone gets the message, "Jennifer Andrews and Richard Miller wish to announce that both will keep their present names for all legal and social purposes." Or "Jennifer Andrews announces that she will take the surname Miller after her marriage on June 5, 1999."

Jennifer Andrews's name will be changed to Jennifer Miller as of May 27, 2000.

Chapter 12

Places Please: The Wedding Rehearsal and Rehearsal Dinner

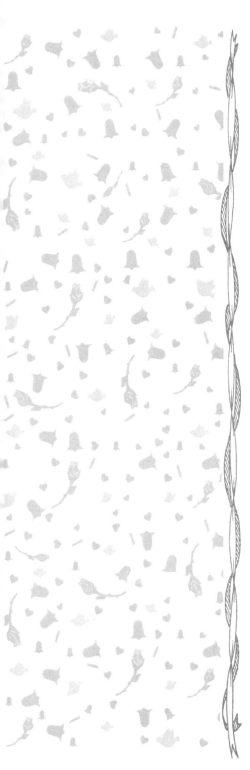

If you're expecting your wedding rehearsal to go something like the final dress rehearsal for a Broadway play, you're likely to be disappointed. Sure, you'll probably have jitters that beat an opening night panic attack, but at least you won't have to worry about your officiant ordering the wedding party around like a director, screaming, "You're all going out there as rookies, but you've got to come back as stars." As anticlimactic as it sounds, the rehearsal is mainly a chance for the officiant to meet your wedding party and acquaint everyone with the basics of the ceremony.

The rehearsal is usually held the night before the wedding at the ceremony site itself. If that time is inconvenient for any of your key players, reschedule for another time, preferably during the week before the wedding. (If it's too far before the wedding, people may forget what they learned.)

Who (besides you and your groom) should attend? The officiant, every member of the wedding party, the father of the bride (to practice dragging her down the aisle, of course), Scripture readers and candle lighters, and any children taking part in the ceremony. Invite the florist to discuss final issues of flower placement. You might also want to arrange for featured soloists or musicians to attend the rehearsal as well. Your readers should check with the officiant to make sure the version of Scripture they've been practicing in front of the mirror at home is in fact the one being used in the ceremony. (Sometimes the wording differs from Bible to Bible depending on the version; only the officiant is likely to know which version will be used in the ceremony.)

Remember, this is your chance to iron out last-minute details and resolve any remaining questions. Though it may not be enough to truly calm your nerves, get everything straight at the rehearsal. Make sure that everything is ready and that all of the participants know what's expected of them.

Sit Back, Enjoy the Show!

Take a moment during the rehearsal to clear up any confusion about seating wedding guests. Although it's not mandatory, the bride's family usually sits on the left side of the church for a Christian ceremony, while the groom's family sits on the right. The reverse is true for Reform and Conservative Jewish weddings. If one side has many more guests than the other, you may dispense with this custom and seat everyone together to achieve a more balanced look. However, men and women are usually segregated in Orthodox Jewish ceremonies. Your siblings should sit in the second row, behind your mother and father. Grandparents sit in the third row, and close friends and relatives sit in the fourth.

Guests are seated as they arrive, from front to back. The mothers of the bride and groom should be seated just before the ceremony begins. Late-arriving guests are not escorted to their seats by ushers. They should take seats near the back of the church, preferably via a side aisle.

Special Seating Arrangements

Divorced parents

Typically, parents are seated in the first row (or in the second if the attendants will be seated during the ceremony). In the case of divorce, the bride's natural mother has the privilege of sitting in the first row, and of selecting those who will sit with her, including her spouse, if she has remarried. If your divorced parents have remained amicable, your father may sit in the second row with his spouse or significant other. If there is some acrimony between the two parties, however, your father should be seated a few rows farther back. However, if you have been raised by your stepmother and prefer to give her the honor, she and your father may sit in the first row, while your mother sits farther back.

"In the ribbons"

In some ceremonies, the first few rows of pews or chairs are sectioned off by ribbons, meaning they are reserved for family and very special friends. No one else should be seated there.

The Processional

After a brief overview of the ceremony, the officiant will talk everyone through a quick practice runthrough, beginning with the processional. This time, at least, you won't have to worry about walking down the aisle "very slowly"; run, skip, and turn cartwheels if you'd like.

In a Catholic processional, the bridesmaids walk down the aisle, one by one, while the ushers and best man wait at the altar. Who goes first is usually determined by height, from shortest to tallest. For large weddings with more than four bridesmaids, bridesmaids walk in pairs. The honor attendant is next, followed by the ring bearer and flower girl. The

"Oh, No, I Forgot the...!"

You might want to bring along items you'll need for the wedding to the rehearsal. This way, you won't have to worry about carrying them with you in the limo ride to the ceremony.

- ♥ Wedding programs
- ♥ Unity candles
- ♥ Marriage license
- ♥ Fee for site
- ♥ Fee for officiant
- ♥ Practice bouquet
- ♥ Aisle runner
- ♥ Toasting goblets for reception
- ♥ Cake knife and server
- ♥ Guest book
- ♥ Seating cards for the reception
- ♥ Maps or written directions
- ♥ Wedding day transportation information

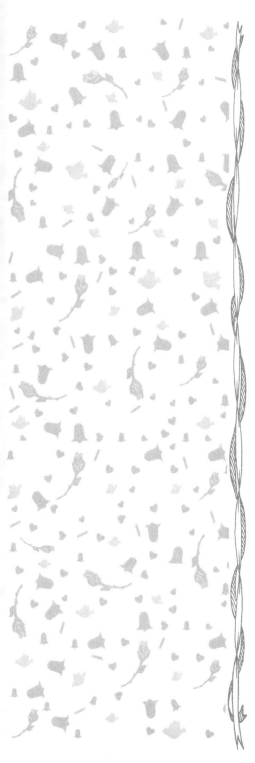

bride then enters on her father's right arm, followed by pages (if any), who carry the bride's train. The Protestant processional is the same, except ushers may precede the bridesmaids in pairs, according to height.

Jewish Orthodox, Conservative, and Reform processions vary according to the families' preferences, devoutness, and local custom. A traditional religious Jewish processional may begin with the rabbi and cantor (with the cantor on the rabbi's right), followed by the ushers walking one by one, and the best man. The groom then walks between his mother (on his right) and his father (on his left). The bridesmaids then walk one by one, followed by the maid of honor, the page, and the flower girl. The bride is the last to enter, with her mother on her right and her father on her left.

If your church has two side aisles instead of a single center aisle, your officiant will most likely advise you to use the left aisle for the processional and the right aisle for the recessional.

Giving the Bride Away

Traditionally, the father of the bride gives the bride away. But sometimes death or divorce has changed the circumstances.

If your father has passed away, do whatever feels most comfortable to you. If your mother has remarried and you are close to your stepfather, he may be a good choice. Otherwise, a brother, a grandfather, a special uncle, or a close family friend could do the honors. Some brides walk down the aisle with their mother or with their groom. Others choose to walk without an escort. Keep in mind that whomever you choose will sit in the front pew with your mother during the ceremony (unless you choose your groom, of course).

If your parents are divorced, and both parents are remarried, your decision will depend on your preference and family situation. To avoid risking civil war, take care to somehow include both men in the proceedings. If you've remained close to your father, you may prefer that he fulfill his traditional role, while your stepfather does a reading. Or they may both escort you down the aisle. Often in Jewish ceremonies both divorced parents walk the bride down the aisle.

Many second-time brides walk down the aisle with their grooms, or with one of their children. However, it's also appropriate for the bride's father to escort her again, or for her to walk alone.

You may decide to do away with this tradition altogether. If so, there are options which you should discuss with your officiant. Instead of asking, "Who gives this woman . . . ?" he or she may ask, "Who blesses this union?" Your father may respond, "Her mother and I do," and take his seat next to your mother. It is also entirely appropriate for both parents to respond, "We do." In this case, your mother should stand up when the officiant asks, "Who blesses this union?"

The Recessional

You've kissed, you've been pronounced husband and wife, now how do you get from the front of the church into your limousine? Arm in arm, you and your new husband (well, tomorrow he will be—remember, this is only the rehearsal) lead the recessional, followed by your child attendants. Your maid of honor and best man are next, followed by your bridesmaids, who are paired with ushers. The order of the Jewish recession is as follows: bride and groom, bride's parents, groom's parents, child attendants, honor attendants, and bridesmaids paired with ushers. The cantor and rabbi walk at the end of the recession.

By the end of the rehearsal, everyone's bound to be feeling giddy with anticipation. Time for another party!

The Rehearsal Dinner (a.k.a. Your Last Single Supper)

The majority of wedding rehearsals are merely warm-ups for the truly important event of the evening: the rehearsal party. The rehearsal party gives everyone involved in the wedding a chance to eat, drink, and be merry, and hopefully to relax and forget about the stresses of the big day to come. Make the most of it. (It wouldn't be surprising if the idea for holding the dinner on the eve of the wedding arose because it's a convenient way to keep the bride and groom from being home alone, nervously climbing the walls in their respective rooms.)

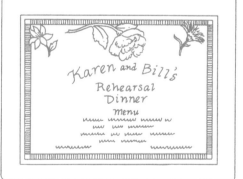

Traditionally, the expense of the rehearsal party is borne by the groom's parents, but these days anyone who wishes may sponsor the party. A very informal affair, the rehearsal party usually takes place in a restaurant or a private home; a simple phone call is the usual means of inviting the guests.

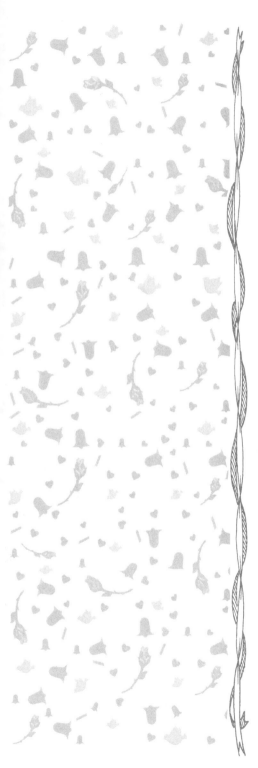

And Who Should Your Host Be Inviting?

♥ All members of the wedding party, along with their spouses or significant others
♥ The parents of the bride and groom
♥ The ceremony officiant, along with his or her spouse or significant other if this is applicable
♥ Any special friends and family members
♥ Grandparents of the bride and groom
♥ Godparents of the bride and groom
♥ Out-of-town wedding guests

Of course, you can invite anyone else you want, but try to keep the party on the intimate side. Remember, the goal of this party is to let everyone relax and give you and your groom some additional time with loved ones who may only be in town for a few days. You'll have plenty of time to party with your other wedding guests on the big day.

A note on children at the rehearsal: their parents should be invited to the rehearsal party. But unless you are counting on a temper tantrum from an overtired child to be part of the reception entertainment, you should make sure the parents get the children home in time for them to get a good night's sleep.

If any of your out-of-town guests will arrive in time for the dinner, you should invite them as well. This way, you'll get to spend more time with people you probably don't see that often, and they'll feel that distance hasn't kept them from being a part of the festivities. Similarly, if you have any close friends that you couldn't manage to fit into the wedding party, you might want to invite them.

The rehearsal dinner is usually when the bride and groom hand out their gifts to the attendants, parents, and anyone else they may have bought presents for. If you follow tradition, you will make a few toasts during the party: the best man to the couple, the groom to his bride and future in-laws, and the bride to the groom and her future in-laws. But if you prefer to skip the toasts, do so, because your dinner doesn't have to include any ceremony at all. Remember, there'll be enough formality come the morning. Feel free to just sit back, relax, and enjoy it all.

Part Three:

The Reception and Beyond

Chapter 13

Your Reception— or The Biggest Cash Drain of the Whole Deal

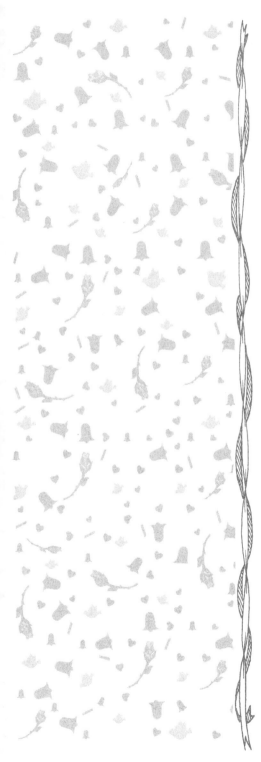

What makes a marriage ceremony a real wedding? Why, the reception afterwards, of course!

If a wedding meant just standing before a religious or civic official and saying "I do," there would be precious little to have a nervous breakdown about. Brides wouldn't have to pull their hair out over every detail, and parents wouldn't have to start putting aside money to pay for their daughter's wedding on the day she was born. (If eloping is beginning to sound pretty good to you right about now, skip this chapter. If not, read on.)

In all but a very few cases, there is some form of party after the ceremony. But this party isn't just any party, it's a reception. With a party, you get chips and dip, some hors d'oeuvres, beer, and wine, and maybe a stereo providing background music. But a traditional reception has flowers, finery, protocol, photographers, caterers, cakes, DJs, and dances. Time to ask your parents where they hide the bankbook.

When, Where, and How

The first thing you have to do is find a place to have your reception. That place has to be available on the day of the ceremony—unless you feel comfortable telling wedding guests to go home and come back the next week for the reception. Religious officiants will tell you to set the ceremony date first and then find a reception site. Many couples try to make the ceremony date conform to the date their desired reception site is open. Of course, it all depends on whether you have a dream reception site or really don't care where it is as long as it's nice.

During peak wedding months (April–October), competition for reception sites can be heavy. If you're marrying in this time frame, plan on looking for a site at least a year in advance.

Oh, the Places You'll Go

While function halls, country clubs, and hotel ballrooms are still the most popular sites for receptions, these days there's no limit to where you can go. As long as people can gather there to eat, drink, and be merry, it will do. Here's a list of potential sites to consider.

Castles, estates, or historic mansions
Museums/art galleries
Scenic mountain resorts
Beaches
Gardens
Ships, boats, or yachts
Country inns
Farmhouses

Public gardens or parks
Luxury hotels
Historic hotels
Historic villages
Concert halls

Observatories
Ranches
Lighthouses
Pier or waterfront restaurants
Historic battleships
Plantations
Indian reservation or memorial site
Apple orchards
College or university chapels, halls, or courtyards
Traditional chapels
Beach clubs
Greenhouses
Aquariums
Theaters

There are also baseball parks, football fields, tennis courts, and other spots connected to hobbies or anything of common interest.

Odds are you'll pay more to secure one of these nontraditional sites than you would for a standard venue, but weigh the cost against all that you'll get for your money. In settings like these, your surroundings won't be part of an insignificant background. They'll say something unique about you and your new husband. Estates and manors are stately and elegant; they offer opulence, style, and often the ambiance of an era gone by. Many have expansive grounds for the guests to stroll—there may be room for a tent for outdoor festivities. The works of art hanging in museums and art galleries can certainly compete with any centerpiece a caterer might provide; add a little music and you've got a reception to remember. Or what about a reception in late fall in an apple orchard—complete with chairs, tables, and a string quartet?

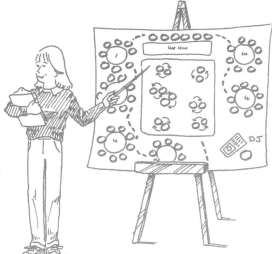

Granted, some of these options will depend on the season and the weather, but if Mother Nature cooperates, sites like these can make for a beautiful and memorable wedding day. (For outdoor sites you will, alas, need to establish a backup site elsewhere—or incorporate a large tent into your plans—as a precaution against inclement weather.)

Theme On

A theme wedding is another step away from the traditional that will make your wedding something special. Depending on the theme you choose, you can live out your fantasies of living in another time or another place—or in a whole new way. Here are some ideas. (Be sure to share whatever theme idea you have with your guests so they can dress appropriately.)

A period wedding. This theme emphasizes the traditions, costumes, music, and customs of an earlier period. Though the 1920s through the 1960s are the most popular periods, you could opt for Colonial America or Victorian England if you prefer—as long as you can find the costumes.

An ethnic wedding. Perhaps you and your fiancé would like to highlight the culture and costumes of your ethnic backgrounds.

A Western-style wedding. Cowboy hats abound here, as do fiddles, square dancing, horses, barbecue fare, and anything else about the wild frontier you want to incorporate.

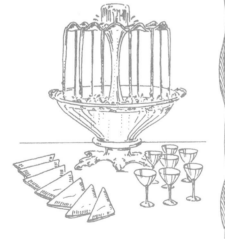

A holiday wedding. A wedding during a holiday season can take advantage of the decorations and spirit of that time. Valentine's Day, with its emphasis on love and romance, is a popular wedding time; Christmas is right up there, too. Easter and Passover are less popular because of certain religious restrictions, but a patriotic motif complete with fireworks might be a good idea for the Fourth of July. If you really want to go out on a limb, how about a Halloween wedding, with the wedding party and guests coming in costume and with pumpkins for a centerpiece?

The all-night wedding. This is a wedding celebration that's planned to last through the entire night. In some cases, the group rents an additional hall after the first reception. In others, the festivities continue at a private home. The wedding usually comes to a close with breakfast the next morning. Coffee, anyone?

A weekend wedding. You've heard of an all-nighter? Well, this is an all-weekender. Usually, a weekend wedding is set up like a mini-vacation for you and your guests, and takes place at a resort or hotel.

The honeymoon wedding. Not everyone's cup of tea, but then again not as bad as it sounds. The honeymoon wedding is akin to a weekend wedding. Guests are invited to a romantic "honeymoon"-type locale such as a resort or an inn, where they can stay with the new couple for a few days. After the honeymoon wedding is over, the bride and groom depart for the real (and much more private) thing.

A progressive wedding. Like to travel? In this variation, the bride and groom attend a number of wedding festivities carried on over a period of days—and located in different places! Depending upon your budget, your love of travel, and the availability of friends and relatives to celebrate, you might start with your ceremony on the Eastern Seaboard, have a reception in the Midwest, and wrap things up in California. (Not all progressive wedding celebrations are that far-flung; many stay in the same state, even the same city.)

A surprise wedding. The wedding is a surprise not to you (you hope), but to your guests. Invite people to a standard-issue party, and if those in the know can keep a secret, your guests will be completely surprised when they arrive at a wedding.

A Memory Lane wedding. Stroll down Memory Lane with your groom, family, and friends by having the wedding at a place of special significance to you as a couple. Perhaps you want to return to the college where you two met, or the park where he proposed.

Or anything else that strikes your fancy! What about a wedding with a sports theme? A wedding that moves from car to car on a train? A beach party wedding? Let your imagination run wild!

No Frills

After all these grand suggestions, it's easy to forget that sometimes the most beautiful and enjoyable weddings are the ones that are the simplest at heart. Without frills and thrills, the meaning of the marriage celebration becomes clearer, and you realize that no matter where you are, it is who you're with that is important.

Home-Sweet-Home Reception

For many couples, this is the perfect solution to the reception dilemma. If you're lucky, you, your parents, or someone you know will have a house and yard big enough to accommodate your reception. The informal, relaxed atmosphere of this kind of celebration can be a lot of fun. What better way to celebrate the most important day in your life than in the house you grew up in or the

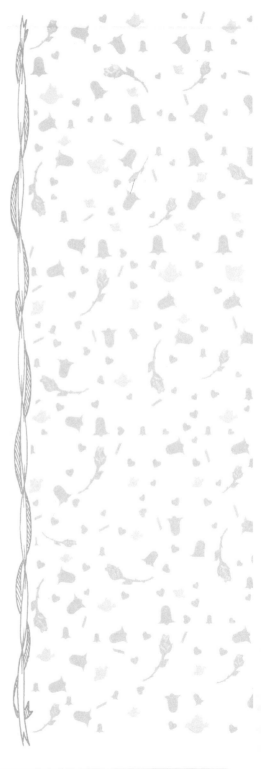

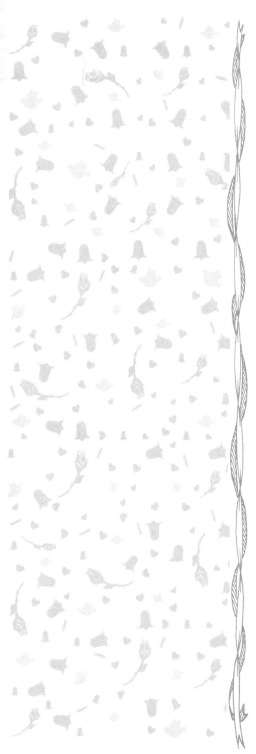

backyard you played in? Placed in a unique context, and surrounded by family and friends, you'll have a memorable reception experience.

Don't assume that having a home reception means your parents have to sweat in the kitchen all day preparing and serving food. If you're expecting more than fifty guests, it's best to bring in a professional caterer for the job.

Because a home or backyard reception is so informal, you won't be tied down to traditional entertainment and menu items—or even a dress code. You can play homemade tapes on your stereo; if the festivities are in the backyard, have a barbecue or a clambake—and tell the guests to wear shorts.

Stay Right Where You Are!

Some receptions are held on the same grounds as the ceremony—the ultimate in convenience for you and your guests. Most churches and synagogues have a function room somewhere on the premises which you can rent without much fuss, and for a much cheaper rate than a commercial site. The reception is typically small and informal; the menu usually a light buffet rather than a big sit-down dinner. (Bear in mind that a site with a religious affiliation may not allow alcohol, and may put restrictions on the kinds of music you can play at the reception.)

While You Wait

You've found the perfect place for your ceremony and the perfect place for your reception. The only problem is, the reception site is booked until two hours after your ceremony ends. Relax. There's no law that says receptions have to occur immediately after the ceremony. However, if a delay is inevitable, make sure that your guests, especially those from out of town, are entertained between the ceremony and the reception. Set up a hospitality suite at a nearby hotel, or ask a close friend to have cocktails or hors d'oeuvres at his or her house. (If the reason for the delay is that you planned to have photographs taken during that time, consider taking photographs before the ceremony or at the reception.)

That's All, Folks!

Despite the many options, there are some couples who will forego the reception. They simply mingle with their guests briefly at the end of the ceremony, and the wedding is over. This arrangement is perfectly acceptable as long as you notify the guests ahead of time (preferably on the invitations).

Interview Your Reception Site

Now that you know about all of the wonderful reception options open to you, it's time to pick some places and put them through the wringer. The reception is the part of your wedding you will most likely spend the most amount of money on. Take the proper steps from the very start to make sure you get every penny's worth. Here's some questions you should ask.

- ♥ How many people can the facility comfortably seat? How big is the dance floor?
- ♥ Is an in-house catering service offered? If it is, and if you don't wish to use it, can you bring in your own caterer? (See section on catering for more details.)
- ♥ Are tables, chairs, dinnerware, and linens supplied? What about decorations?
- ♥ Is the site an appropriate one for live music? Is there proper spacing, wiring, and equipment?
- ♥ Does the site coordinator have any recommendations for set-up and decorations? Are there florists, bands, or disk jockeys he or she can recommend?
- ♥ Can you see photos of previous reception set-ups?
- ♥ How many hours is the site available for? Is there a time minimum you must meet? Are there charges if the reception runs overtime? How much advance notice must you give if you decide to extend your reception?
- ♥ Is there free parking? If there is valet parking, what are the rates and gratuities? (If you pay for everything up front, post a sign informing your guests that the tip has been taken care of.)
- ♥ Will there be coatroom and restroom attendants? A bartender? A doorman? What are the charges?

Words to the Wise

Consult with your caterer about obtaining tables, chairs, and other furniture for a home or backyard reception. (See the section on catering for details.) There are plenty of stores out there that rent everything from decorative arches to grandiose champagne fountains—even portable dance floors!

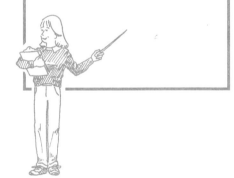

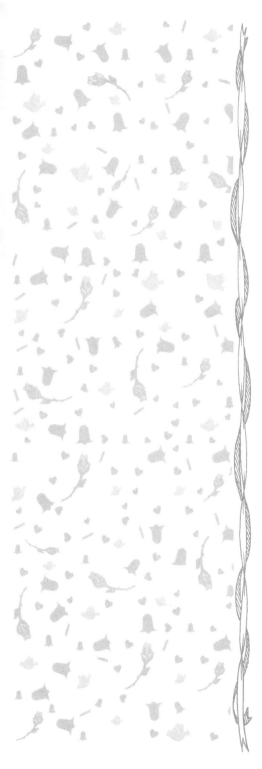

♥ If you've arranged for an open bar, do you have to bring the alcohol or does the site provide it?

♥ If you've arranged for a cash bar, what will the prices be?

♥ Does the facility have more than one reception site on the premises? If someone else is occupying another room at the site, will there still be adequate parking available? Is there enough space between the two rooms to ensure privacy? (You don't want your jazz quartet drowned out by the heavy-metal band playing at the graduation party next door.)

♥ Is yours the only reception happening at the site that day or is there one before or after?

♥ Will the site coordinator be available to advise you on decorations? Layout? Seating?

♥ Is there a separate room where photographs can be taken? Where you can change into your going-away clothes?

♥ Who pays for any police or security that may be required? (It is customary for a policeman to be present at public function sites where alcohol is being served.)

♥ What is the layout of the tables? How many people can sit comfortably at each table?

♥ Will your deposit be returned in the event of a cancellation?

Comparison Shop

You can start your search for the ideal reception site by recalling weddings you have enjoyed recently and by asking friends for their suggestions and comments. Visit the places you are considering, go through all the questions listed above in your preliminary conferences, and *write down the answers*. And note carefully whether the people you will be dealing with are courteous and responsive to your wishes.

If you like a hall and the prices quoted, go back to see a wedding or a formal dinner in progress, especially if you have never been to a party there. If you are considering a restaurant or a country club, it is a good idea to have dinner there on a Saturday or Sunday, when presumably the kitchen and staff are setting forth their best, at their busiest. Check—How crowded are the public rooms? Will your party have adequate privacy and quiet if the rest of the place is full? What ambiance is projected by the clientele the place draws, the physical setting, and the quality of service?

Carefully check the maintenance of the restrooms on a busy evening.

If a place seems like a good possibility, have the site manager give you a preliminary estimate in writing, spelling out the details of menu, service, and everything else you've discussed. Then compare your various estimates and impressions before you commit yourself.

That Costs HOW Much?

Make sure you are aware of all reception-related charges up front. Sales taxes, an item sometimes overlooked, add a hefty amount to the already large reception cost. Cancellations, changes, and last-minute additions will cost additional money. You don't want to come home sunburned and relaxed from your honeymoon, only to turn even redder at the site of unexpected bills.

A deposit, usually a hefty one, will reserve the site you want. Many sites won't refund this deposit if you decide you don't want them anymore. Before you sign on the dotted line, review the agreement carefully, and get references from people who have used the facility for a wedding reception. As always, make sure every part of your agreement, including date, time, services, and policies, is in writing.

All in a Day's Reception

You're probably already familiar with all of the reception traditions: the receiving line, the first toast, the first dance, the cake cutting, and the garter and bouquet throwing. But just in case you're a little foggy on them, here's a refresher:

The receiving line

The receiving line receives a fair amount of bad press these days, and it's usually the first tradition to get the ax. No one will be offended if you choose to lose this formality; in fact, some will probably cheer. But a receiving line doesn't have to take up an agonizing chunk of time, and can be a lot of fun for you and your guests. The receiving line enables you, your groom, and key members of the wedding party to meet and greet your guests—which is very important, since you probably will not have time to socialize

Unexpected Fees

Watch out for escalating fees, especially if you are booking a site a year or more before your wedding. If you reserve a site in August for a wedding the following July, the site may try to charge you at the next year's rates—which are, you guessed it, higher—unless you have a written agreement stipulating otherwise.

with everyone at the reception. Imagine painstakingly choosing the perfect gift and traveling for hours to attend a wedding, and not even having the opportunity to congratulate the bride and groom!

The receiving line should form after the wedding ceremony but before the reception. If you're worried about the line taking up too much time on your big day, or if you and your groom are not immediately proceeding to the reception (because you're taking photos, for example), you should have the receiving line at the church or synagogue. Be sure to check with your officiant first; some have restrictions as to where the line may be formed. The most convenient spot is often near an exit or outside, where guests can move through easily on their way to the reception. If you choose to have the line at the reception site, have refreshments and entertainment available for guests while they're waiting.

Although your bridesmaids traditionally join your families in the receiving line, this often makes for a slow and tedious process. Your best bet is to keep the receiving line small—your guests and attendants will thank you! The order from the head of the line is: bride's mother, bride's father, groom's mother, groom's father, bride, and groom. Your honor attendant may also join you on your left, but the best man does not usually join in the receiving line. It's optional for fathers to stand in line; they may prefer to mingle with their guests. If your parents are divorced, this may be a simple solution to an awkward situation. If you would like to include your father (particularly if he's hosting the celebration), the order is: your mother, your groom's parents, you and your groom, and your stepmother (if your father remarried) and father.

You should welcome your guests, thank them for coming, and introduce them to the other members of the wedding party. If a guest is unknown to you, your groom or someone else in your wedding party may introduce you. Be friendly but brief, otherwise the line may become too long—and everyone, including you, will have much longer to wait until the reception begins!

The first toast

After the receiving line and after the wedding party and guests have been seated, everyone is served a glass of champagne or another sparkling beverage. Toasts, whether serious or joking, are an important part of the wedding reception. Like any other ritual,

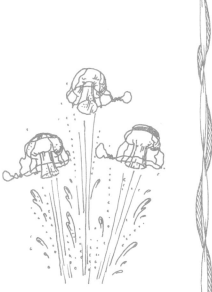

toasting has its etiquette. It helps to sort things out in the midst of merrymaking. For example:

- ♥ To make a toast, stand up, tap on your glass to get the crowd's attention, and go to it—saying something like "Ladies and gentlemen, I have a toast to make," or "I have a few words to say."
- ♥ The "toastee"—the person being toasted—does not drink at the end of the salute, but simply smiles at the toaster.
- ♥ A wedding toast shouldn't take longer than three minutes—more than that and it's overdone! The tone can range from serious and sentimental to humorous.

The order of the toasting can be:

- ♥ Best man toasts the bride
- ♥ Groom toasts the bride
- ♥ Bride toasts the groom
- ♥ Father of the bride toasts the couple
- ♥ Bride toasts her groom's parents
- ♥ Groom toasts his bride's parents
- ♥ Father of the groom toasts the bride
- ♥ Mother of the bride toasts the couple
- ♥ Mother of the groom toasts the couple
- ♥ Everyone else who has a wish to offer

And so on, as long as the champagne and the goodwill hold out! All toasts except the best man's toast are strictly optional. Once the toasting is over, the dancing is started and dinner is served.

The Opening Dances

The bride and groom's first dance is often one of the most romantic parts of your reception. You and your new husband dance or sway to a song the two of you have carefully chosen for its senti-mental value, while your guests look on. Only the most hardened cynic can't help feeling nostalgic at the sight of a bride and groom dancing their first dance together as husband and wife.

After the first dance, the bride dances with her father, and then the groom dances with his mother. Afterwards, the bride and

Words to the Wise

If you choose not to have a receiving line, be sure to make the rounds at your reception to greet your guests. The best time to do it is after the meal, when the dancing has started to heat up. You may want to hand out favors, such as decorative bags of mints, small candles wrapped in ribbons, or a cut flower (for the women only), along with a few words of thanks to your guests for their attendance.

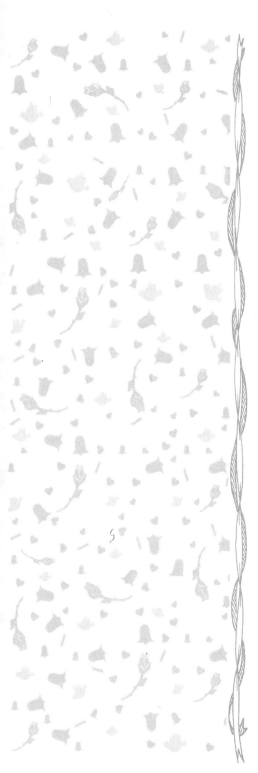

groom's parents dance, the bride dances with her father-in-law, the groom dances with his mother-in-law, and the bridesmaids and ushers dance with each other. Then open dancing begins. Of course, you may eliminate or combine some or all of these dances if you choose, and simply have the bandleader or master of ceremonies announce that open dancing will begin immediately.

The Cake-Cutting Ceremony

Aside from being a tasty dessert, the wedding cake performs a very important function: it is the centerpiece of the ever-popular cake-cutting ceremony. This is when the bride and groom cut the first piece of cake together and feed each other a bite. In some parts of the country, this ritual is accompanied by the tune "The Farmer in the Dell," with the guests singing lyrics modified for the occasion. ("The bride cuts the cake," "The groom cuts the cake," "The bride feeds the groom," and so on.)

At a sit-down reception, the cake is cut right before the dessert (if any) is served. The caterer or baker then cuts the rest of the cake and distributes it to the guests.

The bouquet and garter toss

The bouquet and garter toss are examples of once widely accepted traditions that have gradually lost favor. Today, many brides find the tradition—in which the bride throws her bouquet to a group of single women, while the groom removes the garter from the bride's leg and then tosses it to a group of single men—to be... well, degrading. As a result, many brides decide to eliminate it, in whole or in part. Others still enjoy the bouquet and garter toss and the fun that ensues. Whether or not you choose to include this tradition in your wedding is up to you.

That's Entertainment?

If you want your reception to be a "really beeg sheew" (and you have a really beeg bank account), you might consider having more than just dancing for entertainment. Karaoke, the "sing-along" music machine, has become popular. Guests consult a music play list, select a tune, then stand up in front of the crowd and, accompanied by the soundtrack, belt out their favorite song (hopefully in key and at the right tempo!).

For laughs, have a comedian; for variety, hire a mini-vaudeville troop. If your reception is outdoors, have a skywriter spice things up. And if you don't care whether the guests start a riot, how about a mime? Whatever entertainment you settle on, be sure to get references from satisfied customers before you commit to anything.

Turning the Tables

Unless you're planning a cocktail reception with hors d'oeuvres or an informal buffet, a seating plan is a must. Guests, especially those who don't know many people, often feel uncomfortable without assigned seating. Though trying to come up with a seating plan that pleases everyone isn't impossible, it may very well seem so at times. It's best to realize early on that no matter how hard you try, someone—your mother, your fiancé's mother, your cousin Marta—is bound to be unhappy with some aspect of the seating plan. Don't lose any sleep worrying about who Aunt Sue should sit with. The easiest way to approach the seating plan is to get input from your mother and future mother-in-law; if possible, the three of you should sit down and come up with the plan together. If you all have equal input, coming up with a seating plan should go (relatively) smoothly.

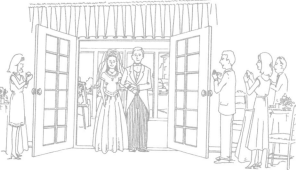

If you're planning a very formal wedding, place cards are necessary for all guests. At less formal receptions, place cards are used only at the head table. For everyone else, table cards are sufficient. The easiest way to alert guests to their table assignments is to place table cards on a table near the reception room entrance. Table cards simply list the name of the guest and their table assignment. Another option is to set up an enlarged seating diagram at the reception entrance.

But instead of these typical methods, why not take this opportunity to show your guests how clever and imaginative you can be? Decorate the tables with centerpieces and other goodies that go along with different themes, and name the tables accordingly. If you put a different type of floral arrangement at each table, you can tell your guests that they'll be sitting at the Daisy table or the Rose table. Don't limit yourself to flowers, either; consider sports, cities, types of cars, types of drinks, pastry, exotic vacation locales, or anything else as an inspiration for table decorating ideas.

At the head of the class

The head table is wherever the bride and groom sit, and is, understandably, the focus of the reception. It usually faces the other tables, near the dance floor. The table is sometimes elevated, and decorations or flowers are usually low enough to allow guests a perfect view of you and your groom.

Traditionally, the bride and groom, honor attendants, and bridesmaids and ushers sit at the head table. The bride and groom sit in the middle, with the best man next to the bride and the maid of honor next to the groom. The ushers and bridesmaids then sit on alternating sides of the bride and groom. If your reception site doesn't have tables big enough to accommodate your wedding party, you and your groom can sit alone at the head table. Or you could sit with your honor attendants at the head table and seat the rest of your attendants together at a smaller table. Child attendants should sit at a regular table with their parents. Spouses of attendants don't usually sit at the head table with their husbands or wives.

Parents usually sit at separate tables with their families. There's no single correct seating arrangement for the parents, however. The bride and groom's parents can sit together with the officiant and his or her spouse at the parents' table, or each set of parents can host their own table with family and friends. If your parents decide to include separate parents' tables, be sure that one of them includes the officiant and his or her spouse.

Not-so musical chairs

By this point, you have probably already realized that planning a wedding requires a little extra maneuvering if you have divorced parents. If you're lucky, your parents either get along or have agreed to declare a truce for a day. If you're not so lucky, seating arrangements can be a bit tricky. But as always, these problems can be solved easily through communication and flexibility.

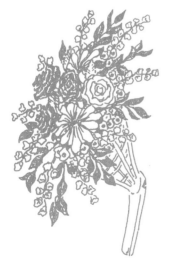

You Oughta Be in Pictures

Give your guests a real treat by having a picture display of you and your groom set up by the guest book table. Include baby photos, school shots, candids of the two of you growing up and when you first began dating, anything that will give your guests an at-a-glance look at what you were and what you've become.

That's Really All, Folks!

After the guests have been whooping it up at your reception all day (or all night, as the case may be), it's sometimes tough for them to stop all the fun and go home to stare at the walls. That's why the parents of the bride or groom usually host a small afterparty for very close family and friends; this way people get to wind down (or continue on with the fun they were having). The afterparty is usually at the parent's home, but these days it is also common for the family to rent another reception site, or extend the time at the one they're at. A rented site has its advantages. Parents don't have to worry about people messing up their home, and there's room for a lot more guests (assuming they want them).

Words to the Wise:

If you are responsible for decorating the hall, check out the details of the decor and service at the reception site. Find out what color napkins and tablecloths will be used; then you can color-coordinate centerpieces and other decorations. And of course, find out when the hall will be available for decorating and give yourself plenty of time to do it right.

Chapter 14

Food, Glorious Food: The Catering Game

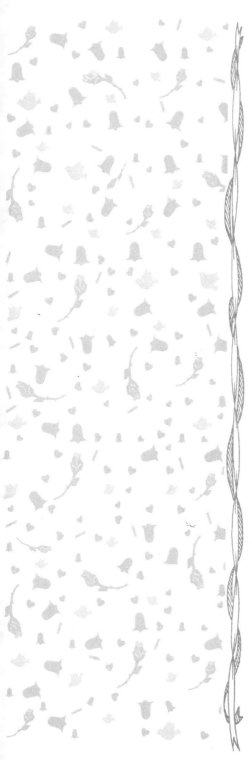

Although you and your groom will probably be too excited to eat much on your wedding day, it would be wrong to assume the same about your guests. You two will be dining on love, excitement, and romance; your guests would prefer beef, chicken, a sandwich—anything, in short, to stave off starvation. That's where the caterer comes in. The mission is a simple one: to keep the guests from gnawing each other's arms off.

Catering can be basic or complex: two people in a kitchen making sandwiches and hors d'oeuvres for an at-home reception; a traveling company complete with cooks and a waitstaff, who serve you at your rented reception site; or a full-service caterer supplying tables, chairs, linens, dinnerware, and a full bar, and coordinating your whole reception for you, from flowers to photos. In between, there are a great many variations on these three approaches. The room may begin to spin as you consider the options, but if you don't want your guests' heads spinning from hunger, settle down and take stock of the situation. The type and location of your reception (along with your budget) will help you determine the kind of caterer you need; after that, all that's left is to find out who can do it best at a price you can afford?

Passing the Taste Bud Test

A caterer can be friendly, inexpensive, cooperative, and every other good adjective under the sun, but if his food doesn't taste good, he might as well be Bozo the Clown for all the good he'll do your reception. Don't subject your guests to rubber meatballs for the sake of a great deal. You don't have to serve an extravagant dinner of prime rib, but you do want food that's worth the money you'll pay for it. Don't hire anyone without tasting the food first; if no samples are available for you in the initial consultation, ask to visit an actual reception site. You'll get to sample the cooking and see the whole troop in action.

Caterer Choices

In-house caterers

If you're lucky, the reception site will have an in-house caterer that fits your budget, serves great food, and knows how to work with you. All hotels offer such services, as do most country clubs. There are several advantages to an in-house caterer, the main one being that you don't have to go through the trouble of finding one yourself. The in-house caterer is already familiar with the particulars of the room, which can carry many advantages (for instance, linens and dinnerware that really complement the overall atmosphere).

But the in-house picture is not all roses. In-house catering is usually more expensive than independent catering, often charging you for lots of little extras (read: things you don't want or need) as part of one all-inclusive package. So—to get the best value, you just shop around and bring in your own people, right?

Unfortunately, it's not always that simple. Some reception sites that offer catering may allow you the option of bringing in your own, but with others, it's the house brand or nothing. If the food is good and the price reasonable, you may be able to live with this. However, if during your taste test you find yourself gagging on something that may be chicken (but may not, considering that gray coloring), consider moving your reception somewhere else.

Independent caterers

Independent caterers come in a number of shapes and sizes. Each offers a different degree of services; each has a different price. Here are some of the main types you're likely to encounter.

Bare-bones caterers

Some caterers specialize in keeping it simple—they provide food and food only. Everything else—beverages, linens, dinnerware, glasses, even waiters and waitresses—has to come from you. Sometimes this can work out to your advantage; they may offer good food at a low price, and you can shop around to get the other elements yourself.

It is true that you can save quite a bit of money this way. If you purchase alcohol in quantity, for instance, you'll avoid the outrageous markups that usually accompany an open bar.

The disadvantage, of course, is that this is very inconvenient for you. What you could be getting in one fell swoop from a complete catering service, you're going to have to go out and do yourself, and chances are your schedule will be pretty full already. There are businesses that specialize in renting party goods and equipment, but

What Your Caterer Needs to Know

Before you go searching for a caterer, find out what your reception site does and doesn't provide. Some sites offer linens, glass and dinnerware, tables, chairs—everything but the food. Others provide nothing, not even a place to sit. Know what you need ahead of time so you'll know what to look for.

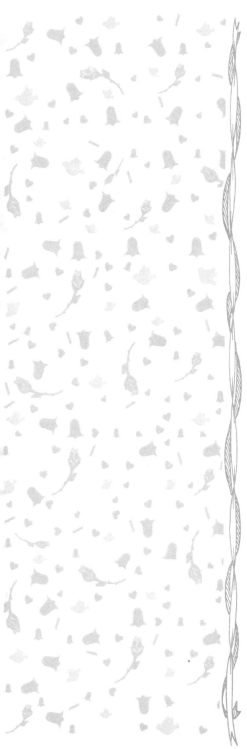

even if you do know the right places to shop, buying or renting everything separately can be a logistical nightmare. If your reception site doesn't provide tables and chairs, for example, you're either going to have to become an instant expert in rental furniture... or think up some fascinating party games that will keep your guests from realizing that they have to eat cross-legged on the floor.

Some-meat-on-their-bones caterers

This type of caterer, which most people associate with a wedding reception, provides food, beverages, a waitstaff, and bartenders. Most also offer linens and dinnerware. If you need tables and chairs, this type of caterer will usually do all the leg work for you and simply add that to the cost of your total bill. If you're lucky, they'll charge you exactly what the rental agency charged them, but it's not uncommon for them to add a fee for their trouble, so get a written estimate before you authorize anything. Some of these caterers will let you supply the alcohol, but others prefer not to worry about the potential liability (or their loss of liquor revenue).

FAT CAT(erer)S

As you would expect, this type of caterer offers just about every item and service you could imagine, as well as a few you probably couldn't. Many of these caterers have branched out into the reception coordinating business. Basically, if you choose to pay them for it, they'll take on the entire responsibility of planning your reception: music, flowers, photographer, the whole nine yards. This may sound like a dream come true, but unless you're careful, it has the potential to become quite a nightmare.

First, there are the costs—this kind of service doesn't come cheap. Second, you're flying blind. How are you to know whether you'll get a high-quality photographer—or a close (amateur) friend of the chef who has a nice camera? Third (and most important) is the question of quality. With so many irons in so many fires, even seasoned veterans can make horrendous mistakes. If you find a "fat" catering service that really appeals to you, consider contracting them for the traditional catering services—but keep tight control over everything else.

Interview Your Caterer

No matter what type of caterer you need, there are a few key questions you should ask before you make a commitment.

♥ What is the final food price? Caterers usually quote you an estimated price based on food prices at that time. About ninety days before the wedding (or perhaps later), they should give you the final price, reflecting current food rates. Early on, ask for an estimate of how much the price will change between the estimated figure and the actual cost. (You don't want to be charged $30 per meal if the estimate was $18.) Ask about price guarantees.

♥ What types of meal service are offered? Sitdown? Buffet? Stations? Russian? Sitdown and buffet are the most common, but at an extremely formal affair you might want Russian-style service where the food is brought out on large platters by trained waiters. The waiters either serve each person from the platter or hold the platter while guests serve themselves. No matter how simple or fancy the service, if you want it, you'd better make sure your caterer can deliver.

♥ Are there several meal options? Do they specialize in any particular cuisine?

♥ Is the catering service covered? If you are counting on them to provide liquor, do they have liability insurance to cover accidents that could occur after the wedding as a result of drunk driving? (It should go without saying that the caterer must have a liquor license if liquor will be served by staff!)

♥ What will the ratio of staff to guests be? Will there be enough people to man the tables? Will those people be dressed appropriately for the occasion?

♥ Will they make provisions for guests with special dietary needs? Try to plan ahead for guests on vegetarian, low-cholesterol, or kosher diets.

♥ Will meals be provided for the disc jockey (or band), photographer, and videographer? They get hungry, too.

♥ Does the caterer offer hors d'oeuvres? At what cost? What is the price difference between having them served by waiters and waitresses and displaying them on a buffet table?

Words to the Wise

Find out up-front whether or not your caterer is going to charge you a "cake-cutting fee." Some caterers will try to hit you with this charge (often as high as $3 per person), which supposedly goes to cover the labor cost of slicing the cake, plus forks and plates. It is an outrageous idea! You are already paying mandatory labor and gratuities fees for the staff. Do your very best to negotiate your way out of this cost. Show the caterer this page. Take along big, tough friends if you have to. But don't get socked with this ridiculous fee.

- ♥ Can the caterer provide a wedding cake? How about a sweet table (with lots of cavity-causing desserts)? At what price?
- ♥ Can you inspect linens, dinnerware, and related items? You don't want brown tablecloths unless you ask for them.
- ♥ Does the caterer's fee include gratuities for the staff, or will you be hit with that bill later? What about the cost of coat room attendants, bartenders, and others who may be working at the reception?
- ♥ What is the refund policy, in the unlikely event you should have to cancel? Better safe than sorry.
- ♥ What does the caterer do with leftover food? Since you're paying for it, you may wish to have it boxed up for yourself—or perhaps given to a local charity.

When you decide on a caterer who meets your budget needs and who has answered these questions to your satisfaction, get every part of your agreement in writing. Don't leave any stone unturned—you might get tripped up later. If you are not familiar with a caterer's work, or he or she is new in the business, ask for references—the names of those who have used the facilities recently. This is most important when you are planning almost a year ahead. You will be asked to give a sizable deposit, and you'll want to make sure the caterer is still in business when the date arrives!

The Food You Want, and How You Want It Served

"Chicken or roast beef?" "Sitdown or buffet?" These are the two most common dilemmas in planning your reception menu. Let's tackle the food question first.

Chicken is the least expensive of the two options; what's more, in this time of diet and health awareness, chicken is probably the healthier option. (A lot of people out there won't eat red meat anymore.). On the other hand, some people feel they're being cheap if they don't serve roast beef—although it's doubtful that choice will make or break your wedding. If you're really concerned, offer your guests a choice of several meals. Guests can pick their meal at the reception—but without any kind of advanced notice, you'll have a hard time estimating the costs. (If everybody orders roast beef, it

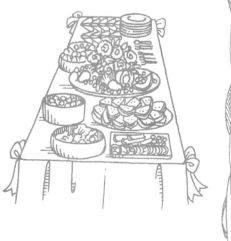

will be more expensive than if only half do.) Your best bet is to put the dinner options on a form and include them with your invitation package; that way, you'll know that you'll be paying for, say, 105 chicken dinners and 63 roast beef.

There's a bit more to consider in the sitdown vs. buffet debate. A sitdown meal is generally considered more formal than a buffet. In addition, many people feel they're treating their guests better by not making them stand in line for their food. Buffet service does, however, have its advantages: it's less expensive to serve than a sitdown meal, because it eliminates the need for waiters and waitresses. A buffet meal can add a relaxed touch to a morning or afternoon wedding.

If you do decide to go with a buffet, consider having two lines going instead of one. You're guests will get to the food twice as fast, an especially nice touch if you're planning a rather large wedding. Though buffet service saves you the cost of a waitstaff, it does require more food than a sitdown meal, since portions are not controlled. You will want to have plenty of food visible so that no one will feel shy about taking enough to eat. The caterer should assign a few staff members to watch the table and replace any food that starts to run low.

Semi-buffet service is another option. With this service, the tables are already set with plates, flatware, and glasses. The waitstaff clear the tables and serve drinks; the only thing the guests pick up at the buffet table is the food. Since many people believe a table set with coffee cups is too "dinerlike," a separate table is usually set up with cups, coffee, cream, and sugar.

A third option, called "stations," is gaining popularity with the buffet crowd. Rather than presenting your guests with warming trays of food that could start to look unappetizing once the bulk of the line has attacked, this option calls for several manned food stations to be set up around the reception hall. Some ideas on types of stations:

Pasta station: This favorite offers a variety of freshly made pastas tossed with a choice of sauces. Tortellini or fettuccine are good pasta choices, with marinara, pesto, and alfredo sauces covering most appetites. A stack of small plates or shallow bowls sits on the table. Waitstaff ask guests their choices, then scoop a small amount of the pasta into a saucepan, add the sauce, and toss it all together. The guests get just the kind of pasta they want, and know it's hot and fresh. A word of warning: pasta

What to Eat When

Luncheon wedding—between 12:00 and 2:00

Tea reception—between 2:00 and 4:00

Cocktail reception—between 4:00 and 7:30

Dinner reception—between 7:00 and 9:00

Of course, these are just guidelines; you can be creative if you wish. It's unlikely you would want to schedule a luncheon reception at 7:00 at night, but if you want a sitdown dinner at 2:00, go ahead and serve one.

Be sure that all the guests are aware of the type of reception you are planning. If you schedule a cocktail reception for 7:30, many guests will assume, unless told otherwise, that you will be serving dinner. Specify all the details on the invitation.

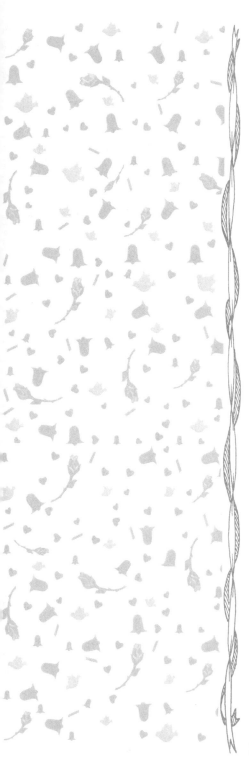

stations are popular, so consider having more than one set up in different locations!

Carving station: Pasta alone will not suffice at a wedding reception. The carving station offers a selection of meats carved right from the bone. Large roasts of turkey, beef, or ham are good choices. Guests are given a slice of their choosing, and again, because it's carved right in front of them, they know it hasn't been sitting under a warming lamp for an hour.

Skewer station: The best combination of vegetables and meats or seafood, this station might require an open flame. Guests watch as their skewer of chicken, beef, or scallops, onion, pepper, mushroom, and zucchini is flame-broiled to perfection, then laid on a bed of rice. A little more time-consuming (and potentially hazardous!) than the pasta or carving stations, the alternative is to have the skewers pre-flamed then presented buffet style.

Salads, fresh fruit, steamed vegetables, breads and rolls, and other side dishes can be laid out on a separate table and self-served with plates provided. Tables are set with silverware and linens so guests have to carry only their plate of food. Condiments that complement the pasta, meats, or skewers such as grated cheese, cranberry sauce, and au jus should be placed near the foods they accompany, but far enough away so that the line moves steadily along.

The beauty of the stations buffet arrangement is that guests get the hot, fresh food they want prepared by a professional. Make certain to arrange a serving time frame with your caterer and agree that when that time is up, the food stations will be cleared; the last thing you want is a platter of meat scraps lying around while your guests are dancing.

If you do decide to have a buffet at your reception, be sure to set aside a head table for the wedding party. No guest really expects the bride to stand in the buffet line in her wedding gown, so it's perfectly acceptable for everybody at the head table to get plated service. Just make sure your caterer can provide both plated and buffet service.

Come On to My House

You may decide to have your wedding at a private home—in a backyard, say. Unless you're a professional caterer by trade, though, it's not wise to cater your own wedding if there will be more than fifty people attending. You probably never had your heart set on doing it anyway; what bride actually wants to have that extra worry and work added to everything else she has to worry about and work on? More to the point, what bride pictures herself with an apron wrapped around her gown serving a meal on her wedding day?

If you bring a caterer into your home (or anyone else's) make sure the catering service checks out the kitchen, the appliances, and the storage and electrical capabilities to ensure that everything is adequate in size and power. Your mother's tiny kitchen may be fine for the family, but how will it handle ten people trying to pre-pare and serve massive quantities of food? Don't take any-thing for granted. When searching for a caterer to bring into your home, apply the same rules and standards you would if you were evaluating caterers for a rented site.

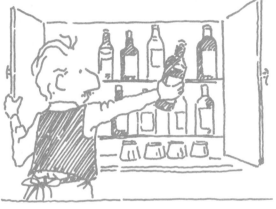

Liquor May Be Quicker, but It Ain't Cheap

The biggest controversy today surrounding alcohol and weddings is whether to have an open or cash bar. At an open bar, guests drink for free; at a cash bar, they drink for cash. Some people will tell you that it's not polite to force your guests to pay for their drinks; after all, the argu-ment goes, they've already spent money on shower and wedding gifts, new outfits, and baby-sitters. How much more are you going to ask of them?

On the other side of the debate is the sobering (as it were) fact that open bars can get extremely expensive! Let's face it. People tend to be wasteful with liquor they haven't bought. A man can order a drink, take one sip, go off to the men's room, forget his drink or assume that it's gotten warm, and go order a new one. Why not; he's not paying for it!

And consider this. With an open bar, not only will there be a lot of half-full glasses left about, there are also likely to be some pretty intoxicated people wandering around. Perhaps the biggest argument against an open bar (even if you can afford it) is that in these times of increased awareness, tougher drunk-driving laws, and

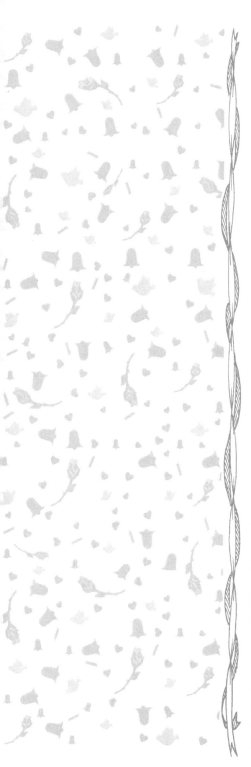

heavy liability issues, no one wants to endanger family and friends, or other drivers. Your best bet is to stick with a cash bar.

If you still feel guilty about making your guests buy drinks, here are a few things you can do to ease your mind:

Have an open bar for the first hour of the reception only. This will ease your guilt, help your guests pass the time pleasantly while you're off taking pictures, and minimize any problems with guests.

Offer tray service. Your guests don't have to pay for their drinks, and you don't incur the massive expense of an open bar. How does tray service work? You choose a few drinks that you feel will be popular with the majority of your guests (include beer and wine for sure bets). The waitstaff pass these selections around on a tray and offer them to your guests. The servers do not float around with drinks all night, but serve them on a schedule to keep down costs (and overconsumption). You might send the servers around before dinner, when dinner is being served, and at other times during the course of the reception. It's wise to stop serving well before the end of the reception to give people a chance to sober up. Tray service obviously will cost you more than a cash bar, but at least you can regulate how much liquor gets consumed.

Serve free champagne punch. A punch like this is fairly light, alcohol-wise, and people just aren't likely to pound down glass after glass. Maybe it's an image thing.

Place bottles of wine on the tables. A typical bottle of wine holds four to five glasses. At a table seated for eight, a bottle of red and a bottle of white ensures that everyone gets a glass or two with their meal. You control the expense and consumption by purchasing a set number of bottles of the wines of your choice, and your guests get a free glass of wine to raise in your honor.

Serve beer and wine only. If your reception site allows it, you may be able to save some money by purchasing a few kegs or several cases of high-quality beer plus some cases of good wine. Guests can drink either for free; any other kind of alcohol can be had for cash.

You may not care if you have a lot of liquor left over at the end of the reception; somehow, some way, you'll probably find something interesting to do with it, no matter how hard it may be. (Actually, liquor stores usually buy back unopened bottles of alcohol, but not loose cans or bottles of beer.) But if you run out of alcohol

Set 'Em Up

If you're having a reception at home, or bringing the alcohol to your reception site, you'll need to know what to bring and how much. In addition to liquor, you'll need . . .

Soft drinks, juices, and other mixers	Cocktail fixings
Cherries	Ice
Lemons	Soda water
Limes	Tonic water
Olives	Milk

Now for the hard stuff:

Beer	Rum
Wine	Tequila
Vodka	Vermouth
Gin	Blended whiskey

With these, you should have something to please everybody, even if you miss a few favorites. But only you know your crowd; if it's mostly brandy or schnapps drinkers, adjust your shopping list accordingly.

Important note: if you are serving alcohol at a home reception, you must have an open bar. Selling alcohol without a license is against the law.

during the reception, you'd best be prepared to put on your track shoes, hijack a truck, and head to the nearest liquor store to get some more.

To save yourself from such an eventuality, the people who know about these things have figured out some standard guidelines of consumption.

On average, each guest will have 4 to 5 drinks in an evening. From a fifth of liquor you'll get 25 drinks, providing you're making them with one ounce of alcohol each (using a one-ounce pony); using 1½ ounces of alcohol (a 1½-ounce jigger), you'll get 18 drinks per fifth. A single case of liquor contains 12 bottles. Assuming that you're using one ounce of alcohol to make every drink, then a case will yield 300 drinks.

For the beer drinkers in a crowd, one-half of a keg will give you 260 8-ounce glasses. (If you're serving beer in bottles and cans instead of on tap, seven cases is the equivalent of one-half of a keg.)

(Note: For those swing-from-the-chandelier wine drinkers, figure that each one will drink the equivalent of one full-sized bottle.)

Make Your Own Bar

If you're having a home or backyard reception, there are stores that will rent you a bar for the day. If you don't want to spend the money, see if you or anyone you know has a table that would suffice.

Make sure that any table you use is sturdy and steady. Draping the table with a nice white tablecloth that extends all the way to the ground not only dresses things up, but also hides excess bottles and trash stored underneath.

The Soft Stuff

Always make sure there are nonalcoholic options on hand for guests who prefer to steer clear of the hard stuff. Every bar should stock soft drinks, but you might also add a nonalcoholic punch. (Punches look very inviting when served in an elegant bowl or fountain.) Don't think you're restricted to that bright red stuff you drank as a kid. There are plenty of delicious nonalcoholic options, including a sparkling grape juice, that look just like champagne!

Champagne or Not Champagne?

Though we commonly refer to any sparkling white wine as champagne, only the wine made in the Champaign region of France deserves this title. As you might expect, you'll pay more for the real thing (how does $60 or more per bottle sound)—whereas you can pick up a decent sparkling wine for around $10. Unless you have a champagne connoisseur on your guest list, nobody will know the difference, and you'll be saving yourself a bundle by buying "fake." If you're like most people, you'll only want enough "champagne" to fill everyone's glass once for the opening (best man's) toast. If your caterer is responsible for procuring the champagne and other liquor, all you have to worry about is the bill; if you have to buy it yourself, assume that each bottle of champagne will yield seven glasses.

Safety First

A menu tip for anyone concerned about guests having a little too much to drink: don't serve salty foods. They only make people thirstier. Do serve meat, fish, cheese, and other high-protein foods; they restore blood sugar which is depleted when someone drinks alcohol, and help sober someone up. Coffee, however, does no such thing; it only wakes the person up, leaving you with someone who is still very drunk and probably a little edgy. If you or anyone else is trying to sober up some guests, have them drink water instead to flush out their systems.

Take Care of Yourself

Have you ever been to a wedding where the bride or groom was incoherent because he or she had had too much to drink? Such a situation is embarrassing for guests to witness, and nine times out of ten the drunken person regrets that they got out of control. The explanations they offer later probably sound familiar: they were nervous and figured a drink (or two) would help them relax; they were in the mood to celebrate; well-wishers kept giving them refills they felt they shouldn't refuse. All these excuses are understandable, but imagine how much better (and smarter) you'll feel if you don't have to give them the next day. If you do drink, be sure to eat something and drink nonalcoholic beverages, too (water is best). It's

Uncorking the Corkage Fee

This fee may be leveled at you if you have your reception in a restaurant or hotel, but intend to bring your own liquor. The corkage fee is meant to make up for the loss of drink revenue. If you are planning on bringing your own liquor to a place like this, find out the price of the corkage fee in advance; it may be so high that it negates the savings you made by BYOBing. (Again, some establishments simply won't allow you to bring your own liquor, so this fee may not even be an issue.) Unlike the similarly absurd cake-cutting fee charged by caterers, this one's got a long tradition and is going to be difficult, if not impossible, to wiggle out of.

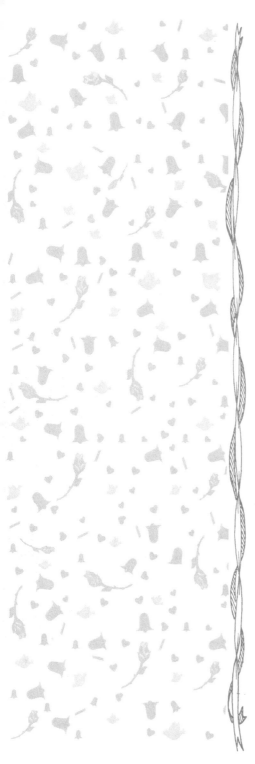

up to you to know when you're about to cross the line from happy newlywed to obnoxious drunk—and to stop yourself in time.

Your Liability as a Host

Rejoicing with the bride and groom does not have to mean drunken reveling. But it does sometimes happen that a few guests go beyond the limits of common sense and wind up really smashed. With recent court decisions, this has become a serious problem for both hosts and caterers. Be aware of your responsibilities.

Liquor may not be served to anyone under age, even at a home party. Courts have ruled that hosts were financially liable when teenagers served liquor at parties in their homes became involved in auto accidents or criminal matters. Caterers and restaurants have been held to the same rule.

Adult guests who are too drunk to drive but do so, and have an accident after being served drinks at your party, are also your responsibility and liability. As a good friend you should call a taxi or find someone else to drive the car in these cases. Caterers and bartenders as well are liable in this situation.

To avoid these situations, discuss with your caterer ways to limit alcohol consumption at your reception. Reliable caterers are happy to cooperate and to suggest options, especially since they are even more accountable than you are should there be an unfortunate accident, be it a bad fall or an auto crash.

Not at My Wedding . . .

If you suspect some friends or relatives may want to consume substances that get them happy but can also get them arrested (read: illegal drugs), take steps to ensure that it won't happen at your wedding. You don't want your big day tarnished by drugs or trouble with the law. Tell everyone in advance: no drugs whatsoever, not even in a quiet stall in the restroom. At the very least, it may offend other guests. At the very worst, it may provide you with the kind of "memorable wedding event" everyone would rather forget.

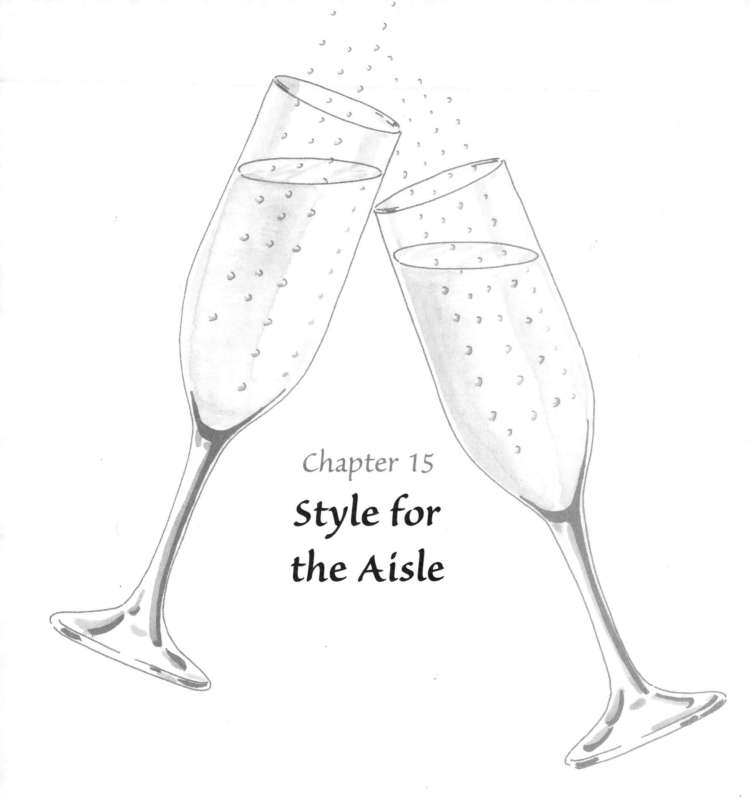

Chapter 15

**Style for
the Aisle**

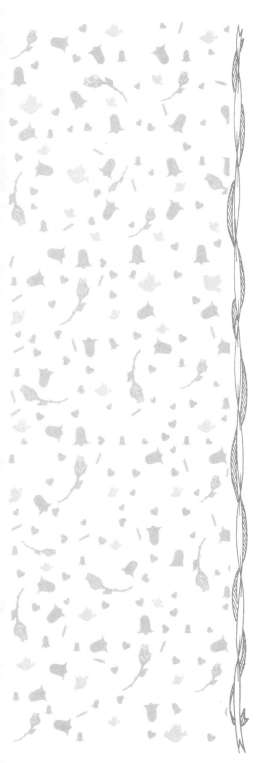

Imagine you're a contestant on the new game show, "Let's Make a Wedding Deal." After you solve the puzzle correctly, the game show host directs your attention to the prize stage. Behind Door Number One are all the components necessary for the most formal of weddings: a date at an ornate cathedral, white tie and tails, an elegant sitdown reception dinner with strolling violinists. Behind Door Number Two, the makings of a quaint, cozy wedding: the sunny backyard garden, bright yellow tent, luncheon buffet. Which door would you pick?

In the real world, of course, you have a much broader range of choices, but the way you answer that question will go a long way toward dictating the style and formality of your wedding attire.

Granted, selecting the right wedding gown is essentially impossible, but when it comes to picking attire to match the formality or informality of the occasion, brides actually have it a little easier than grooms. As long as her gown fits in with the overall style of the wedding (and looks good on her), the bride doesn't have much else to worry about.

On the other hand, a man's wedding attire is much more subject to the degree of formality, the season, and the time of day. This may seem like cause for cheer—finally, something that's more complicated for men than women! But, alas, things aren't as bad as they seem for your groom. Once he knows the answer to the "Let's Make a Wedding Deal" question, just about any formalwear shop can point him (and his attendants) in the right direction.

What the Groom and the Guys Should Be Wearing When

Informal wedding

Business suit
White dress shirt and tie
Black shoes and dark socks
(For the winter, consider dark colors; in the summer, navy, white, and lighter colors are appropriate.)

Semiformal wedding (daytime)

Dark formal suit jacket (in summer, select a lighter shade)
Cummerbund or vest   Four-in-hand or bow tie
Dark trousers   Black shoes and dark socks
White dress shirt

Semiformal wedding (evening)

Formal suit or dinner jacket with matching trousers (preferably black)

Cummerbund or vest   White shirt

Black bow tie   Studs and cufflinks

Formal wedding (daytime)

Cutaway or stroller jacket in gray or black   White high-collared (wing-collared) shirt

Waistcoat (usually gray)   Striped tie

Striped trousers   Studs and cufflinks

Formal wedding (evening)

Black dinner jacket and trousers   Waistcoat

Black bow tie   Cummerbund or vest

White tuxedo shirt   Cufflinks

Very formal wedding (daytime)

Cutaway coat (black or gray)   Striped trousers

Wing-collared shirt   Cufflinks

Ascot   Gloves

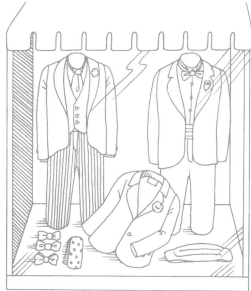

Very formal wedding (evening)

Black tailcoat   White waistcoat

Matching striped trousers trimmed with satin

Patent leather shoes

White bow tie   Studs and cufflinks

White wing-collared shirt   Gloves

So, as it turns out, the men have it easy once again. Lead them to the proper rack, and all they have to do is pick out the right size and stand around for a few minutes getting measured for alterations (and perhaps stuck with a few stray pins). All that's left for them to do is to remember to pick up the suit in time for the wedding. After being spoiled by such simplicity, what man wouldn't fall to pieces if he had to undertake the search for the right wedding gown?

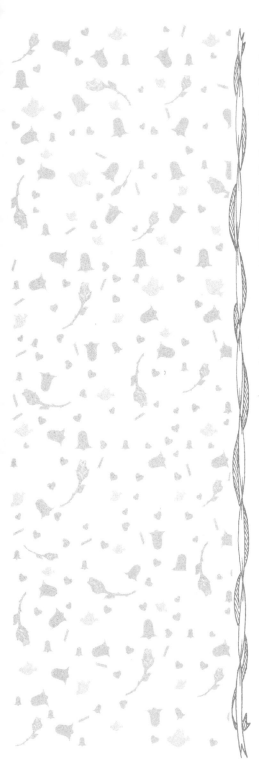

Your Wedding Groan, uh, Gown

You thought finding a bathing suit you liked was tough? Well, you ain't seen nothing yet. Just imagine the pressure you'll put on yourself (and every bridal salon in your immediate vicinity) to find the perfect gown for the most important day of your life.

Is your wedding gown really the single most important piece of clothing you'll ever wear? In the overall scheme of life, no. Only after the wedding is over and you're boxing up the gown for storage will you realize that. Then you'll kick yourself for having spent so much time and money to find an outfit that's only going to sit in a box for the next fifty years. But prior to that moment, yes. Your gown is the make-or-break wardrobe choice that puts all of your past clothing dilemmas in a new (and much more pleasant) light.

Style Guidelines

Brides, too, have style guidelines to help them; these guidelines depend on the type of wedding they're having.

Informal wedding

Formal, lacy suit or formal street-length gown
Corsage or small bouquet
No veil or train

Semiformal wedding

Chapel veil and modest bouquet (with floor-length gown)
Shorter fingertip veil or wide-brimmed hat and small bouquet (with tea-length or mid-calf-length gown)

Formal daytime wedding

Traditional floor-length gown
Fingertip veil or hat
Chapel or sweep train
Gloves
Medium-sized bouquet

Formal evening wedding

Same as formal daytime except:

Longer veil

Very formal wedding

Traditional floor-length gown (usually pure white or off-white) with
cathedral train or extended cathedral train

Long sleeves or long arm-covering gloves

Full-length veil

Elaborate headpiece

Cascade bouquet

Use these ideas as a starting point. Remember, you are by no
means tied to these style guidelines. Your wedding is your big day, so
don't let your decisions be dictated by somebody else. That goes for
your groom's attire, too.

Starting from Scratch

Handy with a needle and thread? Got enough time (and discipline) to
whip yourself up a wedding gown?

Making your own dress can save you a ton of money—a homemade
dress can cost from one quarter to one half the price of a store-bought
one—and allow you to create the design you want to your exact specifi-
cations. Even if you're not up to a do-it-yourself gown, don't despair
completely; maybe you (or a relative or friend) know of a seamstress
whom you trust to make your gown for you. Of course, unlike sewing it
yourself, you'll have to pay labor costs, but it is still likely to be less
expensive than a store gown, and you'll have the "luxury" of complete
design control (that is, you'll have no one else to blame if you don't
like the style of your dress).

Dresses made from scratch can take even longer to make than
manufactured gowns (from six months to a year), so be sure you give
yourself (or your seamstress) plenty of time to work.

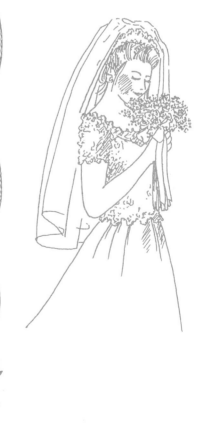

Bridal Salon Shopping: The Easy Way Out?

If you're like most nonsewing brides, you'll be hitting the bridal salons in your area to find your dream gown. Most salons require an appointment; you can usually get one a day or two after you call. Making appointments is worth the trouble, as they ensure that the staff will give you the proper attention. Don't be surprised if you feel like Cinderella being fitted for the magic slipper. The salon people are hoping lavish treatment from them can turn into lavish amounts of money from you. Be careful. Smiles, compliments, and free coffee and tea do not necessarily translate into quality dresses or reputable business practices.

Bridal Salon Bewares

Even if you have an unlimited amount of money to spend on a gown, you want to be sure you're shopping at a reputable shop, one that won't leave you standing at the altar in your slip come your wedding day. Unfortunately, there are a large number of bridal shop operators out there who will try to get as much money out of you as they possibly can; in exchange, they provide little or no quality. Some tricks of the trade to be aware of:

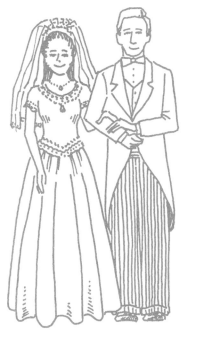

- ♥ The majority of salons require a deposit equal to half the price of the dress. Rather than order the dress from the manufacturer right away, they'll hold your deposit and use the money for other things (like earning interest in the company checking account). They end up ordering your gown at the last possible minute, which means it may not be ready in time for the wedding.
- ♥ For both wedding gowns and attendants' dresses, a shop may grossly overestimate the size a woman takes in order to charge a hefty fee for alterations. Petite women who normally take a size four may find themselves being told to order a size twelve dress. (Believe it or not, this actually happens.)
- ♥ If it sounds too good to be true, it probably is. A salon may offer a great price on a dress, only to charge a small fortune in alteration fees. These rip-off artists get their money one way or another.

How can you survive in this war zone? Arm yourself with these weapons:

- ♥ Always talk to the manager, or even better, the owner. Find out how long the shop has been in business; one would hope that a disreputable establishment would not be able to survive for long. Ask if you can speak with a former customer to get her impression of the shop.
- ♥ Always ask in advance about the price of alterations. Establish a flat rate, so you can't be hit with additional bills later on.
- ♥ Find out exactly when the shop plans on ordering your dress. Ask for verification of the order, and call periodically to check on progress.
- ♥ Get every aspect of your gown's purchase down in writing, including the delivery date. Find out the store's policy regarding late or damaged gowns. If (God forbid) something should go seriously wrong, don't be afraid to take legal action.

Now, the Fun Can Begin

Wedding gowns can take up to six months or more after the order is placed to arrive in your hands, so start wading through that sea of satin, silk, taffeta, chiffon, brocade, shantung, and organza as soon as you can. Leave yourself time for alterations and unforeseen glitches. No book can tell you what style and fabric are best for you; only you can know. In the haze of fabric and design, your instinct will pull you through; when you find the right dress, you'll know.

Second Opinions

You'll want to take along one person (your mother or a close friend, for instance) to consult with on matters of style and appearance, and to fight with when you get frustrated because you don't like any of the fifty dresses you've tried on. It's wise not to take more than one lucky person with you; the situation is stressful enough without inserting the opinions of five other people. If you try to please everyone, you'll never find anything, so stick with one person you trust.

Words to the Wise

Wear a button-down shirt when getting your hair styled. There's nothing worse than suddenly realizing you're going to have to cut yourself out of your favorite shirt, or ruin your hair pulling your shirt off over your head.

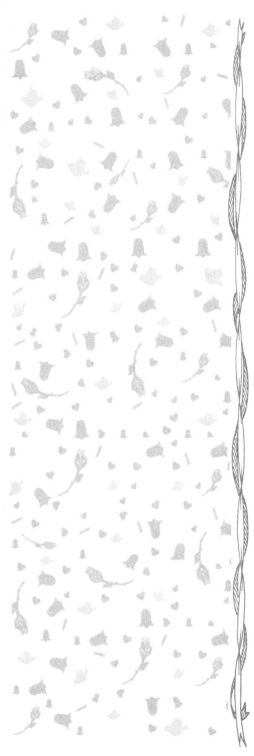

Taking a camera along when you try on gowns would seem like a good idea, wouldn't it? You could take pictures of yourself in your favorite gowns, then look at them in the privacy of your own home, without salespeople breathing down your neck. You could also get a few more opinions, free from the tension of the salon. Yes, it sounds great, but it's not likely to happen. Bridal shops are brutally competitive with one another, and each one guards its supply of goods as if it were a matter of national security. They don't want you to have a picture of yourself in a dress that you can take to another salon. If you did, you'd be able to compare quality and price, and they don't want that.

Hmm, What Else Do I Need?

You've found the perfect dress. Perhaps you're thinking, "No more anguished searching; goodbye to the bridal shop until my dress comes in." If this is what you're thinking, stop. You're still missing something. Hint: it's what the groom lifts in order to kiss you at the end of the ceremony. (Most brides don't wear veils that completely cover their faces anymore; still, it was a good hint.) You need a veil and headpiece—and other accessories besides. Read on.

Topping it all off: the veil

Lifting a "blusher" before the kiss has gone out of style; however, some religions do require that the face be covered at some point during the ceremony. Check with your officiant before deciding against a blusher veil. If he or she gives you the go-ahead to do without, start looking for the perfect piece. Your headpiece and veil should complement the style of your dress; don't pick something so ridiculously elaborate that it overpowers you and your dress. You want all eyes focused on you, the complete package, not you, the little body and tiny head under a massive headpiece.

Today's wedding veils are benefiting from one of our most popular modern conveniences: Velcro! Thanks to Velcro, veils can now be removed from the headpiece after the ceremony, which frees the bride from worrying about ripping her veil during close encounters with family and friends. It may not sound classy, but talk to a bride who has had her head almost snapped off because a hand or ring got caught in her veil and you'll gain a new appreciation for the concept.

Although a headpiece takes only eight to ten weeks to arrive after you order it, try to give yourself more time than that. Having the headpiece well in advance gives you a chance to go through one or two trial runs with your hairdresser.

The bride's handbag

You will not be carrying a handbag during the procession or the ceremony, but you will need a bag, perhaps even two: a small, dressy white bag (a beaded one is especially pretty) in which to carry your personal things—lipstick, mirror, comb, tissues for the tears of joy. Leave this in the bridal room during the ceremony.

Some bridal dressmakers will make up a drawstring bag that matches your gown to hold the many envelopes containing money gifts that will be presented to you at the reception. If you don't fancy this, pass all the gifts you receive along to your father or your husband for safekeeping in an inside jacket pocket.

Shoes

Decide on your shoes early on. They should be silk or satin, dyed to match the dress exactly (not all whites are the same). Choose a pair you can dance and stand in comfortably (you'll be on your feet for hours!), and break them in by wearing them around the house before the wedding.

When it comes to hose, beware of white stockings! They never look right because, once they're on your legs, they never match the dress and shoes. Instead, go for the sheerest champagne, nude or pale blush color you can find and have an extra pair to take with you on the big day, in case of disasters just before the ceremony.

Jewelry

You'll probably want the perfect pair of earrings or a necklace to accent your gown. But before you start hitting the jewelry sections of department stores or specialty jewelry shops, subtly ask your groom if he has any thoughts about getting you a bridal present. If so, you might drop hints as to the type of jewelry you'd like for your wedding day.

If you and your groom decide not to give each other gifts (perfectly understandable, considering how much money is already being spent for that day), maybe there's a special family piece your mother would be thrilled to loan you. Not only would it be more meaningful for you to wear something she, or your grandmother, or her grandmother, wore at her wedding, it would also fulfill the "something borrowed" and/or "something old" requirement.

Wedding Emergency Kit

Make up a wedding day emergency kit and put someone reliable in charge of bringing it everywhere you go. What goes in such a kit? Extra makeup, nylons, needles, thread, any bridal shop–recommended stain treatment, aspirin (and other necessary medications), hairspray, a brush or comb, and some breath mints—just in case.

If all else fails, start hunting through stores, catalogs, and even your own jewelry box. For earrings, remember to keep your wedding day hairstyle in mind; if you plan to wear your hair up or if your hair is short, you may want to go with a simple pair of earrings that won't pull attention away from your face. If your hair will be down and full, you could experiment with something flashier.

Necklaces and bracelets will be dictated by your gown's style. Consider waiting to purchase or borrow these pieces until your dress is nearly ready.

Gloves

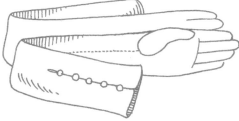

Before you purchase gloves to wear with your dress, ask your salon if they rent them. Chances are, you'll never wear them again, and unlike your wedding dress, gloves aren't worth altering. Make sure gloves fit snugly but are easy to remove for the exchange of rings.

Intimates

Now's the time to toss away your favorite pair of panties and splurge on a new pair! Seriously, you'll want to purchase undergarments that work specifically with your gown. Such garments may include a strapless or pushup bra, a merry widow (i.e., corset), special tummy reducing underwear, and a slip. If your gown requires a petticoat, ask your salon if they could rent you one. (It's unlikely you'll ever wear it again, unless you like to square dance or wear period dress costumes.)

Bridal Bargains

If you're in the market for an inexpensive dress, head for the discontinued rack at the bridal salon. Discontinued dresses are samples that are no longer being made by the manufacturer. These gowns are perfectly good, just not this year's models. Each season, the salons separate these dresses from the rest and offer them at considerably reduced prices. With a discontinued gown, you get a new dress and bridal shop pampering at a price you can (almost) enjoy.

Although salons offer slips, nylons, bras, and shoes, these items are often overpriced and better found elsewhere. As long as your slip doesn't require a hoop or any other fancy stuff, you should be able to find a reasonably priced one at a lingerie shop; don't forget to look at bras and nylons while you're there. You can save a great deal on shoes by buying yourself a simple white (or whatever color best matches the dress) pair at a regular shoe store and decorating them yourself with lace and buttons. Why pay a fortune for shoes that no one will even see?

Heirloom/antique gowns

With the price of most antiques these days, you wouldn't think an antique (or heirloom) gown would be a bargain, but it can be. Antique and heirloom gowns can be significantly less expensive than new ones, and the added style and nostalgia they provide is beyond price. Unless you're fairly petite you may have a hard time finding one that will fit you. Apparently, women were a lot smaller all those years ago.

Used/consignment gowns

Another way to get an inexpensive gown (provided you don't care if you're not the first and only person to wear it) is to shop the consignment stores and other bargain outlets for previously worn gowns. These gowns can be bought for as little as $100, and can be taken home with you that day. Of course, finding a quality wedding gown on consignment may require some tenacity, as well as a little detective work, since they don't come down the pike every day. If you're serious about taking the previously worn route, check the classified section of the local newspaper. You might even ask a newly married acquaintance if she feels like selling you her gown (at a huge discount, of course).

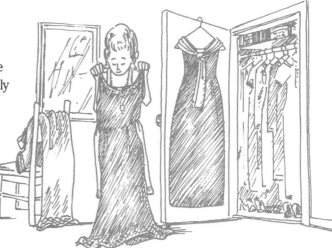

Like any gown you buy, check for quality: there should be no stains, rips, or other flaws. The downside to previously worn gowns: finding someone to alter the gown for you. Bridal salons won't work on gowns that are not bought at their store, so you'll have to search for a reliable seamstress to do the alterations for you. Talented seamstresses who can do the work you require in time for your wedding do not grow on trees. Unfortunately, the expense of these alterations may nullify the money you saved buying the used gown. If possible, get a written estimate of the costs from your seamstress first.

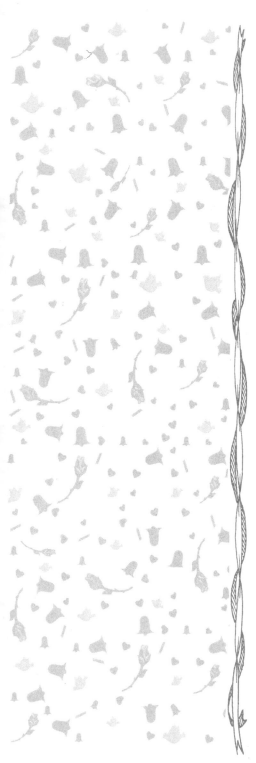

Outlet/warehouse sales

Perhaps you've seen TV news coverage of a local warehouse's one-day wedding gown sale. Brides-to-be line up as early as six o'clock in the morning to get first crack at wedding gowns, many boasting top designer names, marked down as low as $100 each. When the doors open at nine, it's as if a dam has burst. A flood of women cascades through the store to maul the inventory. In this frenzy, women grab as many dresses as they can handle, regardless of size, to increase the odds of finding something they like. No one bothers much with dressing rooms; they try the dresses on right next to the rack. If a woman doesn't like a gown, you can bet there's someone standing next to her ready to grab it.

The obvious advantage of these sales is financial: you can get a new gown for the price of a previously worn one. You save an incredible amount of money, and you still get to be the first one married in the dress. You still have to hustle to find a seamstress to do the alterations, and she won't come cheap. And it goes without saying that you won't get the pampering of a bridal salon; you'll be lucky to get space at the mirror! Shopping this way for a wedding gown is not for everybody, but if you can endure the madhouse atmosphere, and if you do find the gown for you, getting up early to be in line at six o'clock can be worth it.

Renting a gown

Another increasingly popular way to find a gown is to rent one. Again, this option is not for someone who cares about being the first to wear the gown, or who wants to keep it to treasure forever. Like a tuxedo rental, the gown is yours only for the wedding, then it's back on the rack for someone else. Through rental, the average gown can be had for as little as $100; a famous-maker extravaganza that would cost thousands to purchase can be rented for only a few hundred.

The major kink in the rental game: if the gown you choose requires drastic alterations, they may not let you rent it. A great deal of material would be lost trying to make a size twelve dress fit a size four woman; after that, the dress could only be rented to very small women, a prospect the shop isn't likely to welcome.

They're not just for bridesmaids anymore

If you're feeling creative (and are a little more handy with a needle and thread than the average person), an inexpensive alternative to a formal bridal gown is to get an elegant bridesmaid's dress in white. All you'll have to do is dress it up a bit with some lace, buttons, and the like. It probably won't satisfy you for a formal wedding, but for a less formal occasion it can be a thrifty and inventive way to go!

When You're Expecting

These days, the social pressures that once limited attire options for pregnant brides to dresses that disguise their condition are relatively rare. There is no shortage of styles for the pregnant bride to choose from. Obviously, the style you choose will depend upon how far into the pregnancy you are, and how far along you expect to be at the time of the wedding. Brides-to-be in their first trimester will, of course, have a much broader range of choices than those in their second or third.

Train, Train

When talking trains, there are two things you'll want to keep in mind: length and style. The three most common lengths are Sweep, Chapel, and Cathedral. The Sweep train, best known for semiformal occasions, falls around six inches on the floor. The most popular choice these days is the Chapel train, which can fall as much as twenty-two inches on the floor. If you want the type of train that finishes entering the room five minutes after you arrive, the Cathedral train is for you; falling twenty-two inches or more, it's usually reserved for very formal affairs.

Now that you know the lengths, a word about how trains can look. The attached train flows out from the back end of the gown skirt. A Wateau flows from the back yoke, the Capelot from the back shoulder. The detachable train (by far the most conducive to dancing the night away) falls from the waistline and can be, you guessed it, detached.

If you don't remember ever having seen a bride tripping over her train during a dance with her groom, it's because most trains are bustled (if not detached) after the completion of the ceremony to give the bride freedom of movement.

Words to the Wise

As mentioned before, because most wedding gowns are made of delicate material, brides should consult with their bridal salon about what to use to protect the fabric from under-arm perspiration. Protective shields between under-arms and the dress can prevent deodorant from ruining the fabric. If your dress is cut in such a way that protective shields would be seen or would interfere with the style, consult your bridal salon for other options.

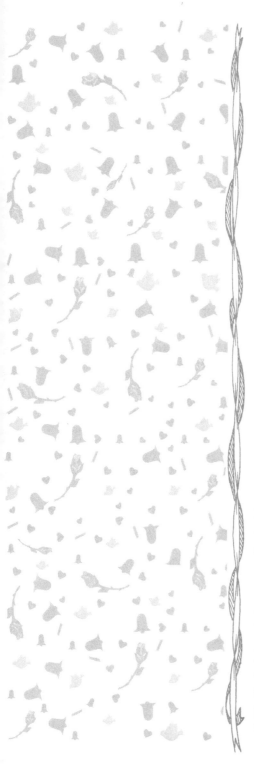

Wedding Day Beauty Tips

Hair prep before your wedding day

Have you ever been warned never to get your hair cut before getting your picture taken because "you'll look like a stranger in your own hair"? True, you usually do feel a little self-conscious after some serious scissor work, and you don't want that feeling translated forever onto film. If heeding that warning is prudent in everyday life, the advice quadruples in value when talking about your wedding. Never never get a haircut or change your hairstyle right before your wedding. Not only do you run the risk of looking like "a stranger in your own hair," but you could absolutely HATE the new do, depressing you to the point where you can't truly enjoy the big day.

The same rule of thumb applies to highlighting, coloring, perming, or straightening your hair. If you want to have an updated look for your wedding day, try it out well in advance—and have it professionally done.

It's only natural to want to try a new hairstyle for your wedding; perhaps after wearing your hair down for 1,257 days in a row, you'd like to try it up, or vice versa. Or maybe you're looking for a style that really complements your headpiece. This is fine. As most politicians will tell you, change is a wonderful thing—don't be afraid of it. Just allow enough time to get acquainted with your new hair before the wedding or to attend to any disasters.

Start experimenting with your hairdresser six months or so before the wedding. After you find the look you want, visit the shop periodically for maintenance. As mentioned when discussing headpieces, you'll want to bring yours to your hairdresser to go through at least one trial run before the big day. Through all this you may get a little sick of the sight of your hairdresser, but feeling that you look the best you ever have for the biggest event of your life is miraculous medicine.

Hair prep on your wedding day

If you feel confident in your ability to style your hair to your liking, there's no need to take a trip to the salon on your wedding day. But if you're like most women, you'll reach for the security of the stylist on that day, either because you feel no one can make you look better or because your hands are too busy shaking to wield a brush. Brides walking out of a salon, hair all done up, headpiece in place, wearing a t-shirt and jeans are a humorous but not uncommon sight. If you don't want to be seen in public this way, see whether your hairdresser would be willing to make the trip to your home, or wherever you may be getting ready that day. This might also save you the trouble of exposing your perfect hairdo to the wind and rain. Of course, we hope it never rains for anyone's wedding day; not only does it put a damper on the occasion, it's a virtual guarantee of a bad hair day.

Putting your face on

If you've always wanted to sit down at one of those department store cosmetic counters and tell the attendant, "Go for it, make me beautiful!" (that is, more beautiful than you already are), this is the time to fulfill that urge. Like your hairdresser, a cosmetologist can help you feel more confident in your appearance, or give you a completely new look. Even if you're completely happy with your daily makeup selection and application skills, you may want to try something different, something special for your wedding day. Consider your face a blank piece of paper (lovely thought, isn't it), and your cosmetologist a renowned artist. She can show you just what colors to apply, what angles to apply them at, and other tricks to make your face into a real work of art.

A department store cosmetologist will gladly give you a consultation and a makeover, especially if it induces you to buy some of her products. If you are completely impressed by her abilities and her advice, buy whatever items you want or need and go home and practice. (You may be spending more on makeup than you ever dreamed, but it's your wedding, so pamper yourself.) Don't be afraid to ask questions, or to go back if you find that it just doesn't look the same. If you're unhappy with the treatment you get, don't despair; try another counter or even another type of store. There is a wide range of product lines out there, from trendy new shades to earthy, classic tones, and plenty of cosmetologists who are more than willing to meet your needs—and get your business.

The alternative to a department store cosmetologist is a professional cosmetologist, whose business it is to make people over, not sell a product. Do a couple of test runs at his or her place of business. The real bonus is that, come your wedding day, you're not left to your own devices; he or she will come to your home and do it all for you.

Best Face Forward

You want your skin to look its clearest, cleanest, and most radiant for your special day. What better way to achieve this than getting a facial the morning of your wedding, right? Wrong! Most professional facials are not given with a light touch. They involve rigorous cleansing methods that can leave skin looking blotchy, reddened, or even damaged. If you do want a facial, be sure to schedule it at least a week or two in advance.

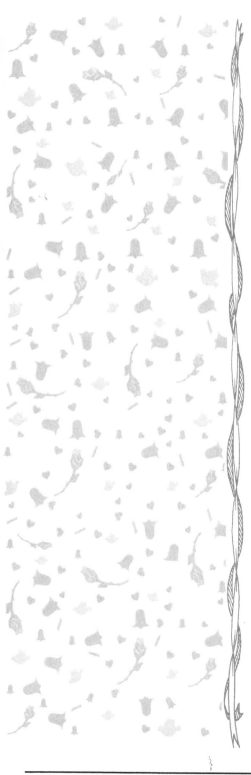

"You're soaking in it"

Does your concept of a manicure include Madge dipping your hand in Palmolive? Having someone file your nails and attend to your cuticles may seem frivolous, but consider this: after admiring your dress, your hair, and your new husband, friends and family are going to want to see your ring finger. Or, your photographer might suggest a "ring shot," where you and your groom clasp left hands over your bouquet. How are you going to feel with all those eyes staring at your fingers?

If your regular toilet routine includes caring for your nails, then you shouldn't need any special attention. But if you're worried your fingernails will look misshapen, bitten, or just plain unattractive, you might want to splurge and get a manicure. A French manicure accents the white half moons at the tips of your nails and gives them a high buff; a standard manicure shapes and polishes the nails. If you decide to have your nails painted, be sure to ask for a subtle color such as sheer pink or off white. Fire-engine red might be fun for the honeymoon, but it would probably raise eyebrows during the ceremony.

Want to experience real pampering? Add a pedicure to the list. No one will see your feet on your wedding day, but there's always the wedding night...

The nose knows

You have a favorite perfume you know drives your fiancé wild—and that will mask any body odor problems you may have as you nervously walk down the aisle. So of course you should wear your perfume on your wedding day, right? Maybe not. If the scent is a light one, okay. But many people are sensitive to strong perfume odors. Perhaps your officiant, or your maid of honor, or your fiancé's best man is one of them. A sneeze just as you're saying "I do" would ruin the romantic moment for sure. A better choice is to save the strong scents for the wedding night and opt for a light dusting of body powder in addition to your regular deodorant/antiperspirant to make you feel fresh and odor-free.

Remember, after all the hair styling, makeup, manicures, and other beauty aids, the thing that truly makes a bride most beautiful is the glow she wears that comes from inside, from all the love and joy she's feeling on her wedding day. That's the one thing you don't have to worry about buying or creating: you already have it.

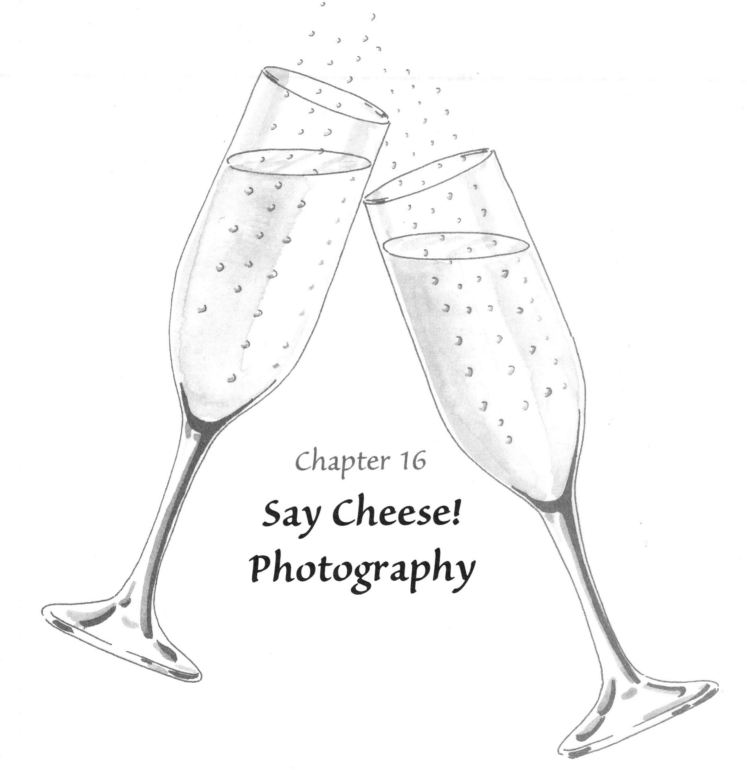

Chapter 16

**Say Cheese!
Photography**

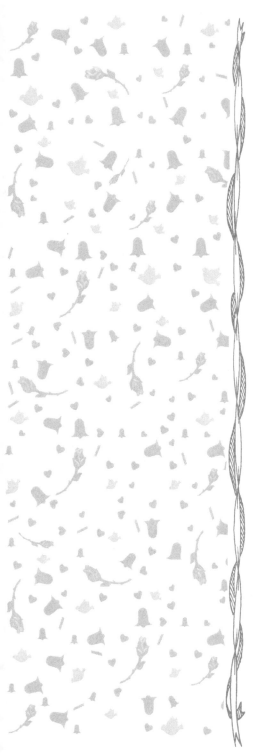

"A picture paints a thousand words." At no time in your life will this statement seem more appropriate than on your wedding day. You'll be feeling things you can't even recognize, never mind describe. And thanks to the art of photography, you won't have to. A good set of wedding prints will go a long way toward capturing and preserving all the emotions, excitement, and memories for you and your family.

Good photography is not just clicking on the auto-focus and shooting away with the family Instamatic. It's an art requiring skill and planning. Needless to say, you don't want to put this huge responsibility in the hands of just anyone, so be very careful about whom you choose. Beware of "professional" photographers who really aren't—yet. Imagine how you'd feel after finding out the entire ceremony was photographed with the lens cap on. A drastic example, but not unheard of. There are countless stories of couples who have received less than quality work for their money: photos that are blurry, ill-composed, and made up of colors that don't appear in the natural world, and definitely didn't appear at the wedding; shots of family and friends with demonic red dots in their eyes. Don't shell out your hard-earned cash for work like that. Take the time to find a photographer who will do you and your wedding justice.

Only work with a reputable photographer—there is no substitute for the education and experience of a professional. Finding such a professional may not be that easy, however. It's quite common for the best people to be booked a year or more in advance, so begin your search early. Start with the word-of-mouth approach: ask your friends, family, coworkers, or anyone else you know who's been married or who has coordinated a wedding recently. Their opinions and their wedding albums will go a long way toward helping you find some options.

Be sure to ask about their overall experience with the photographer or studio in question. The pictures may have come out like a dream, but the person behind the lens could have been a nightmare: rude, pushy, sloppy. If that's the case, keep looking. Your aim is to hire someone who takes great photographs, and does so in a way that makes everyone feel at ease. If you've ever been to a wedding where the photographer has fallen drunk into the punch bowl or made a pass at the maid of honor, you already know that you don't want this happening to you.

You're looking for someone who makes you feel comfortable, someone who is willing to work with you every step of the way. A good photographer who relates well with you, your groom, and your families can bring out the best in everyone and preserve it forever on film.

It also goes without saying that you're looking for someone who's very talented. How can you assess the photographer's talent if you don't even know how to load film into a camera? For starters, look for crispness and thoughtful composition. Did the photographer make good use of lighting? Were a variety of backgrounds and settings used, or is everyone always standing in front of the cake? Is there a good balance of formal and candid shots? This should give you an idea of what to look for, but if you have a friend or family member who knows photography, try bribing them into going along with you.

In addition to the look of the photographs, find out how the photographer will process them. Many studios these days use chemical laboratories for color processing, but this method pales (no pun intended) to an artist processing the colors by hand. With this method, colors are much more accurate, and the details are plentiful and clear. If this sounds suspiciously like the expensive route, it is, but it's also the best route if you can put aside the extra money in your photography budget.

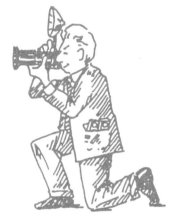

If you can't find a good photographer by word of mouth, go to some bridal fairs and photography shows. Both are likely to yield plenty of good candidates.

When interviewing photographers who haven't worked with anyone you know, make sure you get references and closely examine their work. The photos in the portfolio may be wonderful, but it is possible that the person you're talking to bought them from someone else, and in real life doesn't know an f-stop from a truck stop! Ask for the names of former clients you can contact to get another customer's point of view.

What to Ask Your Photographer

Here is a list of questions that will help you choose the best man, woman, or studio for the job. If the answers you get make you nervous, move on to the next photographer on your list.

- ♥ How long has the photographer been in this business?
- ♥ Does the photographer specialize in weddings? (If he or she isn't a wedding expert, find someone who is.)
- ♥ Is this a full-time photographer? (Part-timers need not apply.)
- ♥ Can you see samples of previous work and speak to some former clients?

♥ What types of photo packages are offered?

♥ What is included in the standard package?

♥ What are the costs for additional photos?

♥ How many pictures does the photographer typically take at a wedding of this size?

♥ In addition to the base package fee, will there be any additional hourly fees? Travel costs?

♥ Will you be charged by the hour?

♥ Does the photographer keep negatives? If so, for how long?

♥ May you purchase negatives if you wish?

♥ Will you be able to purchase extra photos in the future?

♥ Does the photographer use a variety of lighting techniques? A variety of backgrounds?

♥ Will the photographer take a mixture of formal and candid shots?

♥ Would the photographer be willing to incorporate your ideas into the shot list?

♥ Will the photographer provide a contract stipulating services, date, time, costs, and so on?

In the end, you must make your choice based on the individual's talent, your own ceremony and reception needs, your budget, and your gut feeling about the person you'll be working with.

Until you sit down with the photographer to map out a battle plan for the wedding, you will probably be dealing with price ranges rather than concrete amounts. The final price depends on the approach to the wedding you develop with the photographer.

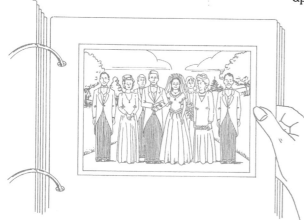

Get the best value you can, but remember: you will do yourself a big favor by opting to pay a little more for a quality job.

After you've chosen the photographer, sit down with him or her and discuss your photographic wants, needs, and expectations. It's important to establish a good relationship well before the wedding so that everyone feels comfortable when the big (and usually nerve-wracking) day comes around.

As you'll soon find out, there are certain photographs that are traditionally taken, so be sure to tell the photographer if you have additional ideas in mind to be captured on film. Give him a list of all the special people you want pictures of, especially people outside of the wedding party. Your photographer may be exceptional, but he's probably not a mind-reader. If your eighty-year-old aunt is famous for her rendition of "the Twist" at family functions, make sure you tell the photographer you want that moment on film!

Similarly, if you don't want some of the standard poses (groom with his ushers, groom with bridal attendants, etc.), let the photographer know. Why waste time and film on pictures you don't want?

Getting Your Money's Worth

Remember to ask how many pictures the photographer plans to take on your wedding day. A good quality studio will take three times as many as you signed up for, to give you the best and broadest selection. If you ask for the thirty-six-photo album, you certainly don't want the photographer taking only thirty-six pictures.

Once the photographer has a pretty good idea of the type of photos you want, as well as how many should be taken, he or she should be able to tell you what package plan or standard deal is best for you. Remember to get an exact price for both the photographs and any additional services the photographer may provide.

Some studios will charge you a basic hourly rate. Others charge a flat fee based on the photographer's time and a certain number of photographs, such as seven hours work and a thirty-six-picture album. Studios may also charge for the photographer's travel time, or for overtime if the job runs longer than expected.

Complete fees for photographers range from $400 to $4,000, depending upon the quality, type, and number of photographs. Get the exact fee in advance. You want to make sure you're not signing on for more than you can handle.

Be sure to find out what the prices are for additional photos you may want to order beyond the original package. The studio may give you a very reasonable price for your package, but charge $100 for every extra photo. Some studios include albums, frames, and special parents' books as part of the deal; ask if yours does too.

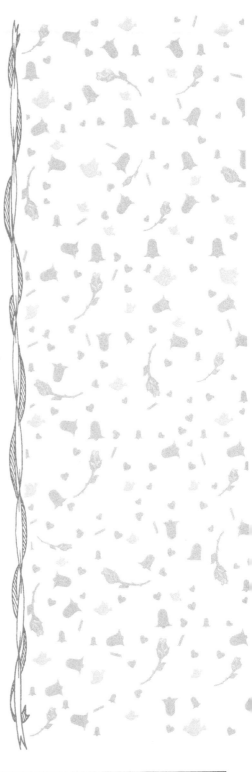

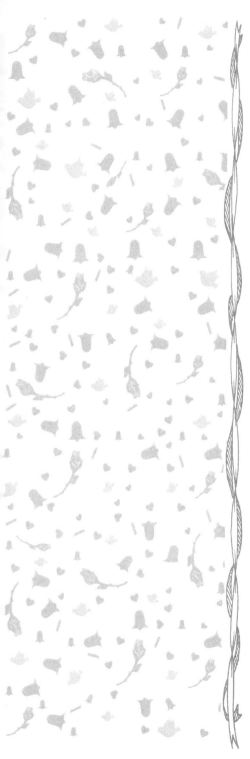

Photographic Extras

Aside from working with you on the wedding day, you may want the photographer to take an engagement photo and/or a formal bridal portrait. If so, you'll want to iron out the details with the photographer in your initial meeting.

The popularity of bridal portraits is not what it used to be. Salons often have trouble getting the gown ready in enough time to take the portrait. Most brides have portraits taken as a gift to their parents; photos can also be used as part of a wedding announcement in the newspaper. If you plan to send a copy along to the paper, be sure to order a 5" X 7" black-and-white shot from the photographer.

Bridal portraits are usually taken either at the photographer's studio or at the bridal salon on the last day of your fitting. Most photographers will meet you at the salon, but you should double-check to make sure.

Photo Thank-you Notes

If your photography budget is overflowing with extra funds, you might consider thank-you notes that feature a picture of you and your groom. You can get one standard photo that goes on every note, or, if you're really ambitious, personalize each one with a photo of you opening the person's gift. These photo-notes are not common practice, but they do add a personal touch and hint at a little extra effort on your part.

Formal Photos Before the Wedding

Although it is considered bad luck for the groom to see the bride before the ceremony, many couples today feel comfortable doing away with this superstition and taking the formal shots before the wedding. Handling the formal photo session this way makes life easier for a lot of people: the photographer doesn't have to rush to get all the shots on your list before hungry guests start a riot; the guests don't suffer from starvation or boredom while they wait for you to pose, pose, and pose again, and you and the wedding party get to enjoy more of the reception.

If seeing the groom before the ceremony is absolutely out of the question for you, try to take as many pictures as you can without him—you alone, you and your parents, you and your attendants, and so on.

At the reception, speed things up by making sure everyone who's going to be in a picture knows where he or she is supposed to be.

Shooting on Location

Some couples opt to take their formal wedding photos at a location other than the reception site. Sometimes the spot they select is of great sentimental value—sometimes it's chosen just because the scenery is gorgeous.

Some on-location photo shoot suggestions are at a beach, lake, or garden (in the spring and summer), near foliage (in the fall), and in a snow-covered wood (in the winter).

If you do plan to take your photo shoot on the road, remember that your guests will have to wait even longer than usual to see you (and their dinner) at the reception. As a way to ease their impatience (and their stomachs), consider offering a first-hour open bar and serving some hors d' oeuvres.

It Can Be All Black and White

Though you may associate black-and-white photos with your parents' and grandparents' weddings, they can add a special touch to yours, too! Color may be brilliant, but black and white is classic. It creates atmosphere and style. Black and white lends itself best to formal portraits; it gives them a timeless feel that is perfect for such an occasion. For candid and action shots, though, it's best to stay with color. How can you show off your ability to color-coordinate the flowers, the dresses, and the cake without color photos to pass around?

For a really distinctive look, the studio can add some hand-colored tinting to your black-and-white photos—the same process used for movie star stills in the 1940s. If you thought you felt special on your wedding day, imagine how you'll feel seeing you and your groom looking like two of the silver screen's greatest lovers!

Of course while you're adding all this style and atmosphere, remember to add a little more money to your overall bill. As odd as it may seem, black-and-white photos (even the untinted variety) cost more than color. While proofs for color shots can be processed by machine, all processing for black and white must be done by hand. Some studios

For Your Bridal Portrait, You Will Need . . .

- ♥ Your gown
- ♥ A hat, veil, or other headpiece you select
- ♥ Gloves, if you plan to wear them
- ♥ Wedding shoes and stockings
- ♥ Jewelry you plan to wear on your wedding day
- ♥ A bridal bouquet (if you can't get one from your florist, the bridal salon or studio can usually provide models)

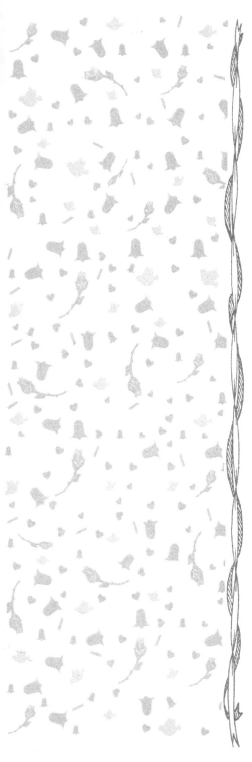

will charge you an additional fee for each roll of black-and-white film shot; others add on a flat amount meant to cover the whole job.

Making the Guests Earn Their Meal

Some of the best photos from your wedding may not even come from the photographer. Place a throw-away camera (you know, the kind they sell at tourist spots and drugstores) on each table. Ask your guests to click away at the people and action around them during the reception. Collect the cameras at the end of the reception and you'll have lots of wonderful candids of people and events the photographer probably wouldn't dream of shooting—and at a fraction of the cost.

Keeping Your Negatives

Ask whether the studio will hang on to your negatives, and if so, for how long. You may want or need a picture from the wedding years later and you'll want to know how to get one made. Most studios will keep the negatives for only a few years; if having them forever is important to you, ask about buying them.

Watch Out!

A photographer's high price tag does not necessarily mean you'll be getting high quality. A low price tag, however, is a pretty reliable sign that you're likely to see low-quality results. Photography is one of the parts of your wedding you should try not to skimp on. You probably won't be dragging your wedding dress out of storage very often, and you may not even remember what kind of flowers you carried, but you can bet that you and your loved ones will be going back to your wedding photographs time and time again. So . . .

Steer clear of part-time photographers who only occasionally handle weddings. They are not likely to have the equipment and experience of an expert in the field.

Make sure the studio you choose specializes in weddings. You may love the studio that did your high school graduation picture . . . but if portraits are all they do, they'll probably flunk out at your wedding. Only experienced wedding photographers know all the nuances of photographing a wedding: how to avoid problems, when to fade into the background, and the best way to compose a moment when working in a crowd.

Be sure to get every part of the agreement with your photographer in writing. Include the date, the agreed arrival time, the length of shooting time, estimates for additional fees or overtime charges, the cost of the package you've selected, and anything else of importance. You don't want to be hit with unexpected bills after the fact.

Avoid very large studios that appear to use the assembly line approach. Often they employ as many as 100 photographers and won't guarantee which one will show up on your wedding day, or how qualified he or she is to do the job. Always ask to see sample wedding photos that were taken by the same photographer who will be working your wedding. If the studio can't or won't supply them, find another one to work with.

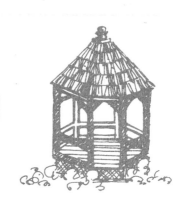

Videography

Despite the clear and present danger of winding up on one of those embarrassing home video shows, videotaping your wedding is pretty much a given these days. Many couples consider their wedding video more valuable than their wedding photographs. This may be because the bride and groom are, ironically, the two people who usually remember the least about their wedding. They're in a fog of emotion and excitement; hundreds of sensory impressions go by in a blur. Still photographs will show them a few staged poses, how things looked; videotape will show how things were.

Unlike a still camera, the video camera records not just images, but time—taking in all the sound and action of a scene. Rather than focusing in on a few key friends and family members, video can capture everybody. You can have a record of the guests as they sing, dance, eat, kiss, cry, laugh. When a bride and groom finally sit down to watch their videotape, it will certainly bring back wonderful memories but it will also show them many things they hadn't seen before.

Your Videographer

When searching for a videographer, apply the same basic guidelines you would for a still photographer. The pictures may be moving this time, but the images should still be crisp and clear, and colors should be cor-

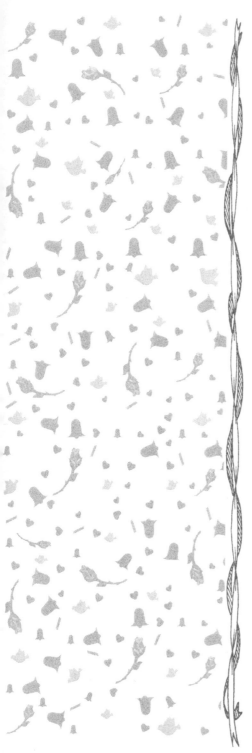

rect. You want to be comfortable with your videographer, and confident he won't be ordering your guests in and out of shots as though he considers himself the next Martin Scorcese.

Remember to confirm that your videographer has up-to-date, quality equipment, not a 25-year-old Super 8 camera. Also ask about editing and dubbing machines, microphones, and lights. Find out how many cameras he or she has, and how many people will be assisting on the job. Some video formats require the simultaneous use of two cameras; one person with one camera will bring you up short.

Ask to view sample tapes. You're looking for smooth editing, clear sound, and an overall professional feel to the tape. With all of the technology today, you don't have to settle for anything short of broadcast quality production values.

If you're lucky, the people at your photography studio will offer video services. If not, they may recommend someone. And don't forget your most precious resource in these situations: word of mouth. Friends, relations, and coworkers should be able to help out with some referrals.

Once you've found someone and verified references, get a written contract stipulating costs, services, manpower commitments, the date, the time, and the place.

What to Ask Your Videographer

Here are some things you'll want to ask your videographer:

- ♥ How long has the person been doing this professionally?
- ♥ Can you see samples of the work and check references?
- ♥ Is the work guaranteed?
- ♥ Can you look at a work in progress in addition to a demo tape? (This way you'll know the videographer is actually doing the work, not buying great demo tapes from someone else.)
- ♥ Is the equipment high-quality, including the editing and dubbing machines?
- ♥ Will the videographer be using a high-quality tape?
- ♥ How many cameras will be used? How big will the videographer's staff be?
- ♥ What special effects are available?
- ♥ Will he or she use wireless microphones during the ceremony so that vows are clearly heard on the tape?
- ♥ How is the fee computed? One flat rate? By the hour?

♥ Is a standard package deal offered? If so, what is it?

♥ Are there ways to cut down on the total price?

♥ How much will it cost to have copies of the original made?

When viewing sample tapes, consider the following questions:

♥ Do the segments tell a story, giving a clear sense of the order in which the events took place?

♥ Does the tape capture the most important moments—such as you cutting the cake and throwing the garter?

♥ Is there steady use of the camera, clear sound, vibrant color, and a nice sharp picture?

♥ How are the shots framed? What editing techniques are used?

♥ Does the tape move smoothly from one scene to the next—rather than lurching ahead unexpectedly?

Money Is (Still) an Object

There are some very elaborate video formats out there, some featuring special lenses and special effects. You could get an Oscar-caliber videotape, but it won't come cheap. Before you get carried away with the idea of seeing your name in lights, remember that nasty little technicality called a budget. The typical wedding video package costs anywhere between $500 and $1,500, depending on the quality of the equipment, the number of hours of coverage, the number of cameras, the amount of editing, and other factors. As always, remember what's most important to you, determine what you can afford, and go from there.

Name That Format

There are various format options for wedding videos. Here are a few you might like to consider.

The nostalgic format. This type of video usually starts with vintage photographs of you and your groom, perhaps as children or young adults. From there, it can show the two of you sharing your lives together. The ceremony, reception, and (sometimes) shots of your honeymoon end this format. Because it takes a little more work to put together, this type of video can be expensive.

Words to the Wise

Ask about the cost of obtaining a few extra copies of your videotape. If a still photo is lost or damaged, you can usually get the negatives from the photographer; once a videotape is gone, however, it's gone for good. If the cost of obtaining multiple copies is too high, check around for a reliable photography store that specializes in videotape dubbing.

The straight shot format. This format uses only one camera, thus making it the least expensive video option offered. No editing is required, but the videographer can still add small touches, such as names and dates, to help spice up the film.

The documentary format. As its title suggests, this format gives you a documentary-style account of your wedding day. It usually starts with you and your groom getting ready, then proceeds to scenes of the ceremony and the reception; sometimes interviews with family and friends are added. The documentary format has become quite popular; prices vary widely depending on the type of equipment used and the amount of editing needed.

If your videographer will be using a format that requires editing, ask if you can have the unedited footage as well. You may not watch this tape as often, but you'll probably want access to the uncut version for those memorable moments that didn't make it onto the "official" tape.

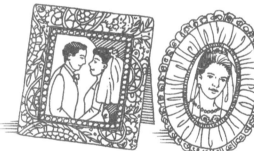

Remember to take your videographer to your ceremony and reception sites ahead of time to check out the lighting, possible angles, and so on. You should also acquaint the videographer with the photographer (if they have not met); this way each person has an idea of whose toes they're stepping on to compete for a shot.

What's Next?

Because videotaping is dependent on technology, there are always new techniques and equipment being advanced. What was not available for a friend's wedding last year might be commonplace today. Ask your videographer about all the options.

Don't have your wedding videotaped by a friend or relative unless you've seen a sample of his or her work and were impressed by it. Your groom's brother may have the best intentions and even own a good video camera, but odds are he won't have the necessary sound and editing equipment to make a tape for posterity. He may miss some key moments if he gets caught up in the excitement. And do you really want those choppy shots of the floor tiles taken while he was leaping to catch the garter?

Chapter 17

Right in Tune: Ceremony and Reception Music

Have you ever been to a wedding that had no music? How about one where the music was so bad you wished there had been none? Let's just say such a wedding is a seemingly endless experience. You certainly don't want anyone to remember your wedding this way, so put some careful thought into this part of the reception. Remember that the right music adds spirit and feeling to any moment; don't pass up the opportunity to let it enhance your big day.

Music for the Aisle

Most marrying couples don't give much thought to ceremony music. With the exception of "Here Comes the Bride" (and a few other stray notes from the organ) there aren't too many songs directly associated with the ceremony. But these days, more and more couples are spicing up their ceremony with a variety of songs, musicians, and singers. And that organ is taking a back seat to horns and strings.

Carefully selected music can provide atmosphere and enhance the mood and meaning of your ceremony. Perhaps some of the songs you pick will reflect the solemnity or the joy you feel as you and your groom begin your marriage.

If additional musicians, singers, and songs are an option you'd like to consider, consult with the officiant in charge of your ceremony. Some religions place restrictions on secular selections during the ceremony, but others may be very open. Ask about this well in advance. You don't want the officiant running you out of the place as the soloist belts out her rendition of Frank Sinatra's "Love and Marriage" during the rehearsal.

Your best bet for finding appropriate ceremony music is to check with the musical coordinator for the ceremony site. Most religious facilities have a staff organist or choir director who can help you choose the best possible music given his or her experience. The coordinator can also recommend singers and musicians who have performed well at other ceremonies. Don't worry if you think you don't know enough about classical or "church" music; the musicians you eventually choose can offer suggestions based on guidelines you set out.

Before you hire a full orchestra to accompany the church choir, though, remember that the cost of musicians and singers for the ceremony must fit into your overall music budget. In other words, you don't hire a $500 string quartet when you have only $700 allotted for ceremony and reception music. It may take some planning, but don't be intimidated; you can have wonderful music for both events with a little compromise and ingenuity.

Most ceremony music is broken up into four parts: prelude, processional, ceremony, and recessional. Each of these sections has its own function and style; you should choose music that is suitable for each. (Note: In the Orthodox Jewish ceremony, there is no music.)

The prelude

The prelude lasts from the time the guests start arriving until all of them are seated and the mother of the bride is ready to make her entrance. The options for music here are very broad: upbeat, slow, or a mixture of both. You want the prelude to establish a mood as well as entertain the guests while they wait.

The end of the prelude, right before the processional, is usually a good time for a soloist or choir to sing a song. During this song, the mother of the bride is seated.

The processional

This is the music that accompanies the wedding party in their jaunt down the aisle. A traditional march helps to set the pace for some nervous feet—and carry the spirit of the day toward the altar.

When it's time for you to make that l-o-o-ong trek down the aisle, you can walk to the same piece as did the bridesmaids before you, or to a song chosen especially for you. Sometimes the piece is the same but played at a different tempo, or with an audience-captivating pause before it begins.

Ceremony music

Music played while the wedding ceremony itself takes place is called, oddly enough, ceremony music. The right music here can enhance the mood and emphasize the meaning of the marriage ceremony. Consider playing a short piece during the lighting of the unity

---

Left Foot, Right Foot

Some processional favorites (and the composers):

"Waltz of the Flowers," Tchaikovsky

"Wedding March," Mendelssohn

Bridal Chorus ("Here Comes the Bride"), Wagner

"Trumpet Voluntary," Dupuis

"Trumpet Voluntary," Clarke

"Trumpet Tune," Purcell

"The Dance of the Sugar Plum Fairies," Tchaikovsky

"Ode to Joy," Beethoven

"The March," Tchaikovsky

"Ave Maria," Shubert

"The Austrian Wedding March," traditional

candle, for example. If Communion is being incorporated as part of the ceremony, this is a good time for another vocal performance.

The recessional

This is your exit music. The song should be joyous and upbeat, reflecting your happiness at being joined for life to the man accompanying you back down the aisle. An up tempo will also help move people along more quickly than a sedate piece—and since everyone knows the reception is following the ceremony, they'll be happy for an excuse to bound rather than stroll out of the church.

Music for a Second Wedding

The only difference in music for a first wedding and for a second or subsequent one is that the recessional tends to be a little less traditional—but even that is not written in stone. Music for a second wedding ceremony is not an issue that breeds much controversy. Just stick to the same basic guidelines.

Reception Music

Your choices for reception music are limited only by your imagination. The only guideline you should be aware of is that you want to entertain your guests, not drive them away. It's an added bonus if the music complements the theme and style of the day. (In other words, for a very formal wedding, a swing group or jazz quartet might go over a bit better than a heavy-metal band.) Whatever type or types of music you do decide on, remember that this form of entertainment is a gift you're giving to your guests, to add to their enjoyment of your wedding. Your best bet is to go with an inclusive song list that covers a broad spectrum of musical tastes: some slow, some dance tunes, some rock, some soul.

Aside from pleasing the guests, you and your fiancé should make sure your own favorites are played. Could you imagine celebrating your wedding without dancing with your new husband to "your song"?

Interludes

Some ceremony music favorites (and the composers):

"My Tribute," Crouch
"The Lord's Prayer," Malotte
"Panis Angelicus," Franck
"Now Thank We All Our God," Bach
"Saviour Like a Shepherd Lead Us," Bradbury
"Cherish the Treasure," Mohr
"We've Only Just Begun," The Carpenters
"The Unity Candle Song," Sullivan
"The Bride's Prayer," Good
"The Wedding Prayer," Dunlap
"All I Ask of You," Norbet and Callahan
"Wherever You Go," Callahan
"The Wedding Song," Paul Stookey
"The Irish Wedding Song," traditional

Silly Love Songs?

There are a few standards that are played as part of the traditional events that take place at the reception: the bride's dance with her father, the groom's dance with his mother, the cutting of the cake, and so on. You should also be prepared to hear plenty of (mushy) love songs.

A Little Ethnic Flair

To add some spice to the usual bag of "wedding" songs, consider featuring some music from your ethnic heritage. If either you or your fiancé is Polish, for instance, play some polkas; if one of you is Italian, a couple of Tarantellas are bound to light up the dance floor. If your guests have strong ethnic ties, they'll appreciate the nostalgia; guests of a different culture will enjoy learning something new.

Who Will Rock Your Reception?

The size, formality, and budget of your wedding should help to determine the type of entertainment you have at the reception. At a very formal affair there may be a strolling accordionist or violinist; or a piano player can provide background music as the meal is served. If you're having your reception in a private home or a backyard, homemade tapes piped through a good stereo system will provide plenty of music to dance to.

Once you decide on the kinds of music you want played at your wedding, it's time to think about who will play it. You may already have someone in mind, such as the DJ who played at your cousin's wedding, or a favorite local band. If you don't have a clue, the word-of-mouth approach is usually reliable. Ask friends, relatives, and coworkers; perhaps they've thrown a wedding recently or have attended one where the music impressed them. Most of the better bands and DJs don't advertise, so word of mouth is probably your only chance to hear about them. If you still come up empty, talk to your reception site coordinator. He or she has probably seen a lot of musical entertainment come and go, and may be able to recommend someone who fits your needs. Another option is to ask

Exit: Stage Left

Some recessional favorites (and the composers):

"The Russian Dance," Tchaikovsky

"Trumpet Tune," Stanley

"Toccata Symphony V," Widor

"All Creatures of Our God and King," Williams

"Trumpet Fanfare (Rondeau)," Mouret

"Pomp and Circumstance," Elgar

"Praise, My Soul, the King of Heaven," Goss

Tear-Jerkers

Some reception favorites (and the people who made them famous):

"Sunrise, Sunset," from *Fiddler on the Roof*
"Daddy's Little Girl," Burke and Gerlach
"You Are the Sunshine of My Life," Stevie Wonder
"Just the Way You Are," Billy Joel
"On the Wings of Love," Jeffrey Osborne
"Here and Now," Luther Vandross
"Truly," Lionel Ritchie
"Hopelessly Devoted to You," Olivia Newton-John
"Endless Love," Diana Ross and Lionel Ritchie
"Up Where We Belong," Joe Cocker and Jennifer Warnes
"Waiting for a Girl Like You," Foreigner
"The Wind Beneath My Wings," Bette Midler
"Pretty Woman," Roy Orbison
"Just Because," Anita Baker
"I Won't Last a Day Without You," Andy Williams
"Through the Eyes of Love," Sager and Hamlisch

"The Glory of Love," Peter Cetera
"Always," Starpoint
"Could I Have This Dance?" Anne Murray
"Lady Love," Lou Rawls
"Just the Two of Us," Grover Washington
"Inspiration," Chicago
"Time in a Bottle," Jim Croce
"Unforgettable," Nat King Cole (or with Natalie Cole)
"Unchained Melody," Righteous Brothers
"Here, There, and Everywhere," The Beatles
"September Morn," Neil Diamond
"Silly Love Songs," Paul McCartney
"The Wedding Song," Paul Stookey
"As Time Goes By," Berlin
"Woman," John Lennon
"Ribbon in the Sky," Stevie Wonder
"Wonderful Tonight," Eric Clapton
"We've Only Just Begun," The Carpenters
"Misty," Johnny Mathis
"I Love You So," Andy Williams
"Beginnings," Chicago
"Theme from Ice Castles," Melissa Manchester

around at music stores, the music departments of local colleges, or local musicians' associations.

Is It Live or Is It Memorex? The Band vs. DJ Dilemma

These days, the big musical decision is whether to have a band or a DJ. When it comes to price, a band is definitely the more expensive way to go, but there are other factors that may influence your choice. Whichever you select, you will want to finalize arrangements approximately six months in advance of your wedding date.

A Live Band

Assuming you can find a charismatic, golden-throated singer, and talented, enthusiastic musicians, there is nothing that can match the excitement and spirit of a live band. If you're lucky enough to find such a band that will work within your budget, snap them up quickly before they sign a record deal and leave town for their world tour.

If you're not so lucky, plan to schlepp around town to bars, lounges, and function halls—anyplace where you might find some decent live music. Get an earful of a number of bands. When you find one that strikes your fancy, go back and listen to them again. Some bands will impress you the first time, but sound like a bunch of cats fighting in a garbage can on an off night. You don't want your reception to be one of their off nights.

In addition to the band's sound, look for a variety of musical styles and tempos in their repertoire. Do they play seven slow songs, one fast number, and two more slow ones—or do they know how to vary the pace? Do they appear to be enjoying themselves—or do they look like someone is holding a gun to their heads?

Once you find a band you like, sit down and talk about exactly what you want from them before committing yourself to anything. Give them a list of songs you have to hear at your wedding. If they don't know the songs already, will they attempt to learn them in time? Ask about their sound system and equipment needs. If your reception site is too small, or doesn't have the proper electrical outlets and fuse power, it's better to know before you hire the band.

Words to the Wise

If you can find out where the speakers are located in the reception room, try to seat your older guests far away from them and from the area where the musicians will be playing. This should prevent most complaints about the sound system. The sound is always too loud for the older generation and never booming enough for the younger! If you can't determine where the noise will be loudest, ask the DJ or band to keep the tunes low through the meal (they should anyway, to promote dinner conversation). Chances are that once the meal is over, anyone who doesn't like their assigned seat will be able to find an open one somewhere else. Until then, they'll just have to grin and bear it!

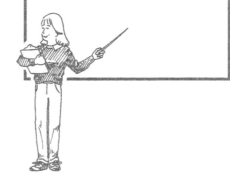

At most weddings, the band leader doubles as the master of ceremonies. If you want your band leader to perform this duty, find out whether he or she will be willing, and if any extra cost is involved. Make sure this person has the poise and charisma to handle the responsibility; you don't want the microphone in the hands of someone who will insult your guests, make jokes as you cut the cake, or mumble your names unintelligibly as you enter the reception site for the first time as husband and wife!

Get It in Writing

Before you sign a contract with the band, make sure the following commitments are stipulated in writing.

The band's attire. You don't want them showing up at a formal wedding in ripped jeans and gym shorts.

The band's arrival time. Make sure the band is set up with instruments tuned before the guests arrive. The band's sound check will probably not make for soothing dinner music.

The exact cost of hiring the band—and everything that price includes. Some bands charge you if they have to add an extra piece of equipment; others charge a fee for playing requests. Find out in advance about everything you'll be expected to pay for.

The band's knowledge of the exact location of the reception. There have actually been instances where the musical talent has shown up at the right hotel, but in the wrong city!

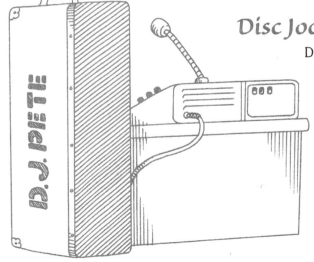

Disc Jockeys

Disc jockeys are fast becoming the wedding music option of choice. DJs can provide more variety than a band, they give you the original version of a song, and they're less of a logistical headache. DJs are seen as slightly less formal than bands, but they're also considerably less expensive, which adds a great deal to their appeal.

It's just as important to see and hear a disc jockey in action as a band. Look for the same things you would look for in a band: balance, variety, a good mix of fast and slow songs, a good personality, and first-rate equipment. Could this person perform the duties of master of ceremonies? Is this included in the total cost?

Find out how big his or her music collection is; your disc jockey should be able to accommodate the majority of your guests' requests. Provide a list of what you want played at the wedding (and if you have some songs you absolutely, positively, upon penalty of death do NOT want played, give him a hit list of those, too!). If some of the music you want isn't available, would the DJ be willing to purchase it? More importantly, would you be charged for the trips to the record store?

Ask about exact cost, including possible extras. Make sure your disc jockey knows the time, the place, the address, and the proper dress.

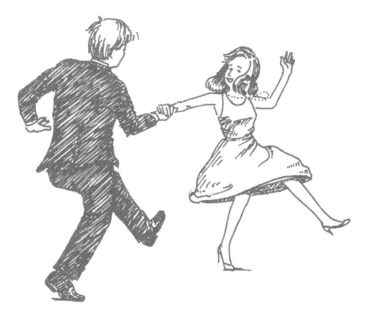

Words to the Wise

Make sure the band you hire is the one that shows up at your wedding. Beware of the following "bait-and-switch" scenario: you are mighty impressed by Bo Beebop and his Boppers, but when your reception rolls around, a totally different (and considerably less impressive) lineup materializes. It seems Bo has several different sets of Boppers that he uses for various occasions, depending on who's available. (Or perhaps Bo himself won't show up because he has another engagement, so the backup band has to play without him.)

Chapter 18

Love in Bloom:
Your Wedding
Flowers

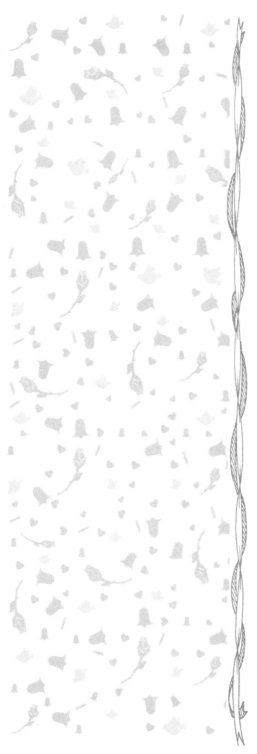

For many women, flowers are the ultimate symbol of love. The beauty, the fragrance, the spirit—everything about flowers, it seems, has captivated the female heart throughout history. Not all men share this passion, but there is one occasion when both men and women agree on the necessity of flowers: their wedding day. Who can say why this is? Perhaps it's because a wedding can bring out the romantic in even the most cynical of grooms. Perhaps the beauty of the day opens his eyes to the beauty of flowers. Whatever the reason, flowers and greenery are an important part of the wedding decor, and their impact shouldn't be undervalued.

Flower Bud(get)

Before you get swept away by all that beauty and romance, determine what your flower budget is. Flowers are one of the areas of your wedding where there is the potential to spend a huge chunk of change almost without trying. You don't have to go broke buying flowers, however. If you're careful (and maybe a little crafty) you can bring your flowers in under budget—without sacrificing any of the beauty or romance.

An honest florist, when presented with a definite budget figure, will steer you in the most practical direction given the dollars you have to spend. Good florists know there's nothing to be gained in making you miserable by showing you things they know you can't afford. But if you don't have (or don't give them) a hint of your budget, many will be quite prepared to tempt you with the most elaborate arrangements in the store.

Once the unpleasant issue of budget has been dealt with, you can concentrate on the actual flowers. Start searching for a florist at least three months before the wedding. Like everything else, word of mouth is the best way to find someone reliable. If you have trouble getting good referrals from friends, consult the Yellow Pages, ask your reception site coordinator, or visit florists' booths at area wedding expositions. Ask for photos of previous displays the florist has done; check references to make sure there is a history of quality work for actual customers. Once you decide on a florist, be sure to get a written contract stipulating costs, times, dates, places, and services. Make sure the florist is set to arrive before the photographer, so everything is ready when picture time comes.

Before you meet with your florist, decide on the color scheme of your wedding. Take color swatches along so the florist can recommend flowers that will either match or complement the overall scheme.

After pointing you in the right direction as to price, your florist can guide you to the flowers that most suit your style and taste. If you're a petite woman, for instance, the florist will probably advise that you avoid carrying an elaborate floral arrangement; it would overwhelm you. He or she will also tell you which flowers will go best in the ceremony and reception locations you've chosen. If the florist has never done work at either site before, make a trip there together so you can both look around and get the feel of things.

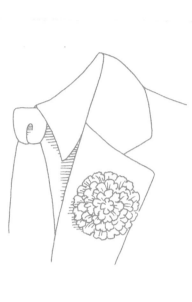

What Do They Mean?

With all the hoopla about a certain flower's appearance, you may have forgotten to consider its meaning:

Amaryllis: splendid beauty
Apple blossoms: temptation
Bachelor's button: celibacy or hope
Bluebell: constancy
Buttercup: riches
Camellia: perfect loveliness, gratitude
Carnation: pure, deep love
Daffodil: regard
Daisy: share your feelings
Forget-me-not: don't forget
    (or true love)
Gardenia: joy
Honeysuckle: generous and
    devoted affection, genuine affection
Ivy: fidelity
Jasmine: amiability (or grace
    and elegance)
Jonquil: affection returned

Lily: purity
Lily of the valley: happiness
Lime: conjugal bliss
Marigold: sacred affection
Myrtle: love
Orange blossom: purity, loveliness
Red chrysanthemum: I love you
Red rose: I love you
Red tulip: love declared
Rose: love
Violet: modesty (or faithfulness)
White camellia: perfect loveliness
White daisy: innocence
White lilac: first emotions of
    love
White lily: purity and innocence
Wood sorrel: joy

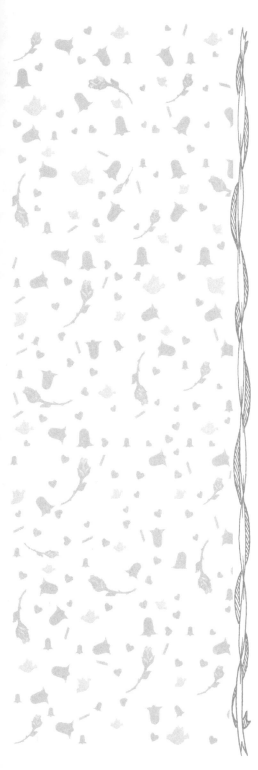

Any Flower, Anytime (Well, Almost)

Years ago, a bride might have been restricted from using certain flowers because they weren't in season at the time of her wedding. Today, most florists stock fresh flowers that have been imported from Europe, the Middle East, South America, and other foreign lands. How does all this importing affect you? It means that "in season" is no longer an issue; all but a few of the most delicate flowers are available at any time of year. (If you do decide to take a chance on one of the delicate flowers, have a second choice to fall back on.)

There are two times of the year that you will still have to plan around carefully: Christmas and Valentine's Day. Flower supplies can get pretty scarce around these holidays, and what is around is likely to be expensive.

This is not to say that you should reschedule your wedding if it's near one of these dates. Both Christmas and Valentine's Day lend a special meaning to the word love; if you want to, take advantage of the season and the spirit for your wedding. Just be sure you've chosen your florist and are in communication with her at least three months before the date, so you can put in advance orders for all the flowers you want. Unfortunately, though, all the added spirit may require a little added dough. Because these two holidays represent two of the most important selling periods of the year, wholesalers hold back the majority of their supplies for these days, then sell them at an increased price to retailers when the time comes. You, the consumer, are part of this chain reaction. Unless you've got contacts within the industry, you're going to pay a little more during these times of the year. But don't go torching the wholesaler yet; although the price differences are certainly noticeable, they aren't really big enough to risk a police record.

Ceremony Flowers

Flowers are an important part of the ceremony because they accent key points and lend atmosphere. If you're being married in a grand cathedral, the odds are that you'll need a few large, elaborate arrangements to compete with the surroundings; small displays would simply be swallowed up. Likewise, small accent displays would be a perfect complement to a quaint country church; large arrangements would overpower the place.

How much of the ceremony site do you want to decorate with flowers? Some couples simply have one large or a few small arrangements placed around the altar. Others also place flowers on the pews, the windows or windowsills, and the doors. If you can, try to arrange a visit to a site your florist has decorated for a wedding. Christmas and Easter are good times to visit, too. Note how the altar arrangements are presented: are they on the floor, or raised up on small tables? Are those tables available to you? If not, can your florist provide something similar? Take photos if permitted. This will give you a record of how the site can look dressed up in flowers.

Presentation

Have you ever received a box of beautiful roses—but been afraid to take them out of the box because you knew that after you tried arranging them in a vase, they wouldn't be beautiful anymore? Let's face it, most of us can pick out attractive flowers in colors that go well together. But most of us could not arrange flowers in a visually appealing way to save our lives. Fortunately, florists can.

Aside from having the talent to arrange flowers in pleasing combinations, florists also know how to present flowers. A good florist would not, for instance, put a beautiful bouquet to water in a Pepsi can. (Even on the odd chance that she were forced at gunpoint to use the can, she'd no doubt figure out a way to make it hold the bouquet as if it were a crystal vase.)

It's doubtful your circumstances will require the use of aluminum in your floral displays. When presenting flowers at the ceremony, your florist may choose to use decorative baskets, glass bowls, or brass vases. Loose flowers can be tied into ribbon for decorating pews and chairs. Ivy can be wound around railings, or placed with bows on candelabras. In season, potted flowers such as lilies, tulips, daffodils, hyacinths, and poinsettias can ornament windows or areas at the front of the church that need a little more flair.

Taking the flowers on the road

Many couples use their ceremony flowers at the reception as well. By using the same flowers, you save yourself the expense of having to decorate both locations. You might even have money left over! All you need to accomplish this feat is a responsible friend or

The Jewish Wedding Canopy (Huppah)

The Jewish wedding ceremony takes place under a wedding canopy, the *huppah*. Among other things, the huppah symbolizes the new home that will be created by the couple. In ancient times it was a specially decorated tent that had been set up in the courtyard of the bride's family. The newlyweds actually lived there for seven days of feasting after the wedding.

Over the years, the huppah evolved into a canopy supported by four poles, which were often decorated with garlands of flowers and greenery. If you decide to use flowers, check with the rabbi to be sure it will be acceptable. Some synagogues do not allow a floral canopy.

If you get the okay, work with your florist to come up with a floral scheme that will complement any arrangement you will hold or wear and that will enhance rather than overpower the canopy itself.

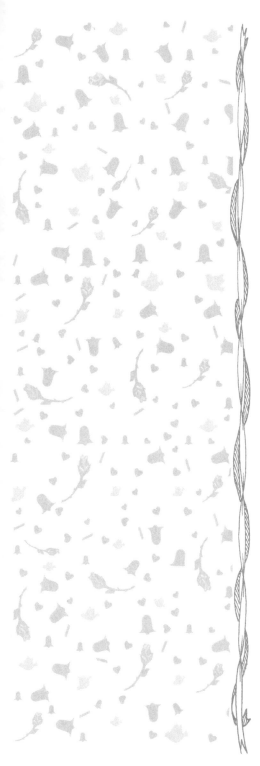

relative to transport the flowers from the ceremony to the reception. While guests are milling around outside of the ceremony and traveling to the reception site, this trustworthy person will be unloading floral displays. By the time everyone arrives, everything should be all set for the photographer and the guests.

If you decide to go this route, make sure the reception site coordinator knows of your plans. Your friend will have enough on his mind, loading and unloading expensive and possibly fragile arrangements into his car; he doesn't need the aggravation of arguing with the reception people about moving furniture, plates, and pianos to make room for the flowers. And be certain your friend knows where you want the arrangements placed. Having them dumped just inside the door probably isn't what you had in mind.

Ceremony flowers aren't the only ones that can be reused to decorate the reception site. If your bridesmaids are willing to part with their bouquets, you could use their flowers to decorate the wedding cake table or the head table. Discuss this possibility with your florist; she may have recommendations on types of bouquets that would work best for this dual purpose.

Flowers at the Reception

The flowers at the reception are meant to highlight the overall design scheme. Place flowers atop the buffet or wedding cake tables; you'll give people something to look at while they think about food. (Flowers can also be used to decorate the cake itself. See the chapter on wedding cake for ideas.)

Depending on the atmosphere of your reception site, hanging plants, small trees, or even topiaries can add a festive air to the proceedings. If your budget allows, consider small flower arrangements for the guest tables; they make wonderful centerpieces. Keep in mind that you want your guests to be able to see one another across the table, so avoid the tall crystal vase with the beautiful flourish of cut flowers and greenery. Keep the arrangements low, especially if your tables are round.

For less formal weddings, small potted plants such as English ivy or philodendrons arranged in decorative baskets make attractive (and affordable!) table decorations. They have the added attraction of being something guests can take home with them and enjoy for years to come.

For a theme wedding or just for fun, you could add a creative element to your table-top arrangements. If your theme is the beach, place a small arrangement in a wide dish of sand, shells, and colorful sea glass. Fall weddings could be dressed up with bright silk maple leaves, assorted nuts in the shell, Red Delicious apples, and tiny gourds. For a Christmastime wedding, arrange flowers in wooden toy sleighs, include gilded or "snow"-covered pine cones, or perhaps place a small decorated wreath flat on the table with a candle in the middle.

After the Wedding

If you use a lot of floral arrangements at your wedding, put someone in charge of dispensing them after the reception. You may want to give the flowers to close friends or relatives, or perhaps to nursing homes or charitable organizations.

You might want to send thank-you flowers to mothers, friends, and relatives as a way of expressing your appreciation for all their help as well.

Flower People

Enough about flowers for places. What about flowers for people? Along with that bouquet you will (or won't) be tossing, you'll have to choose arrangements for the wedding party, for the mother of the bride, and for the mother of the groom.

In most weddings, the bridesmaids carry their flowers rather than wear them. These arrangements can range from elaborate bouquets to simple groupings—or even single long-stemmed roses. (You may decide to add something special to the maid of honor's flowers as a way of making her stand out more.) Communication is key here. If possible, provide your florist with either a swatch of fabric or an accurate color picture of the bridesmaids' dresses. Without a visual reference, your idea of "mostly pink" could vary greatly from your florist's. She envisions a brilliant solid fuchsia and so creates softly toned bouquets of whites and barely pinks. But in reality, the dresses are a floral pattern of barely pinks and whites. A bolder bouquet would have been better; the soft-toned one risks disappearing into the fabric.

Words to the Wise

Here's another way to save money on flowers. Find out whether someone else is being married at your ceremony site on the same day. If so, ask whether they would be willing to share the expense of ceremony flowers. If you do share, you can't very well take the flowers to the reception unless you're the last one getting married (and even then only by mutual agreement).

Floral hairpieces can be a lovely touch for your bridesmaids, and also as part of your veil. Be sure to discuss hairstyles with your bridesmaids and your florist. It would be very frustrating to spend money for flowers that won't stay in your maid of honor's hair because she's decided to wear it loose, or because her hair is too short.

If you're having a flower girl, she'll need a basket of flowers or petals, or a small bouquet. Again, be sure the florist has a good visual reference of what the flower girl will be wearing so she can create a bouquet that complements it.

Who Else?

The mothers of the marrying couple usually receive special corsages just before the ceremony begins. However, if your ceremony includes any readings about the importance of family (or similar elements), you may decide to incorporate the act of passing along these flowers as part of the wedding itself.

Now you won't forget wedding flowers for the mothers (you hope)—but what about grandmothers, great-grandmothers, or Godmothers attending the ceremony who are special to you? You might want to recognize them with a gift of flowers as well.

Flowers for the men are pretty simple. The ushers wear boutonnieres, usually a carnation or a rose. Sometimes the boutonniere is dyed to match the bridesmaids' dresses; sometimes it's white. The groom wears a lapel spray to match the bride's bouquet, or a traditional boutonniere. The fathers usually have boutonnieres similar to those worn by the ushers.

Delivery

Your fiancé is buttoning up the last button on his tux and his ushers are joking with him that now's his last chance to make a getaway. Your makeup and hair would make a movie star jealous, your bridesmaids are admiring themselves in the mirror, and your flower girl hasn't stopped talking about the special basket she's going to carry down the aisle. The only question is, Where is that basket? Not to mention all the other flowers that go with the wedding party.

Say Away from Plastic

Ask your florist to stay away from plastic bouquet holders; they have a nasty habit of dripping all over lovely expensive dresses. All bouquets should be wired and wrapped.

When sewing up the final details with your florist, make sure you're both clear on the delivery schedule. If you plan to take some pictures forty-five minutes before the ceremony begins, chances are you want to be photographed holding your flowers, not standing empty-handed. But unless you tell her, your florist may set up the ceremony site first, then proceed to your place to deliver your bouquets just before you need to leave for the ceremony. Communication is vital: Make sure your flowers are where you want them, when you want them.

Inexpensive Flowers: It's as Smooth As Silk

Well, you thought you could meet your budget. But now you know more places you could use flowers, and the issue of money rears its ugly head again. If you want more than you think you can afford, don't overlook the option of silk. When done well, silk flower arrangements can be as lovely as the real thing—and they even look real. With silk, you get a broader choice of colors (ah, the magic of dye). And while real flowers die quickly, leaving you to lament money spent on something that didn't last, silk flowers can be kept as decorations or keepsakes long after the wedding.

If you can't bear the thought of not being able to smell the wedding flowers, but like the advantages of silk, compromise: use live where it's most important to you and silk in other areas. Some brides have two bouquets made, one real and one silk. They keep whichever they prefer and use the other one for the infamous bouquet toss.

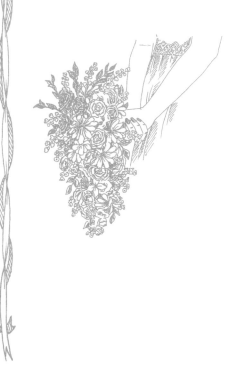

Speaking of That Bouquet

Many brides choose to preserve their bridal bouquet as a memento of the wedding. The odds are very strong indeed that your bouquet will, after a time, end up in storage (which often means "someplace no one remembers"). Keep this in mind if you decide to take your bouquet to the florist for preservation; the process will probably cost you more than the bouquet itself. There are, however, cheaper and more practical ways for you to preserve your bouquet yourself. If you do decide to take advantage of them, you can spend the money on something else. Like your honeymoon.

Pressing

Pressing is the most popular method of bouquet preservation. Your first step is to take a picture of the bouquet; you'll need it to refer to later. Take the bouquet apart (yes, apart) and place the separate flowers in the pages of heavy books, between sheets of blank white paper. (If not cushioned by blank paper, ink from the other pages will ruin the flowers.) The flowers should be kept in the books for two to six weeks, depending on the size. (The bigger the flower, the more time it needs.) When the flowers look ready, glue them onto a mounting board in an arrangement that closely resembles the original bouquet in the photo. Place the board in a picture frame and hang it wherever you desire. (This process works best when it's started soon after your wedding, because the flowers have had less time to wilt.)

Hanging/drying

Again, snap a photo for reference and take the bouquet apart. To preserve shape and prevent drooping, hang the flowers upside down to dry. Some color may be lost in the drying process (the loss is less if the flowers are hung in a dark room). When the flowers are completely dry, spray them with shellac or silica gel for protection. Then reassemble them to match the photo. Like pressing, the earlier you start the process, the more successful it's likely to be.

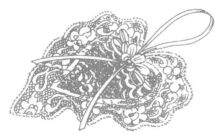

Potpourri

For this method, you'll need to buy some netting or lacy fabric. Dry the flowers and gather the petals together. Place small piles of the petals into four-inch squares of the netting, then tie the squares into little pouches with ribbon. These little sachets can be placed anywhere, filling the air with a little reminder of your wedding day.

Chapter 19

Let Them Eat Cake: Wedding Cakes

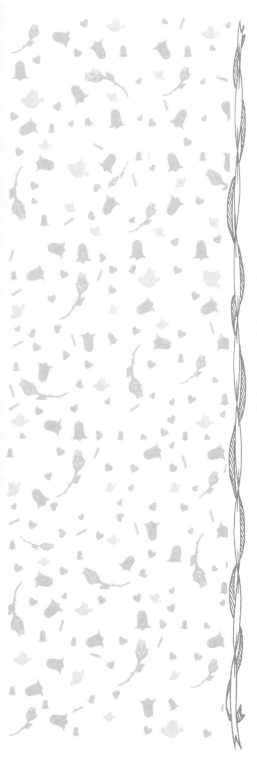

Wedding cakes have been around since medieval times. In Rome, a loaf of wheat bread (*farreus panis*) was broken over the bride's head to symbolize hope for a fertile and fulfilling life. The guests ate the crumbs, which were believed to be good luck. Later, a variant of the custom found its way to England, where guests brought small cakes to the ceremony. The cakes were put into a pile; the bride and groom stood over the pile and kissed. Eventually, someone came up with the idea of stacking the cakes neatly and frosting them together, an early version of the multitiered wedding cakes today. Since then, the cake has lost most of its significance as a fertility symbol, and is seen primarily as a decoration.

Once upon a time, a wedding cake was white inside and out, but today there are countless options for decoration and consumption. The cake can be garnished with fresh flowers or greenery; the icing or trimming can be made to match the wedding colors you've selected. You can even choose a cake because you think it will taste good. The choices for cake flavors, frostings, decorations, and garnishing are plentiful—and tempting. Your cake can be designed any number of ways, too—including multiple tiers, stacked cakes, multiple sections, and even fountains! With so many options, reaching a final decision can be hard.

Cake flavors:

Chocolate	Chocolate hazelnut
Double chocolate	Italian rum
Vanilla	Lemon
White	Orange
Spice	Raspberry
Carrot cake	Strawberry
Cheese cake	Chocolate mousse
Citron chiffon	Chocolate mocha spice
Fruitcake	Banana

Fillings:

Lemon	Custard
Raspberry	Butter cream
Coffee	Vanilla
Strawberry	

Sauces/toppings:

Ice cream/sorbet

Fresh fruit

Sweet fruit sauce

Hot chocolate sauce

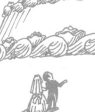

What to Ask Your Baker

Here's a list of questions to ask your baker:

- ♥ What size cake should you have for the number of guests you're having?
- ♥ Can you have different flavors for different layers of the cake?
- ♥ What choices are available in cake flavors and frostings?
- ♥ Does the baker specialize in any flavor, style, or size?
- ♥ Is there a rental fee for tiers or separators?
- ♥ Can a small portion of the cake be prepared with brandy or another form of alcohol? (This makes it easier to eat a year from now—if you decide to follow the tradition of freezing a small quantity of cake and sharing it with your husband on your first anniversary.)

Of course, the really fancy and tasty wedding cakes require a little more time and money. These days the simplest of wedding cakes costs at least $450 if you buy it from a reputable baker (which you probably should).Wedding cake prices are usually based on a per-person basis, plus extra charges for special flavors, icings, and decorations. A typical cake may cost from $2 to $4 per person; add to that $2 to $3 per person if you simply must have that stylish fondant frosting. Colors, decorations, tiers, and fancy extras also add to the cost. Do the math and you'll soon realize that even a very plain cake that is meant as dessert for 300 people will not be cheap.

Don't forget that your cake is in fact edible; it's perfectly appropriate to serve it as dessert. Why spend tons of money and weeks of a baker's time to create the Mona Lisa of wedding cakes, only to have it sit uneaten in a corner of the room? If you feel your cake is not elaborate enough on it's own to constitute dessert, serve it with fresh fruit, ice cream, or a rich sauce. Be sure to taste a sample of

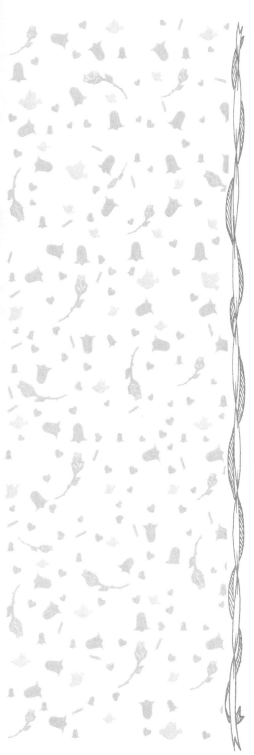

any cake you commission. Your cake could be lovely to look at, but that won't count for much if 200 people can't quite manage to swallow it.

Begin your search for the right bakery at least three months before the wedding. Wedding cakes sometimes require so much time and detail that bakers will work on no more than one per week. The baker should provide you with sample books to help you pick out your cake design; once you've found one you like, you can move on to questions of size and price. If you'd like the colors on the cake to match your wedding colors, bring a sample swatch to the baker.

Rest assured, there are ways to cut costs. Remember, your decorated cake does not have to serve all the guests. Save money by ordering a smaller decorated cake, along with a supplemental sheet cake to feed your guests. On the other hand, if dessert is already included on your wedding menu, there's really no need for a wedding cake except for the traditional cake-cutting ceremony. If that's the case, you can cut costs by making it as small and simple as possible.

How Much Cake Is Enough?

Do you want to serve large slices at a buffet, or smaller slices as dessert? You can cut your cake into three-inch or four-inch slices, with a corresponding change in yield. Finger slices will give you even more. According to one baker, using three-inch cuts you can expect:

Two tiers (14- and 16-inch), 50 servings
Three tiers (12-, 14-, and 16-inch), 75 servings
Four tiers (9-, 12-, 14-, and 16-inch), 125 servings
A sheet cake will yield about 40 servings

Cake That Stands the Test of Time (and a Lot of It!)

Make room in your freezer because you may want to preserve the top layer of your cake for posterity. There is actually a tradition (admittedly less popular than it once was) of freezing a portion of your wedding cake so that on the occasion of your first anniversary, you and your husband can thaw it out and try to eat it. Considering that the cake is a year old, this can be a real culinary experience. Most people freeze the small top layer, which is generally made of a special type of cake (regular wedding cake mixes only last three months or so in the deep freeze). If you think you and your husband would like to participate in this tradition, tell your baker in advance so that he can winterize the top layer. (It should not be surprising that fruitcake is considered the most durable option here; actually, any cake with an alcohol flavoring will hold up pretty well.)

The Groom's Cake

Don't overlook the groom's cake. This represents another opportunity to work fruitcake into the wedding.

In the very old days, the groom's cake was referred to as the wedding cake, and what we now call the wedding cake was known as the bride's cake. Why the terminology was reversed is pretty much anyone's guess. The groom's cake is usually a dark fruitcake reserved for the guests to take home as a memento of the wedding. (You'll notice that no one is actually expected to be seen eating the fruitcake.) The cake slices are packed in little white boxes, often featuring the couple's name and wedding date. According to an old superstition, if a single woman sleeps with the cake box under her pillow that night, she'll dream of the man she is to marry.

Truth be told, groom's cakes are not very popular today. If you decide you'd like to offer one, however, be creative (it doesn't have to be fruitcake any more!). Since the groom is often lost in the shuffle of his own wedding, the groom's cake can serve as a reminder that he is indeed part of things. If he's a hockey player, shape and decorate the cake like a hockey stick or a puck; if he's a tennis buff, commission a racquet cake; if he's a couch potato, have the baker whip up a cake TV.

Inventive designs aren't limited to the groom's cake. It's your wedding, so do something exciting with your wedding cake, too. If you want a big flat square cake instead of a tall round one, or one that looks like a sailboat, talk to your baker about making it happen. As you know by now, these cakes are not cheap, so you might as well get exactly what you want for your money.

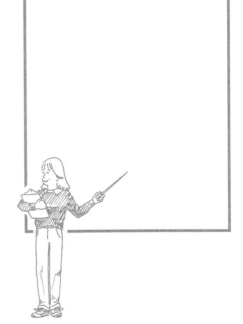

Words to the Wise

Remember to ask if your baker can provide a cake knife. If not, you'll have to buy one of your own.

How to Cut the Wedding Cake

Cut vertically through the bottom layer to the edge of the second layer (1). Then cut wedge-shaped pieces as shown by (2).

When these pieces have been served, do the same with the middle layer. Cut vertically around at the edge of the top layer (3), then cut pieces as shown by (4).

When those pieces have been served, return to the bottom layer and repeat the cuts (5) and (6).

The remaining tiers may be cut into desired-size pieces.

That Singing and Smushing Business

Remember, a wedding cake is not just for eating. Before anybody gets to dig in, the cake performs a very important function: it is the centerpiece of the ever-popular cake-cutting ceremony, when the bride and groom together cut the first piece of cake and take turns feeding one another. Throughout the whole procedure the question is, Will the bride and groom feed each other gently, or smush cake in one another's faces? (Audiences tend to look forward to the latter.)

If I Knew You Were Comin'...

If you're having a home wedding, or a self-catered function in a rented hall, you can make your own cake—if you, your mom, or a friend is a fairly experienced baker. You can work this in easy stages. A few weeks before the date, bake a tier every few days, until you have the three or four you need; wrap each one and store it in your freezer. You can make each tier a different flavor if you like. Unless you have taken a cake decorating course, stay with a good white frosting (Royal, made with egg whites, dries like a hard shell and will keep your cake fresh-tasting, even if you frost it several days ahead). Then decorate very simply, with a few butter cream roses and swirls, or spun-sugar ornaments you can buy at cake decorator supply houses. Simply adding edible silver shots will lend glamour, and leaves and fragrant blossoms (orange blossoms, violets, or tiny roses) will make it even more beautiful.

You can find simple but good recipes in standard cookbooks, with clear directions that explain every step of the process. Cake decorating books show many examples of this art, but most require a great deal of skill and equipment. Use them for ideas only. And let purists howl—you can prepare a very creditable cake with top-quality cake and frosting mixes. A little liqueur improves these short cuts. A helpful booklet on using cake mixes to make a wedding cake is published by Pillsbury Wedding Cakes, P.O. Box 550, Minneapolis, MN 55440, or call 1-800-767-4466.

Taking the Cake (to the Reception)

Make sure the baker arrives at the reception in time to set up the cake before the guests arrive. Multitiered cakes need to be transported in sections and assembled at the reception site; unless you want this phenomenon to be part of the reception entertainment, make arrangements with the site coordinator that will allow the baker plenty of time to get in early and do his thing.

At some weddings, the cake is set up at the head table; at others it's shown off on a table of its own. Whichever you choose, be sure there's enough room for you and your groom both to stand near it, and for the photographer to get good shots of you giving each other a mouthful.

Most people are prepared for the expense of the caterer, the band, the photographer, and so on, but few realize just how much dough (no pun intended) can go into even a modest wedding cake. If you're not going to use your cake for anything but the cutting ceremony with the groom, save yourself some money by making it as small and simple as possible. Of course, you want it to look nice for your guests and your photos, and it can. Just don't set out to feed a small country if your budget won't cooperate.

Chapter 20

Transportation:
Getting There Is
Half the Fun

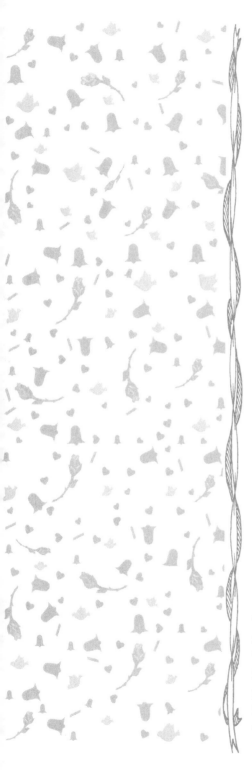

Planes, Trains, Automobiles, or Anything Else That Moves

Picture yourself making the perfect entrance at your wedding ceremony. Are you dropping out of the sky in a hot-air balloon? Trotting to the church via horse-drawn carriage? Rolling by on a parade float? Or panting up to the door in your most comfortable sneakers after an invigorating run? (Okay, maybe the run's not such a great idea.) These days, though, very little is off-limits as far as wedding transportation goes. Innovative couples have been known to use helicopters, boats, hot rods, antique cars, Lear jets, even Harley-Davidsons. As long as it can move you from point A to point B, it's okay for your wedding. Unless it's a pair of sneakers.

Limousines

Limousines are by far the most common mode of wedding transportation. Let's face it, they're what first comes to mind when you think about luxury transportation. Though it may not be as original or exciting as arriving in, say, a Blue Angels fighter plane, showing up in a well-kept limousine is certainly nothing to scoff at. In what other car can you seat ten people comfortably (not that you'd want that many with you on your wedding day), watch TV, serve yourself from the bar, and have a chauffeur at your beck and call, all while sitting in a dress with layers of petticoats? Certainly not the family station wagon. And a big shiny limousine is still impressive enough to instill awe in the occupants of those boring regular cars who are sitting next to it in traffic.

Most couples hire one limousine. Usually this necessitates an intricate series of passenger exchanges on the wedding day. Here's how it works: the bride gets the first ride in the limo; it transports her and her father to the ceremony site. (How the groom makes it to the site is, of course, his problem.) After the ceremony the bride swaps guys and returns to the limousine with her groom, and the two of them ride to the reception. (Alternate scenario: if the ceremony site is close enough to where the bride and bridesmaids are getting ready, the limousine can make its first trip with the bridesmaids, then come back for the bride.) Depending upon the length of the limousine rental, the newlyweds might also be driven in style to their hotel after the reception—or perhaps to the airport to begin their honeymoon.

If your budget has room, you may choose to rent one or two additional limousines to transport attendants and parents. This not only saves you the hassle of coordinating other transportation for them, but also leaves them thinking you're really swell.

The Rules of the Renting Road

Picture this. It's your wedding day. You're all dressed and ready to go; all you need now is the limousine to roll up and get you to the church on time. But it doesn't. Or it does come, but it's covered by a dusty haze and has mud caked on its three remaining hubcaps.

Or it looks snazzy enough on the outside, but inside the TV and bar you requested are not to be found.

You wouldn't mind any of that, would you?

Assuming you don't have that rare constitution that allows you to just grin and bear such a nightmare, you'll want to do everything you can to prevent problems like this ahead of time. A recently married friend or relative may be able to recommend a reliable limousine service with good cars—and thereby save you a lot of legwork. But if you're not that lucky, put on your Consumer Reports hat, by all means get out there, look at the cars, and ask some questions.

Try to find a company that owns its limousines. Owners are more likely to keep track of a car's maintenance (and whereabouts)—perhaps the limo has seen its share of unauthorized excursions. Some limo services rent cars out from another company, which means those cars are probably being shared by several other services. In addition to maintenance and overuse, it's harder for a company that doesn't own its own limos to ensure the availability of any given car, or to supply you with a car of the color and size you want.

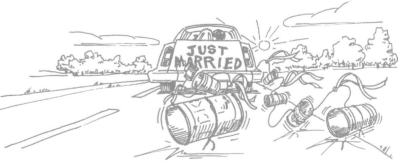

Make sure you verify a service's license and insurance coverage. Get references; verify that its chauffeurs show up on time, are courteous, don't break the speed limit, and don't have a habit of driving into trees.

Inspect all of the cars. Are they good-looking inside and out? Are they what you want? Don't take a company's word that it can supply a white stretch limo with burgundy interior. Get a look at it yourself before you commit to anything.

Most limousine services charge by the hour. Unfortunately for you, the clock starts the second the driver leaves the base, not the moment he or she starts driving you around. (If you can find a service that's based near your home and the festivities, you'll save yourself some money.)

Find out exact costs—and what you'll be getting for your money. Does the limo company provide champagne? Ice? Glasses? Is there an extra charge for a TV and a bar?

Once you decide on a limousine service, get all the details finalized in a written contract. It should specify the type of car, additional options and services you will need, the expected length of service, the date, and the time. It's a good idea to arrange for the limo to arrive at least fifteen to thirty minutes before you're going to need it, just to be on the safe side.

The chauffeur's tip, usually 10–20 percent of the bill, is usually included in the flat fee. But don't take that for granted; check to make sure. You don't want to "stiff" someone who has provided you with good service and who has helped make your day run (or ride) smoothly. By the same token, if you are dissatisfied with the service your chauffeur provides, speak up—and don't be afraid to ask for your money back.

Other Stylish Rides

If you want something less conventional, but don't like the idea of flying, boating, or taking the subway, there are plenty of luxury and antique cars out there available for rental. Are you the white Rolls type? Perhaps a silver Bentley would suit you best. If you've got some extra cash on hand, go all out: snag an Excalibur. It will make for a truly unforgettable shot in your wedding video.

The Best Transportation of All—Free

If for some reason you are unable to rent wedding transportation, look around for family and friends who have nice big cars they'd be willing to lend you. Some car buffs are likely to be horrified at the idea of someone else behind the wheel of their baby; reassure them that if they wish, they are more than welcome to play the part of chauffeur for the day. The only requirement here is that the cars be clean. And be sure to remember your generous friends with a little gift and a full tank of gas. (You should also pay for their pre-wedding car wash.)

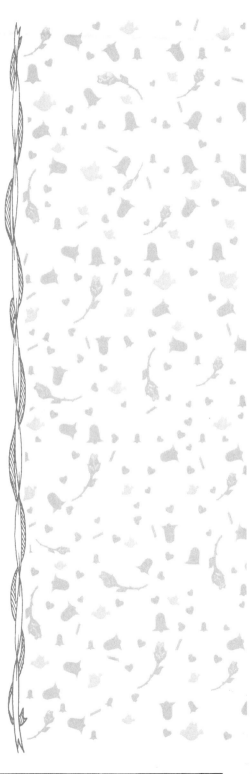

You've Got the Cars, but Where Are the Passengers?

Whether you're renting, borrowing, or using your own, it's important to make sure everyone knows what car is taking whom where. You and your groom, for instance, should make sure you have some way to get to the hotel or the airport after the reception. If you don't have the limo, arrange for a friend to drive your going-away car to the site.

"Trashing" the Going-Away Car

Of course, just because a friend is courteous enough to drive the car to the reception for you, that doesn't mean he'll refrain from enhancing it a bit with some "decorations." Usually the ushers are in charge of this fine art, but other friends and relatives of the groom may offer their services, too. Try to remind people beforehand that safety should come first. Attaching empty tin cans to the rear bumper is fine, but make sure nothing will impair the car's normal motion or in any way interfere with the drive train or motor. Another important item: the driver's field of vision. Be sure anything painted on, draped across, or attached to the windows leaves ample room for the driver to see in all directions. Use washable shoe polish on the windows, not paint!

One inventive group of ushers filled the going-away car with seventy bags of popcorn (taken out of the bags, of course)! Needless to say, the newlyweds had plenty to eat on their honeymoon drive.

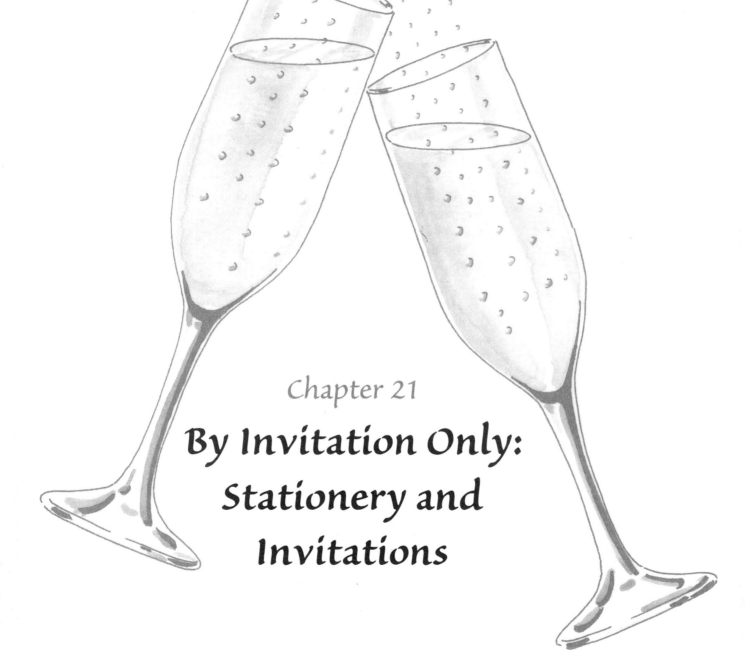

Chapter 21

By Invitation Only: Stationery and Invitations

Invitations

Although nine out of ten people you'll invite to your wedding will probably already know the date, the time, and the place, you still have to sacrifice a bunch of little defenseless trees in order to send out invitations. Wouldn't it be nice if you could just pick up the phone and call the few people who didn't know? It would be less expensive, less time-consuming, and a whole lot easier on those trees. Your tongue wouldn't taste like postage glue for a week, either.

Unfortunately, the powers that be have decreed that you can't skip invitations. In a way, they're probably right: some people do need something to stick on the refrigerator as a reminder of the upcoming event. If they had to write out the information themselves, you might end up with a half-empty church (and a lot of extra reception food). Sending out invitations is also a good way to keep track of who's coming and who's not, provided people pay attention to your request to R.S.V.P. (That's French for "Please call us with a reply so we know how many people are going to show up for this thing.")

The look of your invitation is usually the first hint people get as to the type of wedding you'll be having. If you send out invitations with a colorful bunch of balloons on the front that proclaim "We're having a party!" it's doubtful that your guests will expect a formal affair with top hats and tails. Conversely, an elegantly engraved invitation is bound to give people the message not to show up in jeans.

Where Do You Get 'Em?

The way most brides find invitations these days is by going to a stationery store and browsing through the invitation catalogs. These catalogs contain samples of pre-designed invitations—meaning that the paper color, paper stock, borders, and ornamentation have already been set. You pick out the color of the paper and ink, the style of the script, and the words to use. Some invitations come complete with phrasing; all you do is supply the information for your wedding and the manufacturer does the rest.

These sample catalogs are created by a handful of large printers who currently dominate the invitation market. By printing several lines of mass-produced invitations, these com-

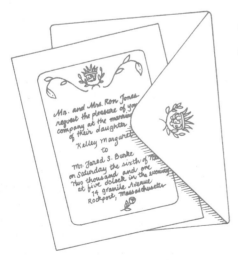

panies are able to offer a greater variety and a cheaper price than a private printer. Because these companies are the main source of wedding invitations, you'll probably see the same sample catalogs in the majority of places you look.

You may have heard about personal stationers or printers, those people who will design a unique invitation for you, then print it. Because of the ease and popularity of the catalog method, doing invitations this way is becoming a thing of the past. Private stationers and printers simply can't afford the overhead costs of offering the broad selection that large manufacturers offer.

If you can't find a catalog invitation you like, or if you want something too specific to be found in a catalog, there are private printers out there who can do the job for you. These printers may be a bit harder to find and a bit more expensive than the big guys, but if you want your invitations to feature lions on roller skates instead of the traditional doves and bells, they're your best bet. Check the business section of your phone directory under "Printers."

Printing Methods

So how do the words make their way onto the paper? There are five main methods.

Engraving. Engraving is the most elegant form of putting ink on paper. The paper is "stamped" from the back by metal plates the printer creates, which raises the letters up off of the paper as they're printed. Unfortunately, you'll be asked to pay extra for all that elegance, so unless you have a very big invitation budget, engraving may not be for you. You will almost certainly have to sign on with a smaller printer (rather than one of the big national operations) if you want to go this route. But read on before you spend the bucks . . .

Thermography. Right now, the most popular way to put the ink on your invitations is called "thermography." By using a special press that heats the ink, the printer creates a raised-letter effect that is almost indistinguishable from engraving. What is distinguishable, however, is the price: about half the cost of engraving. (Most mass-produced invitations are done by thermography these days.)

Calligraphy. Calligraphy (that fancy formal script) is an up-and-coming approach in the invitations world. If you've always admired the style of calligraphy, but didn't think you could afford to have a calligrapher letter your invitations by hand, recent developments may

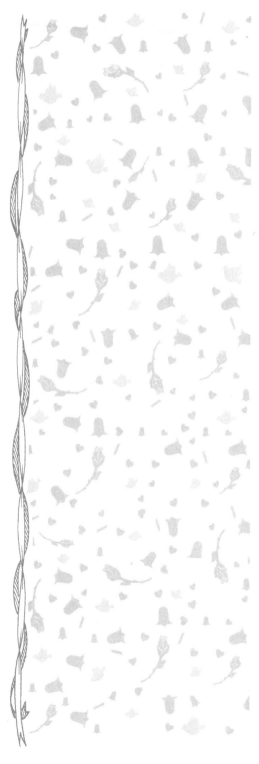

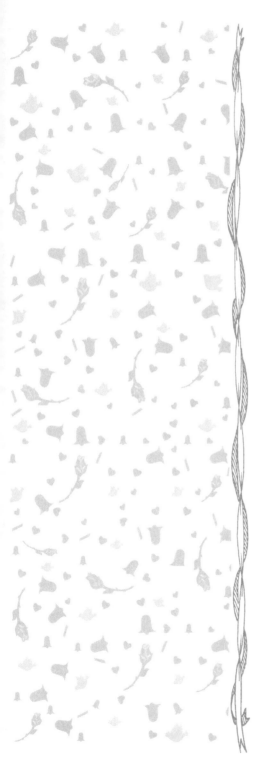

make you reconsider. Some printers are now able to reproduce calligraphy by using a computer program—a method considerably faster (and cheaper) than the human hand. Any sadness you may feel over the computerization of yet another art form is likely to be tempered by your sudden ability to afford it. If you are interested in hiring a human calligrapher, ask your local stationery store for referrals or check the Yellow Pages.

Offset printing. Also known as flat printing, this is the most common form of printing. If you choose to do your invitations this way, you may have to find a small private printer, since most of the big catalog manufacturers are only set up for thermography. While some may consider the offset method boring or unappealing (the letters aren't raised at all), it's the only form of printing that allows you to work with multiple ink colors.

Handwritten invitations. If you're inviting fifty people or fewer, the etiquette gods will allow you to write your invitations out by hand. That may not be good news for your hand, which will probably start cramping after invitation number ten, but it's very good news for your pocketbook. Obviously, this is not a job for someone with lousy handwriting. If yours is suspect, recruit the groom, your mother, or anyone else who's up for the job and can do it well.

What to Say

Having trouble figuring out how to word your invitations? Here are several examples that should fit any situation. Note that in all cases you should include the church's or synagogue's full address; sometimes facilities in the same area have similar or identical names.

Formal/traditional:
Mr. and Mrs. Roger Parker
request the honor of your presence
at the marriage of their daughter
Beth Elaine
to
Mr. Justin Clark
on Saturday, the fifth of August
at two o'clock
Center Street Baptist Church
Fairview, Pennsylvania

Less formal, more contemporary styles:

Mr. and Mrs. Roger Parker
would like you to
join with their daughter
Beth Elaine
and
Justin James
in the celebration of their marriage

When both the bride's and groom's parents sponsor the wedding:

Mr. and Mrs. Roger Parker
and
Mr. and Mrs. Robert Clark
request the honor of your presence
at the marriage of their children
Miss Beth Elaine Parker
and
Mr. Justin James Clark
on Saturday, the fifth of August
at two o'clock
Center Street Baptist Church
Fairview, Pennsylvania

or...

Mr. and Mrs. Roger Parker
request the honor of your presence
at the marriage of their daughter
Beth Elaine Parker
to
Justin James Clark
son of Mr. and Mrs. Robert Clark
Saturday, the fifth of August
at two o'clock
Center Street Baptist Church
Fairview, Pennsylvania

Words to the Wise

Wherever you order your invitations from, be sure to proofread everything before you place the final order. There's nothing quite like receiving a box of 300 invitations on which your name is misspelled—and the date of your wedding is given as "1492."

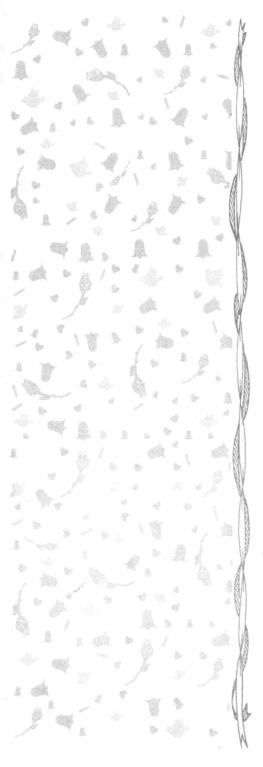

When the groom's parents sponsor the wedding:

Mr. and Mrs. Robert Clark
request the honor of your presence
at the marriage of
Miss Beth Elaine Parker
to their son
Mr. Justin James Clark
Saturday, the fifth of August
at two o'clock
Center Street Baptist Church
Fairview, Pennsylvania

When the bride and groom sponsor their own wedding:

The honor of your presence is requested
at the marriage of
Miss Beth Elaine Parker
and
Mr. Justin Clark

or...

Miss Beth Elaine Parker
and
Mr. Justin James Clark
request the honor of your presence
at their marriage

Circumstances will probably vary when divorced parents sponsor a wedding. Use these examples as general guidelines:

When the mother of the bride is sponsoring and is not remarried:

Mrs. James Parker
requests the honor of your presence
at the marriage of her daughter
Beth Elaine

When the mother of the bride is sponsoring and has remarried:

Mrs. David C. Hayes
requests the honor of your presence
at the marriage of her daughter
Beth Elaine Parker

or...

Mr. and Mrs. David C. Hayes
request the honor of your presence
at the marriage of Mrs. Hayes' daughter
Beth Elaine Parker

When the father of the bride is sponsoring and is not remarried:

Mr. Roger Parker
requests the honor of your presence
at the marriage of his daughter
Beth Elaine

When the father of the bride is sponsoring and has remarried:

Mr. and Mrs. Roger Parker
request the honor of your presence
at the marriage of Mr. Parker's daughter
Beth Elaine

Deceased parents

When one parent is deceased and the sponsor has not remarried:

Mr. Roger Parker
requests the honor of your presence
at the marriage of his daughter
Beth Elaine

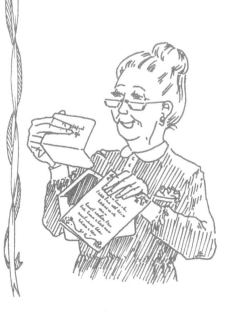

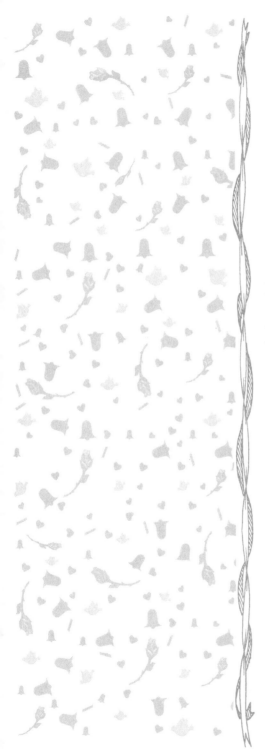

When one parent is deceased and the sponsor has remarried:

Mr. and Mrs. David Spencer
request the honor of your presence
at the marriage of Mrs. Spencer's daughter
Beth Elaine

When both parents are deceased (a close friend or relative may sponsor):

Mr. and Mrs. Frederick Parker
request the honor of your presence
at the marriage of their granddaughter
Beth Elaine Parker

Religious ceremonies

The following are general guidelines for those who wish to emphasize the religious aspect of marriage. If you have any questions, consult your officiant prior to having the invitations printed.

Protestant

Mr. and Mrs. Parker
are pleased to invite you
to join in a Christian celebration
of the marriage of their daughter
Beth Elaine Parker
to
Justin James Clark
on Saturday, the fifth of August
Nineteen hundred and ninety-five
at ten o'clock
St. Phillip's Methodist Church
Fairview, Pennsylvania

Catholic

Mr. and Mrs. Roger Parker
request the honour of your presence
at the Nuptial Mass
at which their daughter
Beth Elaine
and

Justin James Clark
will be united in the
Sacrament of Holy Matrimony
on Saturday, the fifth of August
at six o'clock
Saint Joseph's Catholic Church
Fairview, Pennsylvania

Jewish

(Approaches will differ by ceremony, and by Orthodox, Conservative, or Reform affiliation):

Mr. and Mrs. Samuel Sherman
and
Mr. and Mrs. Jonas Goldsmith
request the honour of your presence
at the marriage of their children
Abigail
and
Daniel
on Sunday, the eleventh of June
at half after four o'clock
Congregation Shearith Israel
Two West Seventieth Street
New York

or...

Mr. and Mrs. Samuel Sherman
request the honour of your presence
at the marriage of their daughter
Abigail
to
Mr. Daniel Goldsmith
son of Mr. and Mrs. Jonas Goldsmith

Military ceremonies

In military weddings, rank determines the placement of names. If the person's rank is lower than sergeant, omit the rank, but list the branch of the service of which he or she is a member.

Jewish Wedding Invitations

The traditional Jewish wedding invitation is written in Hebrew and English. Where can you find a Hebrew text? You can have it hand-lettered with the traditional embellishments by a Hebrew scribe (*sofer*) or a calligrapher, order it from one or two invitation houses that stock Hebrew plates, or have it set up in type for the invitation house to use in your thermographed invitation.

You can take a stab at setting it up yourself if you have computer skills. Many software programs have a set of Hebrew characters in the character map. But this is tricky to use—unless you are familiar with the Hebrew text and agile enough to set it up so that the text reads right to left!

Mr. and Mrs. Roger Parker
request the honor of your presence
at the marriage of their daughter
Beth Elaine
United States Army
to
Justin James Clark

Junior officer's titles are placed below their names and are followed by their branch of service:

Mr. and Mrs. Roger Parker
request the honor of your presence
at the marriage of their daughter
Beth Elaine
to
Justin James Clark
First Lieutenant, United States Navy

Titles are placed before names if the rank is higher than lieutenant; the branch of service is placed on the following line:

Mr. and Mrs. Roger Parker
request the honor of your presence
at the marriage of their daughter
Beth Elaine
to
Captain Justin James Clark
United States Navy

Envelopes

Like the invitations themselves, the envelopes you choose can range from simple, with plain, high-quality paper, to fancy, with foil-laminated inner flaps or flaps with a colorful design. Beautifully packaged invitations are a nice touch, but as you might expect, the more you add to the envelope the greater the cost. Before you break the budget keep in mind that the envelope is a "throw-away" item: once the invitation is opened, the outer envelope is usually thrown away.

Ask yourself if it really makes sense to spend extra on something many people don't keep.

Pre-Printed Return Address

Plan to have the return address pre-printed on the outer envelope and on the response cards. Whose address should it be? Traditionally, whoever is listed as the sponsor for the wedding receives the RSVPs and any gifts that are sent. But if you are the one communicating with the reception site coordinator or caterer, you might prefer to have the responses sent directly to you. That way, you don't have to bug your parents every week (or every day as the big event draws near) to see who's accepted and who hasn't. And if gifts come to your home rather than your parents' home, you don't have to worry about picking them up or having them shipped.

Before you make a decision to put yours as the return address, make sure you tell whomever is sponsoring the wedding. You don't want it to come as a surprise.

Reception Cards

Reception cards tell everyone where your reception is going to be held. If the reception is at a different location than the ceremony, you will need to include these cards in your invitations. Remember to include the full address of the reception site for out-of-town guests. If dinner will be served, be sure to say so—or some guests may brown-bag it.

Sample reception cards
Formal:

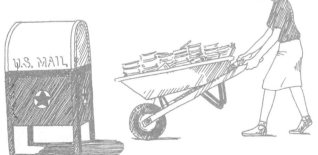

> *Mr. and Mrs. Roger Parker*
> *request the pleasure of your company*
> *Saturday, the fifth of August*
> *at three o'clock*
> *Fairview Country Club*
> *1638 Eastview Lane*
> *Brookdale, Illinois*

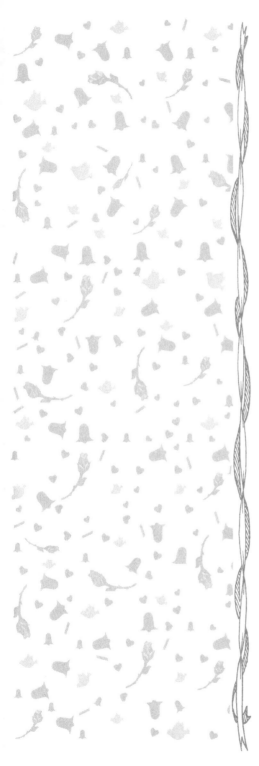

Less formal:

Reception
immediately following the ceremony
Fairview Country Club
1638 Eastview Lane
Brookdale, Illinois

Sample response cards

M_____

_____accepts

_____regrets

Saturday, the fifth of August
Fairview Country Club

or...

The favor of your reply is requested
by the twenty-second of July

M_____

_____will attend

Ordering the Invites

Order your invitations at least three months before the wedding, and always order more invitations than you need. Don't fool yourself into believing you won't make mistakes writing these things out; the last thing you need is a fistfight with your maid of honor because she messed up the last envelope.

Ordering fifty or so extra invitations will lessen the tensions among those writing them out, and will save you the money of having to place a second order. (The majority of charges for your invitation are for the initial start-up of the press and such; adding a few more to your initial order is comparably cheap.) Even if you don't make any mistakes, you will probably like to have a few invitations as keepsakes.

When tallying up the number of invitations to order, don't forget to include all the people who will be at the rehearsal. This includes attendants, siblings, parents, and the officiant, along with their respective significant others. Although a reply is not expected or required, these people may like to have the invitation as a memento.

Plan to mail out invitations about eight weeks before the wedding, with an R.S.V.P. date of about three weeks before the wedding. Be sure to allow yourself some time to address and stamp all those envelopes. If you're planning a wedding near a holiday, mail out your invitations a few weeks earlier to give your guests some extra time to plan. This should also give you plenty of time to give a final head count to the caterer. Also, as regrets come in, you can send invitations to those people squeezed off the original guest list.

Pressed for time? Ask your printer to provide you with the envelopes in advance. That way, you can write them out while the invitations are being printed. Most mass-produced invitation orders are turned around within three to four weeks, so unless you're under some pretty remarkable scheduling pressure, you should have plenty of time.

Writing Them and Sending Them Out

You will need...

- ♥ Several pens (use black ink only)
- ♥ Several friends and/or family members with good penmanship
- ♥ Plenty of food, drink, money, and whatever else it will take to bribe friends and/or family members into helping you
- ♥ Stamps
- ♥ Invitations and envelopes

It's a good idea to have a few people over to help you address your invitations, but don't invite so man y that things become confusing. Make sure the same person who writes the information on the inside of an invitation also addresses its outer envelope. This makes the invitation package look uniform, and lets the person receiving it know that it was put together with care.

There are two big invitation-writing taboos:

1. Never use a typewriter or printed label to address an invitation envelope.
2. With the exception of Mr., Mrs., and Ms., do not use abbreviations.

As If That Weren't Enough...

You can also get napkins, matchbooks, pens, pencils, and almost anything else under the sun with your name and wedding date printed on it. Just remember—you could be spending the money on your honeymoon.

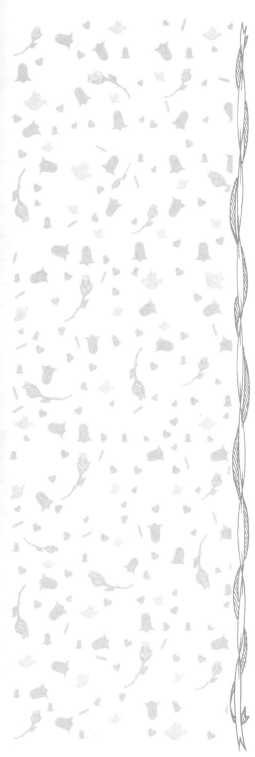

When addressing the outer envelope, include the full name of the person or persons you are inviting; on the inner envelope, you can be more casual.

Outer envelope:
Mr. and Mrs. Stephen Michael McGill
(*or* . . . Ms. Linda Ann Smith and Mr. Stephen Michael McGill)
16 Maple Drive
Chestnut Hill, Massachusetts 02555

Inner envelope:
Mr. and Mrs. McGill
(*or* . . . Stephen and Linda)

If you are inviting the whole family, the approach is pretty much the same:
Mr. and Mrs. Stephen Michael McGill and Family
(*or* . . . The Smith-McGill Family)
16 Maple Drive
Chestnut Hill, Massachusetts 02555

On the inner envelope:
Mr. and Mrs. McGill
Andrea, Paul, and Meg
(Children's names should come after their parents'.)

When you are inviting a single person with a guest, the outer envelope should be addressed to him or her only; the inner envelope includes the phrase, "and guest."

Response Cards and Return Envelopes

It used to be that response cards weren't included in the invitation since etiquette dictated that the receiver of the invitation promptly respond with a phone call or formal note of acceptance. However, even die-hard etiquette mavens acknowledge that today, your invitation package should include response cards and return envelopes because it's easier for all involved.

As mentioned, response cards are a big help in keeping track of who's coming and who's not. Your potential guests fill in their names, indicating whether or not they plan to attend and, if they do, how many will be in their party. They drop the card into the self-addressed stamped envelope you've provided for them, and in a few days (depending on the speed of the mail), you should know whether or not they're coming.

As for those oblivious souls who neglect to return your card... well, try not to be too hard on them. A simple phone call that tactfully passes over their failure to R.S.V.P. will suffice.

Packaging the Invites

Now that you've got everything addressed and ready to go, what's the best way to fit it all into the envelope? Packing up the invitation and its extras can be as frustrating and complicated as making out your seating plan. Here's a method that should make things easier for you.

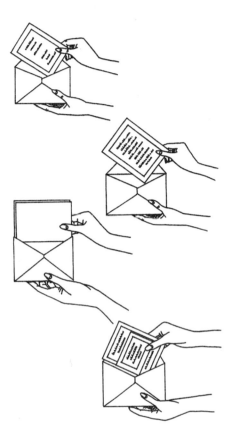

1. Place the response card face-up under the flap of the response card envelope.
2. Place a small piece of tissue paper over the lettering on the invitation.
3. Put any extra enclosures (receptions cards, maps, directions, etc.) inside the invitation.
4. Put the response card and envelope inside the invitation as well. The lettering should be facing upward.
5. Place the invitation inside of the inner envelope with the lettering facing the back flap. Don't seal this envelope.
6. Put the inner envelope inside the outer envelope; again, the writing on the inner envelope should face the flap of the outer envelope.
7. Seal the outer envelope. Make sure the envelope is properly addressed and contains your return address.
8. Stamp and mail.

Postage

Find out in advance how much postage you will need to mail your invitations. Sometimes, with heavy paper and lots of inserts, the whole package requires more than a standard first-class stamp. The

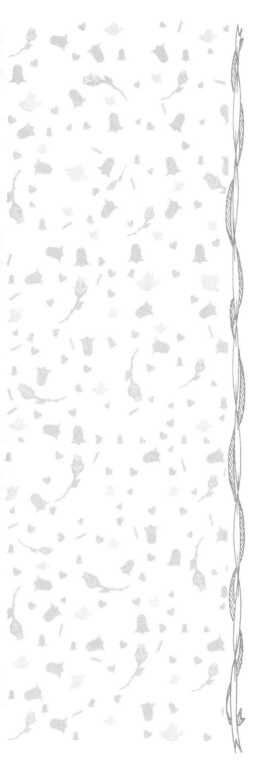

return envelope needs only a standard first-class stamp, which you are expected to provide.

And instead of wearing out your tongue and those of your friends, purchase a few water applicator wands from your local office supply store. These wands are filled with water and stopped with a small sponge that, when pressed to the back of an envelope or stamp, releases a small amount of water. Or, place a damp sponge in a bowl and dab stamps on its surface to moisten. (Not recommended for envelopes since the whole flap might get wet.)

Additional Stationery

Your business with printers and stationery suppliers may not end when you order your invitations. Thank-you notes are an absolute must, but there are other specialty items that you can include if you have the desire and the money.

Thank-you notes

Thank-you notes are sometimes referred to as informals. You can order thank-you notes that match your invitations, or you can choose something completely different. Despite the name, the notes can be as formal or informal as you like. If you already have personal stationery, you might consider using that for your thank-you notes instead of ordering something new. It's perfectly proper as far as etiquette is concerned, and you might save some money.

The following are stationery products that you might (or might not) use, depending on your situation, your budget, and your preference.

Maps

Include directions to the ceremony and reception sites in the invitations you send to out-of-town guests. Maps add to the usefulness of the directions—provided they are drawn by someone whose sole art expertise does not lie in drawing stick people, and they are large enough to be read without a magnifying glass.

Announcements

If you and your fiancé are like most couples, you were not able to invite everyone on your original guest list; business associates, friends and family living far away, and others may have been squeezed off the list due to budget or space constraints. Wedding announcements are a convenient way to let people know of your recent nuptials. They are not sent to those who received an invitation, including those who were unable to come. Note that people receiving announcements are under no obligation to buy you a gift.

Announcements should be mailed immediately after your wedding. You and your fiancé should have them ready before you leave for your honeymoon; your maid of honor or best man can mail them while you are gone.

The traditional wording of announcements is as follows:

Mr. and Mrs. Joseph Moran
proudly announce
the marriage of their daughter
Margaret Ann
and
Mr. Justin James McCann
on Saturday, the third of July
one thousand nine hundred and
ninety-three
Holy Trinity Lutheran Church
Chicago, Illinois

Whoever is named on the invitation as the wedding's sponsor should also be the person or persons announcing the marriage.

Ceremony cards

Ceremony cards (guaranteeing entrance into the proceedings) are not necessary for a traditional wedding site, but if your wedding is being held at a public place (such as a museum or a historic mansion), you may want to have some way to distinguish your guests from the tourists. Aside from the fact that they will be better dressed, you hope.

At-home cards

These cards let people know your new name, your new address, and when you'll be moved in. You can also use at-home cards to let people know whether or not you have taken your husband's name and how you prefer to be addressed. To add to your paper trail, there is an entirely different kind of card dedicated solely to the name issue, known as a name card. If you wish, you can send your address information on the at-home card, and your name preference on the name card, but it really is more sensible—and affordable—to combine the information onto one. (Some people really must hate trees.)

Pew cards

You will need pew cards if you wish to reserve seats at the ceremony for any special family and friends. Have them sit as close as possible to where the action is. Your special guests can pass the pew cards to the usher at the ceremony, who then knows to seat the special guests in the front sections marked off as "Reserved."

Rain cards

If you're having your ceremony and/or reception outdoors, rain cards notify people of an alternate location in the event of rain.

Ceremony programs

Ceremony programs are to your wedding what a playbill is to a concert or play. The program identifies the order of the ceremony, the participants, the music, and the readings. Ceremony programs afford a personal touch. Perhaps you have a favorite poem, quote, or song that can't be included in the ceremony itself, or maybe there's a special memory you'd like to share, such as how you and your groom met. Why not print it on the back of the program to give your family and friends something meaningful to read while they wait for the ceremony to begin?

Programs don't have to be professionally designed and printed to be elegant. If you don't have a great deal of extra money, but you do have a friend with very nice penmanship, artistic talent, or a good personal computer system, you can create the program yourself and photocopy enough sheets for all of your guests.

Hint: if your ceremony site doesn't allow flash photography, be sure to include a polite warning in the program.

Chapter 22

Your Wedding Day: A Possible Scenario

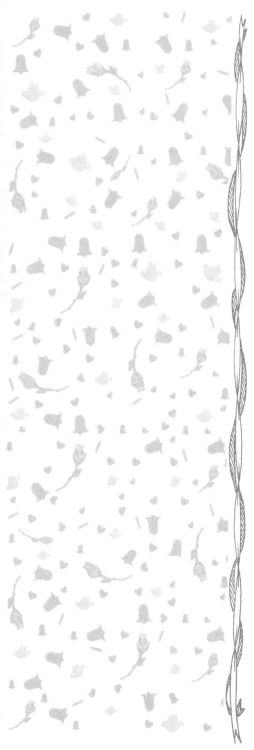

You wake up. Or maybe you don't really wake up, since you never actually fell asleep the night before. In any event, you roll out of bed. If your wedding is at eleven o'clock in the morning, you probably roll out earlier (and faster) than you would if it's at four o'clock in the afternoon.

You hop into the shower and stand in the spray long enough to feel clean, refreshed, and ready to face the day. You don't bother fussing with your hair or makeup too much because you have an appointment with your hairdresser and of course you'll be wearing special makeup applied by a cosmetologist due to arrive later.

You jump into some jeans and a button-down shirt. You try to eat a light meal, even a little tea and toast. You're looking for anything that will give you a little fuel and keep you from fainting as you walk down the aisle. Your maid of honor arrives, right on cue, to drive you to the appointment with your hairdresser. (Don't trust your own shaking hands behind the wheel.) After your hairdresser makes your hair (complete with headpiece if you brought it) look stunning, you jet back home, ready for the next step.

Your bridesmaids and maid of honor have started to assemble. Soon, the cosmetologist you hired is there to put everyone's face on. While being made up, everyone feasts on the cold cuts platter that you picked up at the deli the day before. This is to hold them over, because the reception dinner is a while away. Again, a nibble or two on your part, plus a glass of water or juice, wouldn't be a bad idea. Stay away from caffeinated beverages, though; you'll already be nervous and coffee or soda would just make you jittery.

After your attendants all get their faces, you get yours. You come out gorgeous, of course. By now your bouquet and the bridesmaids' flowers should have arrived. The bridesmaids fight for a turn in the bathroom as they get ready, while your father sulks in his bedroom before changing into his tux, gazing at pictures of you as a little girl.

Around two hours before the ceremony, you start getting dressed. First, a good dousing of light powder, to make you feel fresh. Then you wrestle into your special undergarments, including hose, and call for help getting into your gown.

Everyone else, including your mother, is almost done. You have plenty of hands to fasten any tricky buttons or zippers. You make sure you're equipped with "something old, something new, something borrowed, and something blue."

The photographer arrives at your house about an hour before the wedding to take shots of you alone, you with your family, and you with your attendants. The videographer catches some of the fun, too. Across town, your groom is finally stepping out of the shower and into his tux.

The limo pulls up and whisks your attendants to the ceremony site. The driver will be right back for you and your dad. Your mother fawns over you one last time before getting into the car that takes her to the ceremony.

The limo comes for you. Outside, all of your neighbors are gathered to catch a glimpse of the lovely bride. (Perhaps they wonder how this tomboy turned into such a beautiful woman.) The photographer snaps one last shot, then hurries to his car to beat you to the ceremony site. Your father helps you into the limo and you speed away.

At the ceremony site, everyone is already seated, waiting for you. But they're far from bored, as the prelude music you've selected is entrancing. You gather in the vestibule with your bridesmaids; the processional begins. They're off, walking, as ordered, "very slowly."

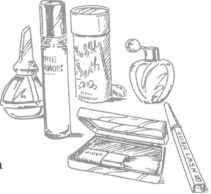

Then it's your turn. As your groom steps out to the altar to greet you, you half float, half quiver up the aisle. When you reach your groom, your father shakes your hand and kisses him goodbye . . . or is it the other way around? From here on in, things could get a little foggy unless you remember a key piece of advice given to you by a past bride: stay focused!

The groom takes your hand in his; the two of you approach the altar and the ceremony begins. It goes without a glitch: talking, reading, rings, giving, taking, kissing. And you're married.

You bounce back down the aisle together to that wonderfully peppy recessional music you chose. The photographer and videographer film every step you take, but in a very polite, talented way. If the weather is good, you have a brief receiving line outside in the courtyard. Or you have it at the reception site. Or you dispense with this time-consuming step altogether.

You and your new husband share some champagne in the limousine ride to the reception. Everyone else gets there via your well-coordinated, well-executed transportation plan. At the reception site, you quickly take your formal photographs and are back at the reception before anyone even has time to get hungry.

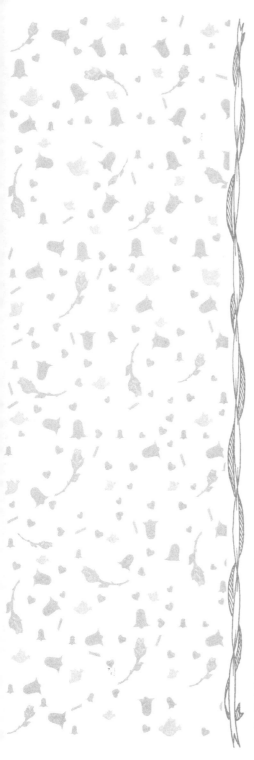

You seat yourself at the head table with your groom and are immediately greeted with the sound of silverware clinking against glasses. (You'll hear this sound a lot that day; it is the signal for you and your groom to kiss.)

Dinner is served. After everyone is satisfied, you and your groom have your first dance. Then you cut the cake. Then you dance with your father. Then the groom dances with his mother. Then everybody pretty much dances with everybody. Toward the end of the reception, the groom removes your garter and tosses it away to all the eligible gents; you toss your bouquet to the single ladies.

Then you and your groom change into your going-away clothes. You say goodbye to everyone, and leave for your wedding night and honeymoon.

No problem.

The Second Time Around: Remarrying

Although Elizabeth Taylor and Mickey Rooney may be the acknowledged experts at the remarriage game, there are some things you may have questions about if you're heading into your second (or third, or fourth) marriage. There are a few rules of protocol to follow, but there isn't as much to worry about as you might think.

The main rule you should try to follow if this is not the first marriage for either you or your fiancé is to not try to duplicate or compete with your previous wedding. You certainly don't want your fiancé to think you're trying to live in the past by having everything be as it was in your first wedding; you want to start fresh.

By the same token, many people believe that if they had a large wedding the first time around, they must keep things very quiet and subdued for a subsequent wedding. This is not the case at all, particularly if one member of the marrying couple has never been married before. In the past, second weddings may have been more hush-hush, but these days they can be treated with the same joy and excitement as a first wedding. The bride may still have her father walk her down the aisle—although she may not wish to wear pure white and a fancy veil if it's not her first trip down. There may still be a receiving line, a wedding cake, dancing, bouquet tossing, and all of the other wonderful reception traditions.

Remembering the Date in Years to Come . . .

Here's what you might be receiving for anniversary gifts through the years:

	Traditional	Modern
1st	Paper	Clocks
2nd	Cotton	China
3rd	Leather	Crystal & glass
4th	Linen	Electric appliance
5th	Wood	Silverware
6th	Iron	Wood
7th	Wool	Desk set
8th	Bronze	Linens & lace
9th	Pottery	Leather
10th	Tin, aluminum	Diamond jewelry
11th	Steel	Fashion jewelry
12th	Silk	Pearl or colored gem
13th	Lace	Textile & fur
14th	Ivory	Gold jewelry
15th	Crystal	Watches
16th	Skips	Sterling or plate holloware
17th	Skips	Furniture
18th	Skips	Porcelain
19th	Skips	Bronze
20th	China	Platinum
25th	Silver	Sterling silver
30th	Pearl	Diamond
35th	Coral, jade	Jade
40th	Ruby	Ruby
45th	Sapphire	Sapphire
50th	Gold	Gold
55th	Emerald	Emerald
60th	Diamond	Diamond

Another point of concern for some couples is the issue of shower and wedding gifts. They feel that if family and friends have already given gifts it is not fair to ask them to do so again. The answer to this dilemma is completely up to you and your fiancé. If the two of you are older and established in your lives, you may wish to include a "no gifts, please" clause on your invitations (see stationery chapter for details). But if this is a first marriage for one of you, or the two of you really would appreciate some help in starting your new life together, it is perfectly acceptable to have a shower and for guests to give gifts for the wedding. (Note: guests are not obligated to give gifts for a remarriage, but many may want to anyway.)

As far as the ceremony itself goes, you should consult with your officiant about any restrictions or requirements surrounding the marriage of a divorced person. Once those issues have been dealt with, the ceremony can pretty much proceed as if it were a first marriage. Granted, some people choose to have less traditional music and Scripture selections, but ultimately the choice is up to you and your fiancé.

The final word

If you're a real stickler for etiquette, you can consult Emily Post—or any number of books dedicated solely to the issue of remarriage. But these days, it really doesn't need to be that complicated. You and your fiancé should handle a remarriage in a way that makes both of you feel comfortable. If it's his second marriage, and he prefers things to be very simple and quiet, but it's your first and you want a wedding with all the trimmings, of course, you will definitely need to compromise. Just don't let yourself worry about gossip and the expectations of family and friends; they should be happy that the two of you have found each other and plan to make a life together.

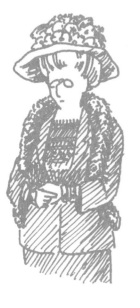

Chapter 23

Into the Sunset:
Your Honeymoon

You'll probably agree that, what with all the frenzied planning, coordinating, organizing, and worrying involved, getting yourself married can be a full-time job—and then some! When it's all over with, you'll need more than just an ordinary vacation to recuperate.

On the surface, a honeymoon is no different from any other vacation you might take. You pack your bags, make your reservations, and leave home for fun in the sun, snow, or wherever. But let's face it, to a pair of newlyweds, a honeymoon is much more than that; it's their first getaway together as a married couple, and perhaps the ultimate romantic experience. Ten years from now, you probably won't remember just when it was you spent that summer week in the mountains, or that long weekend skiing. But you're bound to remember nearly every detail about your honeymoon, wherever you may go.

The Early Bird Catches the Plane

Once you and your fiancé agree on where you'd like to (and can afford to) spend your honeymoon, you should talk to a travel agent and start making your reservations. Some of the more popular tourist and honeymoon spots can be booked solid up to a year in advance, so call early—especially if you've got your heart set on a particular location. Don't get caught napping!

Hand-in-hand into the sunset

Just in case you don't have a dream destination in mind, here is a list of some of the most popular honeymoon spots:

The Caribbean:

1. Aruba
2. Cayman Islands
3. Little Dix Bay, British Virgin Islands
4. Montego Bay, Jamaica
5. Nassau, Bahamas
6. Negril, Jamaica
7. Ocho Rios, Jamaica
8. Paradise Island, Bahamas
9. St. Croix

Mexico:

1. Baja California region
2. Cancun, Quintana Roo
3. Guadalajara, Jalisco
4. Isla de Cozumel, Quintana Roo
5. Puerto Vallarta, Jalisco

South Pacific:

1. The Marquesas
2. Tahiti

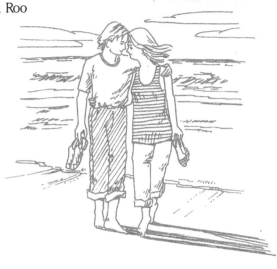

Europe:

1. Greece
2. Spain
3. England
4. France
5. Rome
6. Italy
7. Germany
8. Austria
9. Switzerland
10. Sweden
11. Finland
12. Norway
13. Monaco

United States:

1. Alaska
2. Hawaii
3. Grand Canyon National Park, Arizona
4. Niagara Falls, New York
5. The California Pacific Coast Highway
6. Hilton Head, South Carolina
7. Poconos Mountains, Pennsylvania
8. Disneyland, Anaheim, California
9. Walt Disney World, Orlando, Florida
10. Massachusetts Beach Resorts: Cape Cod, Martha's Vineyard, and Nantucket
11. U.S. Virgin Islands

And don't forget about more exotic locations like Australia, the Netherlands, Japan, and South America!

Ultimately, of course, your budget is likely to have at least as big an impact on the destination you choose as your dreams do. But here's a word of advice: don't despair of your desired trip just because you think it's beyond your means. Research all the details. Consult a travel agent or look through travel sites on the Internet to find low-priced airfares, reduced-rate package deals, and other ways to save money. You may be pleasantly surprised. Perhaps you can afford a trip to Hawaii by staying at a less-than-four-star hotel, or travel Europe via hostels and bed and breakfasts. Remember, however, to confirm that "inexpensive" lodging does not mean "without running water," "dilapidated," or "situated in the red-light district."

Travel Agents

Perhaps you're used to handling your vacation arrangements by yourself, without the help of a travel agent. If you're going out of the country, however, you may wish to work with an agent to help you figure out the nuances of international travel. Because foreign vacations can get very complicated—with connecting flights that have to meet boats that have to meet trains (you get the picture)—putting all the responsibility in the lap of a trained agent may be a good idea. After all, you've already got enough to do with planning the wedding.

Your agent will tell you what paperwork, identification, and other necessities you will need in order to travel abroad. With the exception of Canada, Mexico, and some parts of the Caribbean, you'll need a passport, which takes at least six weeks (and sometimes longer) to obtain. Here are some other documents you will need that may take some time to track down.

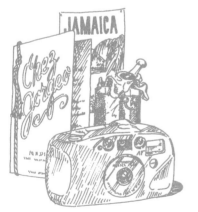

Birth certificate
Driver's license (or other picture ID)
Proof of marriage
Proof of citizenship

The Fine Art of Tipping

When, whom, and how much to tip are often embarrassing and confusing questions. In some situations you can ask your companions at the dining table in a hotel or on shipboard, or the management, but it's better to be prepared with some knowledge of the travel tipping structure. Here are some guidelines.

On board a ship

Room steward: cleans your cabin, makes the bed, supplies towels, soap, ice, and room service. Tip $3.50 per day per person. Tip at the end of the trip. Some also tip on the first day, "to ensure perfect service"—a slogan said to be the origin of the word "tips."

Dining room waiter and busboy: waiter, $3.50 per person per day, half that for the busboy.

Bartenders, wine steward, pool and deck attendants, etc.: check the bar bill. On almost all ships, a service charge is automatically added, making a tip unnecessary. Other service personnel should be tipped when the service is given, at the same rate as for service ashore, usually 15 percent.

Maitre d', headwaiter: in charge of the dining room. No tip is necessary unless he has handled special requests for you.

"No-tipping" ships: some cruise lines advertise a "no-tip" policy. People still tip for special service on such ships, but it is not necessary if you do not ask for anything "above and beyond."

At the airport

Porter: $1 per bag when you check in at the curb or have bags taken to check in for you.

In a hotel

Bellboy: $1 per bag, plus $1 for hospitable gestures—turning on lights, opening windows. Tip on service.

Chambermaid: $1 for each service, minimum $5 per couple per week. Tip each day; a new maid may be assigned during your stay.

Doorman: $1 per bag; $1 for hailing a taxi. Tip on service.

Headwaiter: $5 per week for special service, $2–$3 for regular service—tip on your first day.

Wait staff: 15 to 20 percent of the bill when no service charge is added; some add 5 percent when there is a service charge. Tip at each meal.

Room Service: 15 to 20 percent of bill in addition to the room service charge.

Other service personnel: the general rule to follow is to tip 15 to 20 percent of the bill, unless the person serving you owns the business. Some owner-hairdressers, for example, do not accept tips, but charge more for their services.

What Goes Into Your Carry-on Bag?

Tickets
Traveler's checks
Driver's licenses
Proof of age and citizenship
Passports, visas (if appropriate)
List of luggage contents (for insurance purposes if luggage is lost or stolen)
Name and phone number of someone to contact in case of emergency
Checking account numbers (kept separate from checks)
Eyewear
Any medication
Valuable jewelry
Marriage license
Birth control
List of credit card numbers

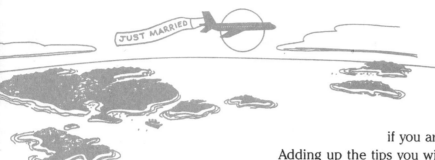

Note that in a foreign country the amount to tip should be calculated in the currency of that country. It may be less or more than you would tip in dollars, depending on the exchange rate. Ask at the hotel desk, or ask the purser (aboard ship), if you are uncertain.

Adding up the tips you will have to pay out leaves you with a rather hefty bottom line. Now you can better understand why you see the pizza delivery cars driving up to swanky hotels and why many people prefer five-star motels, where there are none of the "front-end" tips associated with arriving and leaving.

I'll Just Sleep on the Plane

Everybody has heard stories of newlyweds who party at their reception and post-reception gatherings all night, only to have to drag themselves, physically and mentally exhausted, to the airport for a five a.m. flight the next morning. Fatigue can breed irritability and forgetfulness; add the stress of travel to that and you have the recipe for potential disaster. Even if you get to your destination without mishap, you certainly don't want to risk bickering with your spouse your first full day as a married couple—or looking like something the cat dragged in because you have dark circles under your eyes and didn't have time to take a shower.

If possible, try to arrange your departure to give yourself at least six hours of sleep the night before. You may not wake up totally refreshed (weddings have a way of making you feel like you've run a marathon), but you'll be better off than if you only slept from two to four a.m. Top it off with a long hot shower and a hearty breakfast—perhaps splurge for room service?—and you should have a good start to the first day of your honeymoon.

Traveling Tips (as in Advice!)

You should employ a little basic traveler's savvy on your honeymoon. You will need to give some thought to security and safety, just as you would with any other vacation.

Things You DEFINITELY Don't Want to Forget:

For your suitcase
- ♥ Camera
- ♥ Film (and plenty of it)
- ♥ Batteries (for camera)
- ♥ Cosmetics
- ♥ Deodorant
- ♥ Hair dryer
- ♥ Corkscrew or bottle opener
- ♥ Shampoo
- ♥ Conditioner
- ♥ Toothbrushes and toothpaste
- ♥ Disposable razors (and blades)
- ♥ Q-tips
- ♥ Nail clippers or scissors
- ♥ First-aid kit
- ♥ Feminine hygiene products
- ♥ Pain reliever
- ♥ Antacids
- ♥ Vitamins

For the beach:
- ♥ Bathing suits
- ♥ Sandals
- ♥ Coverups
- ♥ Sunscreen and tanning lotion
- ♥ Sunglasses
- ♥ Beach bag

For the snow:
- ♥ Winter jacket, hat, boots, gloves
- ♥ Sweaters
- ♥ Thick socks
- ♥ Skis (if you have them)

Try to use traveler's checks rather than cash whenever possible. The major brands are accepted in just about every foreign country, and unlike cash, they can be replaced if lost or stolen.

Keep all important items in a carry-on bag; that way you'll have them if the rest of your luggage is lost or stolen.

Confirm all of your reservations the week before you leave. There's nothing quite like dragging all your heavy luggage into a hotel lobby in some exotic locale, desiring only a soft bed—to find that you don't even have a room.

Assuming you do get a room, don't be afraid to complain to the management if the service or accommodations are not to your satisfaction. And don't wait until you're leaving; let people know about any problems A.S.A.P. so the situation can be remedied and you can enjoy yourselves.

Don't Get Caught with Your Pants Down (or Without Your Pants at All!)

You should pack for your trip a few days before the wedding (a week beforehand would be ideal, but, let's face it, that's unrealistic). Don't be caught running around the house in your wedding dress, throwing clothes into a suitcase while you wait for the limo to arrive. Not only is this undignified, it's a recipe for trouble. Haste may make waste, but it can also make for forgetfulness, too. (It's hard to get cozy with your new hubby if you've forgotten to pack the toothbrushes or deodorant.)

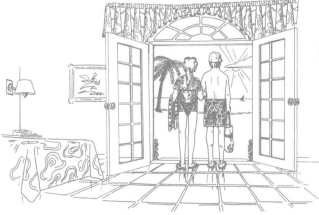

Plan well, and plan in advance, and guess what? Once you're there at your honeymoon destination, your poor, planned-out body and mind won't have to plan anything else.

In other words, you'll be done with everything. So enjoy yourself. You'll have earned it.

Chapter 24

His Home, Her Home—Your Home! Moving into Your First Home Together

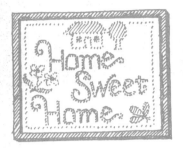

It used to be that an engaged couple never slept in the same bedroom until the wedding night. Nowadays, many set up house before getting married. If the idea of apartment- or house-hunting on top of organizing your wedding sounds like a nightmare, think of how relieved you'll be to have a familiar home to return to after the honeymoon. All you have to do is figure out how, where, what, and when this move from separate to joint should happen.

Before You Begin Packing...

Like the decisions you make concerning your wedding, it's wise—and diplomatic—to discuss plans to live together before you marry with both sets of parents. Plan to talk with them well before you start packing; the last thing either of you wants is to so offend someone with your decision that they refuse to take part in your wedding. While this may sound extreme, remember that what seems natural (and necessary) today may seem immoral to a person from another generation or background. Try to anticipate reactions before broaching the subject, and most importantly, be sensitive to responses.

If the reactions you receive are negative, you may want to rethink your initial plans to move in together. Look for a compromise. If you had hoped to live together for a year before the wedding, maybe you can change that to a month. If that doesn't help, perhaps your fiancé can move into the new apartment a month before your wedding while you stay where you are until after the honeymoon. There's no reason why you can't get the place in shape during that month; you just won't be living there.

Those Left Behind

There may be another person or people who need to know of your future living arrangements: your and/or your fiancé's roommates. While your roommates are undoubtedly happy for your upcoming change in marital status, they may also be concerned that when you move out they're going to be left holding the bag for rent, bills, and finding another roommate to take your place.

Try to give your roommate at least a month's notice before you move. Offer to help find a replacement by asking friends if they know of anyone in need of a place, by putting (and paying for) an ad in the newspaper, or by listing the opening in a roommate locater service. Anticipate that your roommate will show the place to prospective new roomies and keep your space tidy. Transfer any bills in your name to your roommate's name to avoid future confusion or tension.

A few days before you move, settle up unpaid bills. If you are owed a security deposit refund, be sure your roommate knows you've contacted the rental agent for its return. Let your roommate know the date and time you plan to move your belongings. Finally, leave your room in pristine condition for the next occupant—and make sure your roommate knows your forwarding address in case anything comes up.

How, Where, What, and When?

This section doesn't presume to give step-by-step instructions about finding the perfect home. But it should give you a sense of how to begin what can be a difficult, time-consuming, and possibly tension-filled process—and alert you and your fiancé to some possible pitfalls.

How? The financial picture

For the first time in your life, you'll be combining your income with someone else's in a common budget. Though you may have been taught that it's impolite to ask how much someone earns, now is not the time to be delicate. How you and your future husband are going to pay bills affects you; it's best not to be surprised.

You probably have a good idea already of how much your fiancé brings home each paycheck, but do you know how he budgets his money? And vice versa, does he know how you spend your earnings each month? If either answer is unclear, make a date to sit down with

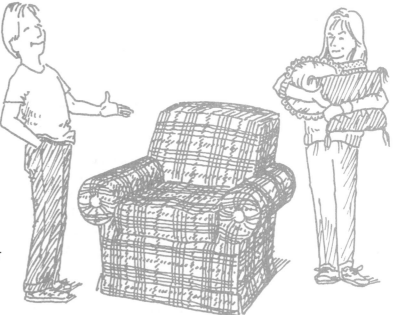

your fiancé and talk frankly about how you might go about setting up a budget you both can live with.

You might also want to discuss the use of credit cards—there's nothing scarier than assuming you're in the black, only to see a lot of numbers in the "balance due" column of the credit card statement.

You can arrive at dollar amounts for many budget expense items by tallying up averages for past bills from your or your fiancé's old apartment. Though those fees will change in your new place, you'll at least have a starting point. To be on the safe side, consider padding the amounts by twenty dollars.

The exception will be rent/mortgage. As a rule of thumb, the amount you spend monthly for rent or mortgage should not exceed two weeks' income from either your or your spouse's job. To spend more would probably stress your income too much—especially if one of you were to suddenly be without employment.

Once you have a dollar amount for rent or mortgage in mind, it's time to begin the search...

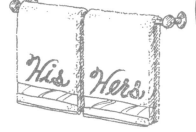

Where?

If you're one of the lucky ones, you or your fiancé already lives alone in a place that's large enough for two and that both of you love. If so, you can skip the advice on "what" and "where" and move right on to "when." But if you're like many couples, you'll want to start fresh. One of the first decisions facing you will be where you want to live.

And miles to go before I sleep...

Your vision of married bliss may be a cozy little house in the country, hours from the hue and cry of the bustling city. But what if your job means commuting to that bustling city five days a week? Chances are, you'd rather spend time with your new husband than on the road between your office and your home. Likewise, if it's your husband that's doing the commuting, you don't want to be stuck at home drumming your fingers on the table as you wait for him to finally walk through the door. Unless you simply can't live without that country house, you'll be better off searching for a place that's more convenient to both your workplaces—and saving that dream home for a time in your life when commuting isn't an issue.

Budget Items

A budget is split into two basic categories: income and expenses. It goes without saying that the intelligent couple will be sure to have more of the former and less of the latter, but sometimes it takes a bit of practice to get the numbers just right. Here are some categories you might include in your budget:

Income:
Your paycheck
His paycheck
Any other regular
    source of income

Expenses:
Rent/Mortgage
Telephone
Electricity
Heating
Groceries
Cable television
Student loan(s)
Car insurance
Home/renter's insurance
Gasoline
Car payment(s)

When choosing a place to live, you'll want to be sure it has at least some of the amenities that are important to your and your husband's daily life. If you like a good game of tennis on the weekends, make sure there are public tennis courts available. Maybe you're a gourmet cook who needs ingredients found only in specialty markets; if so, then the typical supermarket chain probably won't suit you. Do you need a place where you can easily launch your boat? Make sure there's water nearby.

Once you've decided what your town must have, drive through a few possibilities to check them out more thoroughly. Park the car in the downtown area and take a stroll to get a feel for the place. Strike up a conversation with the person who serves your coffee. Pick up a copy of the local paper. Time the commute from the town center to your office.

If you know someone who lives in a town you're considering, pump him or her for information. Do they like what the town has to offer? What are the pluses and minuses? How long have they lived there? Does the community have several housing options to choose from?

If everything seems perfect, it's time to start looking for housing.

What? House, condo, or apartment?

Determining what type of housing you should be looking at usually comes down to two factors: money and time. Comparatively speaking, apartments are the least expensive option and the easiest to find. You go through the apartment listings in the paper, then make some calls to set up appointments to check them out. First month's and last month's rent, plus a security deposit, are the standard up-front financial requirements. You hand over a check, sign some papers, and move in. Unless you choose the most luxurious apartment in the ritziest part of town, chances are your monthly rental costs will be less than any mortgage you would pay for a house or condo.

Condominiums and houses are more expensive for several reasons. First, in order to purchase one you need to come up with a down payment. Three, five, ten, and twenty percent of the total cost are the usual amounts of money buyers must have available to secure a house or condo. On top of that, there are other fees to pay when the final paperwork is processed—fees that can run into

---

Words to the Wise

Some places will rent apartments on a month-by-month, or tenant-at-will, basis, while others demand a year-long lease. Be sure you know which option you're getting before you sign. If you only plan to stay in your apartment while you search for the perfect house, you don't want to be stuck with a year-long lease.

Real Estate Agents

When looking for an apartment, you probably won't have to use a realtor unless you live in a very desirable town where competition for good apartments is fierce. If you do decide to go through an agency, however, be sure you find an agent you like and trust. Word of mouth is usually the best way, though you may be stuck dealing with the listing agent if you find an apartment through the newspaper. And often, agencies will charge you a fee if you take the apartment—sometimes as much as a half or even a whole month's rent.

For houses and condos, realtors are a must. Again, be sure the person you're dealing with is trustworthy and has been in the business for a while. The single most important thing to keep in mind when looking at houses or condos with a realtor is that he or she is representing the seller, not you.

Their goal is to sell the house and make their clients (and themselves) a profit. Realtors are required by law to inform you of this up front; if they don't, it's time to get yourself another realtor.

Remember, just because you start off working with someone, that doesn't mean you have to stick with them. If you don't feel they're serving your needs, move on to the next one.

Buyer's agents are a relatively new breed. Unlike realtors, buyer's agents represent you, not the seller. They listen to your needs, then go through the listings to find just the right place for you. Then they will work with the seller's listing agent to make a deal that you can live with. It will cost you a small fee to get them working, but in the end, it may be worth the price to know you've got an informed professional on your side.

thousands of dollars. Finally, monthly mortgage payments are generally higher than rent. For newlyweds, these costs can be prohibitive, often making a nice apartment more attractive than a house or a condo in the early years of marriage.

Since condos and houses are more permanent residences than apartments, you'll want to spend time finding the perfect place. That can take as little as a month or as long as a year, depending on the amount of inventory available and your personal preferences.

Prioritize wants and needs

Once you've decided what your budget can afford, list what you want your new home to offer. How many rooms and of what sort you'll need is determined by your lifestyles and personalities. If you like to entertain, an apartment with a shoebox-sized dining area and a galley kitchen would not be a good choice. You might opt for a place with a spare bedroom if you hope to have frequent overnight guests or need a separate office space. And everyone has heard stories of how fights for closet and bathroom-counter space have ruined relationships; if you're concerned you and your husband will fall into this category, go for the place with the walk-in closets and the bath and a half.

Don't forget to include your outdoor expectations in the list. If you love to barbeque, you'll want to be sure you have a place to do it. Two cars might not need a garage, but they will need parking. And a yen for gardening probably won't be satisfied with just a window box or two.

In the end, you might have to compromise a few hoped-fors in order to find a good place to start your future together. But if you're armed with a solid idea of what both of you really must have, you can save yourself time and aggravation as you search.

When?

If parental reaction isn't an issue for you, the "when" of moving in together depends solely on what's practical. The most logical time to move is when your current living arrangement changes: your lease is up and it makes more sense to move than to renew it; your roommate is leaving first and you don't want to look for another roommate (or have your fiancé move in); you just have to move out of your parents' house now because you're driving each other crazy.

This last reason aside, unless you and your fiancé are fortunate enough to be going through such changes simultaneously, you'll need to coordinate your move carefully. It would be expensive and wasteful to be paying for your new apartment together if you still have to pay rent on an old place because one of you couldn't get out of a lease. If that's what you're faced with, ask your current rental agent if he'd consider letting you sublet your apartment (it will be up to you to find a suitable tenant, and any problems that tenant causes become your problems). Or, if your lease is up, see if you can remain in your apartment on a tenant-at-will basis until your fiancé is ready to move.

The only instance in which you may want to buck up the extra cash for two apartments is if the date of your wedding is looming nearer than one month. Give yourself time to tie up the loose ends of your wedding without the hassle of tying up boxes at the same time!

What If We Already Live Together?

It may be that you and your fiancé have been living together, or will be living together for some time before the wedding. This can make certain parts of wedding planning a lot less complicated. (For one thing, your fiancé will be readily available for discussions about the wedding arrangements.)

If you're coordinating much of the wedding yourself, you can have RSVPs mailed to you instead of your parents (or whoever is listed as the sponsor) and can keep an accurate running count of who is coming. Living together, you and your partner will have a clear picture of what you should register for. If you see your fiancé using the same ratty towel day after day, you know for a fact that a new set of bath linens will be welcome. Likewise, if your fiancé has listened to you complain about the cookware for weeks, he knows new pots and pans had better be on the register. Guests can send gifts directly to your home so you don't have to arrange to pick them up or have them shipped to you.

Living at the same address for a while before the wedding means you and your partner have a better understanding of each other's finances. You won't have to set up billing procedures for your utilities or cable, or figure out a system for paying those bills.

Plan Ahead

If you've decided to look for a house or condo as your first home, be sure to give yourselves plenty of time to see a wide variety of listings. A house or condo is a major investment—you don't want to feel rushed into making a hasty decision. Also, the actual process of buying a house can be time-consuming. Again, if you hurry through the necessary steps you may find you've overlooked something you wish you hadn't.

With the potential tension surrounding the planning of a wedding, not having to deal with such worrisome things can be a relief.

Distance Makes the Heart Grow Fonder

While living together before the wedding does have its practical side, many couples prefer to stick with tradition. They don't want to experience what it's like to be married before they actually are married. Somehow, the excitement and romance of the first night in their new home is enhanced because they now share the same name. It's as husband and wife that they set up housekeeping, make decisions about furnishings, and organize their finances.

Waiting until you're official can be a wonderfully romantic way to go—just be sure that when the honeymoon's over, you both have a key that opens the same front door!

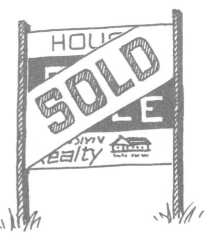

Part Four:

Worksheets

NEWSPAPER ENGAGEMENT ANNOUNCEMENT WORKSHEET

To appear in _____ newspaper on_____.

(name of newspaper)   (date)

Names of the bride's parents:

Address: ....

Telephone number with area code: _____

Mr. and Mrs. _____ of _____

(bride's parents' names)   (their city, if out of town)

announce the engagement of their daughter, _____, to

(bride's first and middle name)

_____, the son of Mr. and Mrs. _____,

(grooms's first and last name)   (groom's parents' names)

of _____. A _____ wedding is planned. (Or, No date has

(groom's parents' city)   (month/season)

been set for the wedding.)

WEDDING STYLE WORKSHEET

Type of Ceremony: ☐ Religious ☐ Spiritual ☐ Civil

Level of Formality: ☐ Very Formal ☐ Formal ☐ Semiformal ☐ Informal

Desired Qualities (circle all that apply):

Artistic	Exotic	Luxurious	Sophisticated
Avant-garde	Family-Oriented	Outdoor	Spiritual
Casual	Fantasy	Personal	Spontaneous
Chic	Festive	Picturesque	Stylish
Community-oriented	Fun	Polished	Theatrical
Contemporary	Glamorous	Private	Traditional
Country	Grand	Quaint	Unique
Creative	Indoor	Relaxed	Urban
Dramatic	Intimate	Romantic	Warm
Elaborate	Large	Sentimental	
Elegant	Lavish	Simple	
Ethnic	Lively	Small	

Ceremony Location:

First choice:

Second choice:

Third choice:

Personalized Elements of Ceremony:

Readings

Music

Vows

Symbolic Ceremonies:

Season/Month:

First choice:

Second choice:

Third choice:

Time of Day: ☐ Morning   ☐ Afternoon   ☐ Evening   ☐ Other: _____

Bride's Attire:

Groom's Attire:

Number of Desired Attendants:

Attendants' Attire:

Number of Desired Guests:

Wedding Theme (if any):

First choice:

Second choice:

Third choice:

Type of Reception: ☐ Cocktail   ☐ Champagne Brunch   ☐ Luncheon   ☐ Tea   ☐ Buffet Dinner   ☐ Weekend Wedding   ☐ Sit-Down Dinner   ☐ Other: _____

Reception Location:

First choice:

Second choice:

Third choice:

Entertainment:

Other:

Honeymoon Ideas:

Notes:

WEDDING BUDGET WORKSHEET

ITEM	PROJECTED COST*	DEPOSIT PAID	BALANCE DUE	WHO PAYS?
Wedding Consultant				
Fee				
Tip (usually 15–20%)				
Pre-wedding Parties				
Engagement**				
Site rental				
Equipment rental				
Invitations				
Food				
Beverages				
Decorations				
Flowers				
Party favors				
Bridesmaids' party/luncheon				
Rehearsal dinner**				
Site rental				
Equipment rental				
Invitations				
Food				
Beverages				
Decorations				
Flowers				
Party favors				
Weekend wedding parties				

*(including tax, if applicable) **(if hosted by bride and groom)

ITEM	PROJECTED COST*	DEPOSIT PAID	BALANCE DUE	WHO PAYS?
Ceremony				
Location fee				
Officiant's fee				
Donation to church (optional, amount varies)				
Organist				
Tip (amount varies)				
Other musicians				
Tip (amount varies)				
Program				
Aisle runner				
Business and Legal Matters				
Marriage license				
Blood test (if applicable)				
Wedding Jewelry				
Engagement ring				
Bride's wedding band				
Groom's wedding band				
Bride's Formalwear				
Wedding gown				
Alterations				
Undergarments (slip, bustier, hosiery, etc.)				
Headpiece				
Shoes				
Jewelry (excluding engagement and wedding rings)				

ITEM	PROJECTED COST*	DEPOSIT PAID	BALANCE DUE	WHO PAYS?
Purse (optional)				
Cosmetics, or makeup stylist				
Hair stylist				
Going-away outfit				
Going-away accessories				
Honeymoon clothes				
Groom's Formalwear				
Tuxedo				
Shoes				
Going-away outfit				
Honeymoon clothes				
Gifts				
Bride's Attendants				
Groom's Attendants				
Bride (optional)				
Groom (optional)				
Reception				
Site rental				
Equipment rental (chairs, tent, etc.)				
Decorations				
Servers, bartenders				
Wine service for cocktail hour				
Hors d'oeuvres				
Entrees				
Meals for hired help				

ITEM	PROJECTED COST*	DEPOSIT PAID	BALANCE DUE	WHO PAYS?
Nonalcoholic beverages				
Wine				
Champagne				
Liquor				
Dessert				
Toasting glasses				
Guest book and pen				
Place cards				
Printed napkins				
Party favors (matches, chocolates, etc.)				
Box or pouch for envelope gifts				
Tip for caterer or banquet manager (usually 15–20%)				
Tip for servers, bartenders (usually 15–20% total)				
Photography and Videography				
Engagement portrait				
Wedding portrait				
Wedding proofs				
Photographer's fee				
Wedding prints				
Album				
Mothers' albums				
Extra prints				
Videographer's fee				
Videotape				

ITEM	PROJECTED COST*	DEPOSIT PAID	BALANCE DUE	WHO PAYS?
Reception Music				
Musicians for cocktail hour				
Tip (optional, up to 15%)				
Live band				
Tip (optional, usually $25 per band member)				
Disc jockey				
Tip (optional, usually 15–20%)				
Flowers and Decorations				
Flowers for wedding site				
Decorations for wedding site				
Bride's bouquet				
Bridesmaids' flowers				
Boutonnieres				
Corsages				
Flowers for reception site				
Potted plants				
Table centerpieces				
Head table				
Cake table				
Decorations for reception				
Wedding Invitations and Stationery				
Invitations				
Announcements				
Thank-you notes				
Calligrapher				

ITEM	PROJECTED COST*	DEPOSIT PAID	BALANCE DUE	WHO PAYS?
Postage (for invitations and response cards)				
Wedding Cake				
Groom's cake				
Cake top and decorations				
Flowers for cake				
Cake serving set				
Cake boxes				
Wedding Transportation				
Limousines or rented cars				
Parking				
Tip for drivers (usually 15–20%)				
Guest Accommodations				
Guest Transportation				
Honeymoon				
Transportation				
Accommodations				
Meals				
Spending money				
Additional Expenses (list below)				

TOTAL OF ALL EXPENSES

WEDDING CONSULTANT WORKSHEET

Name:

Address:

Phone:

Contact:

Hours:

Appointments:

Date: Time:

Date: Time:

Date: Time:

Date: Time:

Service:

Number of hours:

Overtime cost:

Provides the following services:

Cost:

Fee: ❐ Flat ❐ Hourly percentage: _____   ❐ Per guest

Total amount due:

Amount of deposit: Date:

Amount due: Date:

Gratuities included?   Yes   No

Sales tax included?   Yes   No

Date contract signed:

Terms of cancellation:

Notes:

CHOOSING YOUR ENGAGEMENT RING WORKSHEET

Jewelry store #1:

Address:

Telephone number:

Sales representative:

Store hours:

Notes:

Jewelry store #2:

Address:

Telephone number:

Sales representative:

Store hours:

Notes:

Jewelry store #3:

Address:

Telephone number:

Sales representative:

Store hours:

Notes:

STONE	#1	#2	#3	#4	#5
Jewelry store					
Clarity					
Cut					
Color					
Carats					
Other stones					
Setting					
Notes					
Price per carat					
Tax, other charges					
Total price					

Final choice: (stone number from above)   Ring size:

Order date: Date ready:

Deposit amount: Due date:

Balance: Due date:

Notes:

WEDDING JEWELRY WORKSHEET

	BRIDE'S WEDDING BAND	GROOM'S WEDDING BAND	OTHER JEWELRY (IF APPLICABLE)	JEWELRY STORE
Description				
Setting				
Stones				
(if applicable)				
Notes				
Price				
Tax, other charges				
Total price				

BRIDE'S ATTENDANTS LIST

Maid/Matron of Honor:

Name: .... Address: ....

Telephone: .... Special duties: ....

Bridesmaids:

Name: .... Address: ....

Telephone: .... Special duties: ....

Name: .... Address: ....

Telephone: .... Special duties: ....

Name: .... Address: ....

Telephone: .... Special duties: ....

Name: .... Address: ....

Telephone: .... Special duties: ....

Flower Girl:

Name: .... Address: ....

Telephone: .... Special duties: ....

Other Honor Attendants:

Name: .... Address: ....

Telephone: .... Special duties: ....

Name: .... Address: ....

Telephone: .... Special duties: ....

Name: .... Address: ....

Telephone: .... Special duties: ....

Groom's Attendants List

Best Man:

Name: Address:

Telephone: Special duties:

Ushers:

Name: Address:

Telephone: Special duties:

Name: Address:

Telephone: Special duties:

Name: Address:

Telephone: Special duties:

Name: Address:

Telephone: Special duties:

Ring Bearer:

Name: Address:

Telephone: Special duties:

Other Honor Attendants:

Name: Address:

Telephone: Special duties:

Name: Address:

Telephone: Special duties:

Name: Address:

Telephone: Special duties:

WEDDING GUEST LIST WORKSHEET

NAME	ADDRESS	TELEPHONE	RSVP RECEIVED?
1.			
2.			
3.			
4.			
5.			
6.			
7.			
8.			
9.			
10.			
11.			
12.			
13.			
14.			
15.			
16.			
17.			
18.			
19.			
20.			
21.			
22.			
23.			
24.			
25.			

NAME	ADDRESS	TELEPHONE	RSVP RECEIVED?
26.			
27.			
28.			
29.			
30.			
31.			
32.			
33.			
34.			
35.			
36.			
37.			
38.			
39.			
40.			
41.			
42.			
43.			
44.			
45.			
46.			
47.			
48.			
49.			
50.			

NAME	ADDRESS	TELEPHONE	RSVP RECEIVED?
51.			
52.			
53.			
54.			
55.			
56.			
57.			
58.			
59.			
60.			
61.			
62.			
63.			
64.			
65.			
66.			
67.			
68.			
69.			
70.			
71.			
72.			
73.			
74.			
75.			

WEDDING GUEST LIST WORKSHEET (CONTINUED)

NAME	ADDRESS	TELEPHONE	RSVP RECEIVED?
76.			
77.			
78.			
79.			
80.			
81.			
82.			
83.			
84.			
85.			
86.			
87.			
88.			
89.			
90.			
91.			
92.			
93.			
94.			
95.			
96.			
97.			
98.			
99.			
100.			

GUEST ACCOMMODATIONS WORKSHEET

Be sure to give a copy of this to your mother, maid/matron of honor, and anyone else guests may contact for information about accommodations.

Blocks of Rooms Reserved for Wedding at:

Hotel:

Address:

Directions:

Approximate distance from ceremony site: Reception site:

Telephone:

Toll-free reservations number:

Fax number:

Contact:

Number of single rooms reserved in block: Daily rate:

Number of double rooms reserved in block: Daily rate:

Total number of rooms reserved in block:

Date(s) reserved:

Cut-off/Last-day reservations accepted:

Terms of agreement:

Payment procedure:

Notes:

Hotel:

Address:

Directions:

Approximate distance from ceremony site: Reception site:

Telephone:

Toll-free reservations number:

Fax number:

Contact:

Number of single rooms reserved in block: .... Daily rate: ....

Number of double rooms reserved in block: .... Daily rate: ....

Total number of rooms reserved in block: ....

Date(s) reserved: ....

Cut-off/Last-day reservations accepted: ....

Terms of agreement: ....

Payment procedure: ....

Notes: ....

Other Nearby Lodgings:

Hotel: ....

Address: ....

Directions: ....

Approximate distance from ceremony site: .... Reception site: ....

Telephone: ....

Toll-free reservations number: ....

Daily room rate: ....

Notes: ....

Hotel: ....

Address: ....

Directions: ....

Approximate distance from ceremony site: .... Reception site: ....

Telephone: ....

Toll-free reservations number: ....

Daily room rate: ....

Notes: ....

BRIDAL SHOWER GUEST LIST

Name: _____ Address: _____

Telephone: _____ RSVP Number in Party: _____

Name: _____ Address: _____

Telephone: _____ RSVP Number in Party: _____

Name: _____ Address: _____

Telephone: _____ RSVP Number in Party: _____

Name: _____ Address: _____

Telephone: _____ RSVP Number in Party: _____

Name: _____ Address: _____

Telephone: _____ RSVP Number in Party: _____

Name: _____ Address: _____

Telephone: _____ RSVP Number in Party: _____

Name: _____ Address: _____

Telephone: _____ RSVP Number in Party: _____

Name: _____ Address: _____

Telephone: _____ RSVP Number in Party: _____

Name: _____ Address: _____

Telephone: _____ RSVP Number in Party: _____

Name: _____ Address: _____

Telephone: _____ RSVP Number in Party: _____

Name: _____ Address: _____

Telephone: _____ RSVP Number in Party: _____

Name: _____ Address: _____

Telephone: _____ RSVP Number in Party: _____

Name: _____ Address: _____

Telephone: _____ RSVP Number in Party: _____

Name: _____

Address: _____

Telephone: _____

RSVP Number in Party: _____

Name: _____

Address: _____

Telephone: _____

RSVP Number in Party: _____

Name: _____

Address: _____

Telephone: _____

RSVP Number in Party: _____

Name: _____

Address: _____

Telephone: _____

RSVP Number in Party: _____

Name: _____

Address: _____

Telephone: _____

RSVP Number in Party: _____

Name: _____

Address: _____

Telephone: _____

RSVP Number in Party: _____

Name: _____

Address: _____

Telephone: _____

RSVP Number in Party: _____

Name: _____

Address: _____

Telephone: _____

RSVP Number in Party: _____

Name: _____

Address: _____

Telephone: _____

RSVP Number in Party: _____

Name: _____

Address: _____

Telephone: _____

RSVP Number in Party: _____

Name: _____

Address: _____

Telephone: _____

RSVP Number in Party: _____

Name: _____

Address: _____

Telephone: _____

RSVP Number in Party: _____

Name: _____

Address: _____

Telephone: _____

RSVP Number in Party: _____

SHOWER GIFT RECORDER

NAME	DESCRIPTION OF GIFT	THANK-YOU NOTE SENT?

BACHELORETTE PARTY GUEST LIST

Name:	Address:
Telephone:	RSVP
Name:	Address:
Telephone:	RSVP
Name:	Address:
Telephone:	RSVP
Name:	Address:
Telephone:	RSVP
Name:	Address:
Telephone:	RSVP
Name:	Address:
Telephone:	RSVP
Name:	Address:
Telephone:	RSVP
Name:	Address:
Telephone:	RSVP
Name:	Address:
Telephone:	RSVP
Name:	Address:
Telephone:	RSVP
Name:	Address:
Telephone:	RSVP
Name:	Address:
Telephone:	RSVP
Name:	Address:
Telephone:	RSVP

BACHELOR PARTY GUEST LIST

Name:	Address:
Telephone:	RSVP
Name:	Address:
Telephone:	RSVP
Name:	Address:
Telephone:	RSVP
Name:	Address:
Telephone:	RSVP
Name:	Address:
Telephone:	RSVP
Name:	Address:
Telephone:	RSVP
Name:	Address:
Telephone:	RSVP
Name:	Address:
Telephone:	RSVP
Name:	Address:
Telephone:	RSVP
Name:	Address:
Telephone:	RSVP
Name:	Address:
Telephone:	RSVP
Name:	Address:
Telephone:	RSVP
Name:	Address:
Telephone:	RSVP

ATTENDANTS' PARTY WORKSHEET

Location:

Telephone:

Contact:

Date:

Time:

Directions:

Number of Guests:

Menu:

Beverages:

Activities:

Other:

Cost:

Notes:

POST-WEDDING PARTY WORKSHEET

Location:

Telephone:

Contact:

Date:

Time:

Directions:

Number of Guests:

Menu:

Beverages:

POST-WEDDING PARTY GUEST LIST

Name: _____ Address: _____

Telephone: _____ RSVP _____

Name: _____ Address: _____

Telephone: _____ RSVP _____

Name: _____ Address: _____

Telephone: _____ RSVP _____

Name: _____ Address: _____

Telephone: _____ RSVP _____

Name: _____ Address: _____

Telephone: _____ RSVP _____

Name: _____ Address: _____

Telephone: _____ RSVP _____

Name: _____ Address: _____

Telephone: _____ RSVP _____

Name: _____ Address: _____

Telephone: _____ RSVP _____

Name: _____ Address: _____

Telephone: _____ RSVP _____

Name: _____ Address: _____

Telephone: _____ RSVP _____

Name: _____ Address: _____

Telephone: _____ RSVP _____

Name: _____ Address: _____

Telephone: _____ RSVP _____

Name: _____ Address: _____

Telephone: _____ RSVP _____

GIFT REGISTRY CHECKLIST

FORMAL DINNERWARE	DESIRED QUANTITY:	QUANTITY RECEIVED:	MANUFACTURER:	PATTERN/MODEL:
Dinner plates				
Sandwich/lunch plates				
Salad/dessert plates				
Bread and butter plates				
Cups and saucers				
Rimmed soup bowls				
Soup/cereal bowls				
Fruit bowls				
Open vegetable dishes				
Covered vegetable dishes				
Gravy boat				
Sugar bowl				
Creamer				
Small platter				
Medium platter				
Large platter				
Salt and pepper shakers				
Coffeepot				
Teapot				
Butter dish				
Other:				

CASUAL DINNERWARE	DESIRED QUANTITY:	QUANTITY RECEIVED:	MANUFACTURER:	PATTERN/MODEL:
Dinner plates				
Sandwich/lunch plates				
Salad/dessert plates				
Bread and butter plates				
Cups and saucers				
Rimmed soup bowls				
Soup/cereal bowls				
Fruit bowls				
Open vegetable dishes				
Covered vegetable dishes				
Gravy boat				
Sugar bowl				
Creamer				
Small platter				
Medium platter				
Large platter				
Salt and pepper shakers				
Coffeepot				
Butter dish				
Mugs				
Other:				

FORMAL FLATWARE	DESIRED QUANTITY:	QUANTITY RECEIVED:	MANUFACTURER:	PATTERN/MODEL:
Five-piece place setting				
Four-piece place setting				
Dinner forks				
Dinner knives				
Teaspoons				
Salad forks				
Soup spoons				
Butter spreader				
Butter knives				
Cold meat fork				
Sugar spoon				
Serving spoon				
Pierced spoon				
Gravy ladle				
Pie/cake server				
Hostess set				
Serve set				
Silver chest				
Other:				

CASUAL FLATWARE	DESIRED QUANTITY:	QUANTITY RECEIVED:	MANUFACTURER:	PATTERN/MODEL:
Five-piece setting				
Dinner forks				
Dinner knives				
Teaspoons				
Salad forks				
Soup spoons				
Hostess set				
Serve set				
Gravy ladle				
Cake/pie server				
Other:				

CRYSTAL	DESIRED QUANTITY:	QUANTITY RECEIVED:	MANUFACTURER:	PATTERN/MODEL:
Wine glasses				
Champagne flutes				
Water goblets				
Cordials				
Brandy snifters				
Decanters				
Pitchers				
Other:				

CASUAL GLASS/BARWARE	DESIRED QUANTITY:	QUANTITY RECEIVED:	MANUFACTURER:	PATTERN/MODEL:
Water glasses				
Juice glasses				
Beer mugs				
Pilsners				
Highball glasses				
Decanter				
Pitcher				
Punch bowl set				
Cocktail shaker				
Ice bucket				
Champagne cooler				
Irish coffee set				
Whiskey set				
Martini set				
Wine rack				
Bar utensils				
Other:				

ADDITIONAL SERVING PIECES	DESIRED QUANTITY:	QUANTITY RECEIVED:	MANUFACTURER:	PATTERN/MODEL:
Sugar/creamer				
Coffee service				
Serving tray				
Relish tray				
Canapé tray				
Chip and dip server				
Cheese board				
Cake plate				
Large salad bowl				
Salad bowl set				
Salad tongs				
Gravy boat				
Butter dish				
Salt and pepper shakers				
Round baker				
Rectangular baker				
Demitasse set				
Other:				

HOME DECOR	DESIRED QUANTITY:	QUANTITY RECEIVED:	MANUFACTURER:	PATTERN/MODEL:
Vase				
Bud vase				
Bowl				
Candlesticks				
Picture frame				
Figurine				
Clock				
Lamp				
Framed art				
Brass accessories				
Picnic basket				
Other:				

SMALL APPLIANCES	DESIRED QUANTITY:	QUANTITY RECEIVED:	MANUFACTURER:	PATTERN/MODEL:
Coffee maker				
Coffee grinder				
Espresso/cappuccino maker				
Food processor				
Mini processor				
Mini chopper				
Blender				
Hand mixer				
Stand mixer				
Bread baker				
Pasta machine				
Citrus juicer				
Juice extractor				
Toaster (specify two-slice or four-slice)				
Toaster oven				
Convection oven				
Microwave				
Electric fry pan				
Electric wok				
Electric griddle				
Sandwich maker				
Waffle maker				
Hot tray				
Indoor grill				
Crock pot				
Rice cooker				
Can opener				
Food Slicer				

SMALL APPLIANCES
(CONTINUED)

	DESIRED QUANTITY:	QUANTITY RECEIVED:	MANUFACTURER:	PATTERN/MODEL:
Electric knife				
Iron				
Vacuum cleaner				
Fan				
Humidifier				
Dehumidifier				
Space heater				
Other:				

CUTLERY

	DESIRED QUANTITY:	QUANTITY RECEIVED:	MANUFACTURER:	PATTERN/MODEL:
Carving set				
Cutlery set				
Knife set				
Knife block				
Steel sharpener				
Boning knife (specify size)				
Paring knife (specify size)				
Chef knife (specify size)				
Bread knife (specify size)				
Slicing knife (specify size)				
Carving fork				
Utility knife (specify size)				
Kitchen shears				
Cleaver				
Other:				

BAKEWARE	DESIRED QUANTITY:	QUANTITY RECEIVED:	MANUFACTURER:	PATTERN/MODEL:
Cake pan				
Cookie sheet				
Bread pan				
Muffin tin				
Cooling rack				
Bundt pan				
Springform cake pan				
Pie plate				
Roasting pan				
Pizza pan				
Covered casserole				
Soufflé dish				
Rectangular baker				
Lasagna pan				
Pizza pan				
Pizza stone				
Other:				

KITCHEN BASICS	DESIRED QUANTITY:	QUANTITY RECEIVED:	MANUFACTURER:	PATTERN/MODEL:
Kitchen tool set				
Canister set				
Spice rack				
Cutting board				
Salad bowl set				
Salt and pepper mill				
Kitchen towels				
Pot holders				
Apron				
Mixing bowl set				
Measuring cup set				
Rolling pin				
Cookie jar				
Tea kettle				
Coffee mugs				
Other:				

COOKWARE	DESIRED QUANTITY:	QUANTITY RECEIVED:	MANUFACTURER:	PATTERN/MODEL:
Saucepan (small)				
Saucepan (medium)				
Saucepan (large)				
Sauté pan (small)				
Sauté pan (large)				
Frying pan (small)				
Frying pan (medium)				
Frying pan (large)				
Stockpot (small)				
Stockpot (large)				
Roasting pan				
Omelet pan (small)				
Omelet pan (large)				
Skillet				
Double boiler				
Steamer insert				
Wok				
Griddle				
Stirfry pan				
Microwave cookware set				
Tea kettle				
Dutch oven				
Other:				

LUGGAGE

LUGGAGE	DESIRED QUANTITY:	QUANTITY RECEIVED:	MANUFACTURER:	PATTERN/MODEL:
Duffel bag				
Beauty case				
Carry-on tote				
Suitcases (specify quantity and sizes)				
Garment bag				
Luggage cart				
Other:				

HOME ELECTRONICS

HOME ELECTRONICS	Desired Quantity:	Quantity Received:	Manufacturer:	Pattern/Model:
Stereo				
CD player				
Television				
VCR				
Camcorder				
Telephone				
Answering machine				
Portable stereo				
Camera				
Other:				

TABLE LINENS

	DESIRED QUANTITY:	QUANTITY RECEIVED:	MANUFACTURER:	PATTERN/MODEL:
Tablecloth				
Place mats				
Napkins				
Napkin rings				
Other:				

BED LINENS

	DESIRED QUANTITY:	QUANTITY RECEIVED:	MANUFACTURER:	PATTERN/MODEL:
Flat sheets (specify full, queen, or king)				
Fitted sheets (specify full, queen, or king)				
Pillowcases (specify standard or king)				
Sets of sheets (specify full, queen, or king)				
Comforter				
Comforter set				
Dust ruffle				
Pillow shams				
Window treatment				
Down comforter				
Duvet cover				
Bedspread				
Quilt				
Blanket				
Electric blanket				
Cotton blanket				

BED LINENS (continued)	DESIRED QUANTITY:	QUANTITY RECEIVED:	MANUFACTURER:	PATTERN/MODEL:
Decorative pillows				
Down pillows (specify standard, queen, or king)				
Pillows (specify standard, queen, or king)				
Mattress pad				
Other:				

BATH TOWELS AND ACCESSORIES	DESIRED QUANTITY:	QUANTITY RECEIVED:	MANUFACTURER:	PATTERN/MODEL:
Bath towels				
Bath sheets				
Hand towels				
Washcloths				
Fingertip towels				
Shower curtain				
Bath mat				
Bath rug				
Lid cover				
Hamper				
Scale				
Wastebasket				
Other:				

CEREMONY WORKSHEET

Location of ceremony: Address:

Date of ceremony: Time of ceremony:

Officiant's name: Location fee:

Officiant's fee: Recommended church donation:

Wedding program available?   Fee:

PART OF CEREMONY	DESCRIPTION	NOTES
Processional		
Opening words		
Giving away or blessing		
Reading		
Prayers		
Marriage vows		
Exchange of rings		
Pronouncement of marriage		
Lighting of unity candle		
Benediction		
Closing words		
Recessional		
Other		

NEWSPAPER WEDDING
ANNOUNCEMENT WORKSHEET

To appear in _____ newspaper on_____ .
    (name of newspaper)   (date)

Name(s) of sender:

Address:

Telephone number with area code:

_____ and _____ were married at
(bride's first, middle and maiden names)   (grooms's first, middle and last name)

_____ in _____ .
(name of church or synagogue)   (town)

The bride, _____
(optional: name change information, for example, "will continue to use her surname"),

is the daughter of Mr. and Mrs. _____ of _____ .
(bride's parents' names)   (their city, if out of town)

She graduated from _____ and is a/an _____
(optional: name of college or university)   (job title)

at _____ . The bridegroom, son of Mr. and
(name of employer)

Mrs. _____ of _____ , graduated
(groom's parents' names)   (their city, if out of town)

from _____ and is a/an _____ at
(optional: name of college or university)   (job title)

_____ . The couple will live in _____ after
(name of employer)   (city or town)

a trip to _____ .
(honeymoon vacation)

BRIDE'S NAME AND ADDRESS
CHANGE WORKSHEET

INFORMATION TO BE CHANGED	NAME OF INSTITUTION	NOTIFIED OF NAME CHANGE?	NOTIFIED OF ADDRESS?	NOTIFIED OF CHANGE IN MARITAL STATUS?
401k accounts				
Automotive insurance				
Bank accounts				
Billing accounts				
Car registration				
Club memberships				
Credit cards				
Dentist				
Doctors				
Driver's license				
Employment records				
Homeowner's/Renter's insurance				
IRA accounts				
Leases				
Life insurance				
Loans				
Medical insurance				
Other insurance accounts				
Passport				
Pension plan records				
Post office				
Property titles				
Safety deposit box				
School records				
Social Security				
Stocks and bonds				
Subscriptions				
Telephone listing				
Voter registration records				
Wills/Trusts				
Other (list below)				

GROOM'S NAME AND ADDRESS CHANGE WORKSHEET

INFORMATION TO BE CHANGED	NAME OF INSTITUTION	NOTIFIED OF NAME CHANGE?	NOTIFIED OF ADDRESS?	NOTIFIED OF CHANGE IN MARITAL STATUS?
401k accounts				
Automotive insurance				
Bank accounts				
Billing accounts				
Car registration				
Club memberships				
Credit cards				
Dentist				
Doctors				
Driver's license				
Employment records				
Homeowner's/Renter's insurance				
IRA accounts				
Leases				
Life insurance				
Loans				
Medical insurance				
Other insurance accounts				
Passport				
Pension plan records				
Post office				
Property titles				
Safety deposit box				
School records				
Social Security				
Stocks and bonds				
Subscriptions				
Telephone listing				
Voter registration records				
Wills/Trusts				
Other (list below)				

RECEIVING LINE WORKSHEET

(in order, beginning at the head of the line)

Bride's mother:

Bride's father:

Groom's mother:

Groom's father:

Bride:

Groom:

Maid of honor (optional):

Best man (optional):

Bridesmaid (optional):

Usher (optional):

Bridesmaid (optional):

Usher (optional):

Bridesmaid (optional):

Usher (optional):

Bridesmaid (optional):

Usher (optional):

Bridesmaid (optional):

Usher (optional):

Other honor attendant (optional):

Other honor attendant (optional):

Notes:

REHEARSAL DINNER WORKSHEET

Wedding Rehearsal:

Location:

Telephone:

Contact:

Date:

Time:

Directions:

Notes:

Dinner:

Location:

Telephone:

Contact:

Date:

Time:

Directions:

Number of Guests:

Menu:

Beverages:

Notes:

REHEARSAL DINNER GUEST LIST

Name: .... Address: ....

Telephone: .... RSVP Number in Party: ....

Name: .... Address: ....

Telephone: .... RSVP Number in Party: ....

Name: .... Address: ....

Telephone: .... RSVP Number in Party: ....

Name: .... Address: ....

Telephone: .... RSVP Number in Party: ....

Name: .... Address: ....

Telephone: .... RSVP Number in Party: ....

Name: .... Address: ....

Telephone: .... RSVP Number in Party: ....

Name: .... Address: ....

Telephone: .... RSVP Number in Party: ....

Name: .... Address: ....

Telephone: .... RSVP Number in Party: ....

Name: .... Address: ....

Telephone: .... RSVP Number in Party: ....

Name: .... Address: ....

Telephone: .... RSVP Number in Party: ....

Name: .... Address: ....

Telephone: .... RSVP Number in Party: ....

Name: .... Address: ....

Telephone: .... RSVP Number in Party: ....

Name: .... Address: ....

Telephone: .... RSVP Number in Party: ....

RECEPTION SITE WORKSHEET

Reception site:

Address:

Telephone:

Contact: Hours:

Appointments:

Date: Time:

Date: Time:

Date: Time:

Date: Time:

Cost:

Total amount due:

Amount of deposit: Date:

Balance due: Date:

Room reserved:

Date: Time: Number of hours:

Overtime cost:

Occupancy:

Final head count due date:

Reception location includes the following services:

Reception location includes the following equipment:

Terms of cancellation:

Other:

ITEM	DESCRIPTION	COST	NOTES
Reception Site			
Site rental			
Overtime fee			
Other			
Equipment			
Tent			
Chairs			
Tables			
Linens			
Other			
Service			
Servers			
Bartenders			
Valet parking attendants			
Coat checkers			
Other (list below)			
TOTAL			

Caterer Worksheet

Name (if different from reception site):

Address:

Telephone:

Contact: Hours:

Appointments:

Date: Time:

Date: Time:

Date: Time:

Date of hired services: Time:

Number of hours: Cocktail hour:

Overtime cost: Final head count due date:

Menu:

Sit down or buffet?

Includes the following services:

Includes the following equipment:

Cost:

Total amount due:

Amount of deposit: Date:

Balance due: Date:

Gratuities included? ❐ Yes   ❐ No   Sales tax included?   ❐ Yes   ❐ No

Terms of cancellation:

Notes:

ITEM	DESCRIPTION	COST	NOTES
Food			
Appetizers			
Entrees			
Dessert			
Other food			
Beverages			
Nonalcoholic			
Champagne			
Wine			
Liquor			
Equipment			
Tent			
Chairs			
Tables			
Linens			
Dinnerware			
Flatware			
Glassware			
Serving pieces			
Other			
Service			
Servers			
Bartenders			
Valet parking attendants			
Coat checkers			
Overtime cost			
Other			
Gratuities			
Sales tax			
TOTAL			

MENU AND BEVERAGE WORKSHEET

ITEM	DESCRIPTION	COST	NOTES
Appetizers			
Entrees			
Desserts (if any)			
Beverages (nonalcoholic)			
Wine			
Champagne			
Open bar			
Other			
Gratuities			
Sales tax			
TOTAL			

EQUIPMENT RENTAL WORKSHEET

Name of rental company: _____   Address: _____

Telephone: _____   Contact: _____

Hours: _____   Order date: _____

☐ Delivery?   ☐ Pick up?

Date: _____   Time: _____

Special instructions: _____

Total amount due: _____

Amount of deposit: _____   Date: _____

Balance due: _____   Date: _____

Cancellation policy: _____

Damaged goods policy: _____

Notes: _____

ITEM	DESCRIPTION	QUANTITY	COST	TOTAL COST	(QUANTITY x COST)
Ceremony Equipment:					
Aisle runner					
Candelabra					
Canopy/*Chuppah*					
Lattice arch					
Microphone					
Other					
Tents:					
Size					
Size					
Flooring/Carpeting					
Lighting					
Decoration					
Other					

EQUIPMENT RENTAL WORKSHEET (CONTINUED)

ITEM	DESCRIPTION	QUANTITY	COST	TOTAL COST	(QUANTITY X COST)
Chairs:					
Style					
Style					
Style					
Other					
Tables:					
Size					
Size					
Size					
Other					
Linens:					
Table					
Chair covers					
Napkins					
Other					
Dinnerware:					
Dinner plates					
Salad plates					
Bread plates					
Dessert plates					
Cake plates					
Soup bowls					
Fruit bowls					
Cups and saucers					
Other					

ITEM	DESCRIPTION	QUANTITY	COST	TOTAL COST	(QUANTITY x COST)
Flatware:					
Dinner forks					
Salad forks					
Dinner knives					
Steak knives					
Butter knives					
Spoons					
Soup spoons					
Serving spoons					
Meat forks					
Carving knives					
Cake serving set					
Other					
Glassware:					
Wine glasses					
Champagne glasses					
Water goblets					
Highball glasses					
Double rocks glasses					
Snifters					
16 oz. glasses					
8 oz. glasses					
Punch cups					
Other					

ITEM	DESCRIPTION	QUANTITY	COST	TOTAL COST	(QUANTITY x COST)
Bar Equipment:					
Ice buckets					
Ice tubs					
Bottle/can openers					
Corkscrews					
Cocktail shakers					
Stirring sticks					
Electric blenders					
Strainers					
Cocktail napkins					
Other					
Serving pieces:					
Serving trays					
Platters					
Serving bowls					
Punch bowls					
Water pitchers					
Salt and pepper sets					
Butter dishes					
Creamer/sugar sets					
Bread baskets					
Condiment trays					
Other					

EQUIPMENT RENTAL WORKSHEET (CONTINUED)

ITEM	DESCRIPTION	QUANTITY	COST	TOTAL COST	(QUANTITY X COST)
Miscellaneous:					
Coffee maker					
Insulated coffee pitchers					
Hot plates					
Microwaves					
Grill					
Coolers					
Coat racks					
Hangers					
Ashtrays					
Trash cans					
Other					
TOTAL					

SEATING DIAGRAM

Draw a simple, aerial-view diagram of the reception hall below. It should include the head table, parents' tables, guest tables, and any other significant features of the room (dance floor, bar, location of band or DJ, exits, etc.).

Seating Chart

Head Table: Shape of table:

Number of chairs: Order of seating (list or draw diagram below):

Bride's Parents' Table: Shape of table:

Number of chairs: Order of seating (list or draw diagram below):

Groom's Parents' Table: Shape of table:

Number of chairs: Order of seating (list or draw diagram below):

List below which guests you would like to seat at each table:

Table 1	Table 2	Table 3	Table 4

Table 5	Table 6	Table 7	Table 8

Table 9	Table 10	Table 11	Table 12

RECEPTION EVENTS WORKSHEET

Give a copy of this checklist to your reception site coordinator and band leader or disc jockey.

Introduce entire bridal party?   ☐ Yes   ☐ No   Music:

Introduce only bride and groom?   ☐ Yes   ☐ No   Music:

Parent(s) of bride:

Parent(s) of groom:

Grandparent(s) of bride:

Grandparent(s) of groom:

Flower girl(s):

Ring bearer(s):

Bridesmaids: Ushers:

Maid of honor: Best man:

Matron of honor:

Bride's first name:Groom's first name:

Bride and groom as they are to be introduced:

Receiving line at reception?   ☐ Yes   ☐ No   When:

Music:

Blessing?   ☐ Yes   ☐ No   By whom:

First toast?   ☐ Yes   ☐ No   By whom:

Other toasts?   ☐ Yes   ☐ No   By whom:

By whom:

By whom:

First dance: ☐ Yes   ☐ No   When:

Music:

To join in first dance:

Maid of honor and best man?   ☐ Yes   ☐ No

Parents of bride and groom?   ☐ Yes   ☐ No

Bridesmaids and ushers?   ☐ Yes   ☐ No

Guests?   ☐ Yes   ☐ No

Father-daughter dance?   ❑ Yes   ❑ No   Music:

Mother-son dance?   ❑ Yes   ❑ No   Music:

Open dance floor for guests after first dance?   ❑ Yes   ❑ No

Cake-cutting?   ❑ Yes   ❑ No   Music:

Bouquet toss?   ❑ Yes   ❑ No

Garter toss?   ❑ Yes   ❑ No

Last dance?   ❑ Yes   ❑ No   Music:

Other event:

When: Music:

Other event:

When: Music:

Special requests and dedications:

Notes:

BRIDAL ATTIRE WORKSHEET

Bridal Salon:

Address: Telephone:

Salesperson: Store hours:

Directions: Notes:

Wedding Gown: Description:

Manufacturer: Style number:

Color: Cost:

Order date: Deposit paid: Date:

Balance due: Date: Delivery date and time:

Delivery instructions/Pick-up date: Notes:

Headpiece and veil: Description:

Manufacturer: Style number:

Color: Cost:

Order date: Deposit paid: Date:

Balance due: Date: Delivery date and time:

Delivery instructions/Pick-up date: Notes:

ACCESORY	SIZE	COLOR	COST	WHERE PURCHASED (if different from above)	PICKED UP?
Slip					
Bra					
Hosiery					
Garter					
Gloves					
Shoes					
Jewelry					
Other					

BRIDAL BEAUTY WORKSHEET

HAIR STYLIST

Name: Salon:

Address: Telephone:

Hours:

Consultations:

Date: Time:

Date: Time:

Wedding Day Appointment:

Location: Date:

Time: Number of hours:

Services included: Total cost of services:

Overtime cost:

MANICURIST/PEDICURIST

Name: Salon:

Address: Telephone:

Hours:

Wedding Day Appointment:

Location: Date:

Time: Number of hours:

Services included: Total cost of services:

Overtime cost:

MAKEUP ARTIST

Name: Salon:

Address: Telephone:

Hours:

Consultations:

Date: Time:

Date: Time:

Wedding Day Appointment:

Location: Date:

Time: Number of hours:

Services included: Total cost of services:

Overtime cost: Travel fee (if applicable):

Notes:

GROOM'S ATTIRE WORKSHEET

Tuxedo Shop: .... Name: ....

Address: .... Telephone: ....

Salesperson: .... Store hours: ....

Directions: .... Services included: ....

Groom's Attire:

Tuxedo style and color: .... Cost: ....

Order date: .... Deposit paid: ....

Date: .... Balance due: ....

Date: .... Fitting date #1: ....

Time: .... Fitting date #2: ....

Time: .... Pick-up date and time: ....

Return date and time: .... Late fee: ....

Terms of cancellation: ....

Groom's Measurements:

Groom's height: .... Weight: ....

Coat size: .... Arm inseam: ....

Pants waist: .... Length (outseam): ....

Shirt neck: .... Sleeve: ....

Shoe size: .... Width: ....

GROOM'S ATTIRE WORKSHEET (CONTINUED)

ACCESSORY	SIZE	COLOR	COST	WHERE PURCHASED (if different from above)	PICKED UP?
Tie/Ascot					
Cummerbund					
Pocket handkerchief					
Suspenders					
Studs					
Cufflinks					
Formal socks					
Shoes					
Top hat					
Cane					
Gloves					
Other					

BRIDE'S ATTENDANTS' ATTIRE WORKSHEET

Place of Purchase: ....

Address: ....

Salesperson: ....

Directions: ....

Name: ....

Telephone: ....

Store hours: ....

Notes: ....

Attendants' Attire:

Description of dress: ....

Style number: ....

Cost per dress: ....

Total cost of dresses: ....

Sizes ordered: ....

Date: ....

Date: ....

Delivery instructions/Pick-up date: ....

Description of alterations: ....

Description of accessories
(hosiery, shoes, jewelry, etc.): ....

Cost of dying shoes (if applicable): ....

Notes: ....

Manufacturer: ....

Color: ....

Number ordered: ....

Order date: ....

Deposit paid: ....

Balance due: ....

Delivery date and time: ....

Alterations fee (total): ....

Cost of accessories: ....

Color: ....

Maid/Matron of Honor:

Name: ....

Shoe size: ....

Fitting date #1: ....

Fitting date #2: ....

Fitting date #3: ....

Notes: ....

Dress size: ....

Other sizes: ....

Time: ....

Time: ....

Time: ....

Bridesmaids:

Name: .... Dress size: ....

Shoe size: .... Other sizes: ....

Fitting date #1: .... Time: ....

Fitting date #2: .... Time: ....

Fitting date #3: .... Time: ....

Notes: ....

Name: .... Dress size: ....

Shoe size: .... Other sizes: ....

Fitting date #1: .... Time: ....

Fitting date #2: .... Time: ....

Fitting date #3: .... Time: ....

Notes: ....

Name: .... Dress size: ....

Shoe size: .... Other sizes: ....

Fitting date #1: .... Time: ....

Fitting date #2: .... Time: ....

Fitting date #3: .... Time: ....

Notes: ....

Name: .... Dress size: ....

Shoe size: .... Other sizes: ....

Fitting date #1: .... Time: ....

Fitting date #2: .... Time: ....

Fitting date #3: .... Time: ....

Notes: ....

Flower Girl's Attire:

Description of dress: Manufacturer:

Style number: Color:

Cost per dress: Number ordered:

Total cost of dresses: Order date:

Sizes ordered:

Deposit paid: Date:

Balance due: Date:

Delivery date and time:

Delivery instructions/Pick-up date:

Alterations fee (total):   Description of alterations:

Description of accessories (hosiery, shoes, jewelry, etc.):

Cost of accessories:

Cost of dying shoes (if applicable):   Color:

Notes:

GROOM'S ATTENDANTS' ATTIRE WORKSHEET

Attendants' Attire:

Tuxedo style and color: Cost per tuxedo:

Number ordered: Total cost of tuxedos:

Order date: Sizes ordered:

Deposit paid: Date:

Balance due: Date:

Ready date and time: Return date and time:

Late fee:

Description of accessories (socks, shoes, studs, cufflinks, etc.):

Cost of accessories: Notes:

Best Man:

Name: Height:

Weight: Tuxedo style and color:

Coat size: Arm inseam:

Pants waist: Length (outseam):

Shirt neck: Sleeve:

Shoe size: Width:

Fitting date #1:   Time:

Fitting date #2:   Time:

Pick-up date: Time:

Date returned: Time:

Notes:

Ushers:

Name:	Height:
Weight:	Tuxedo style and color:
Coat size:	Arm inseam:
Pants waist:	Length (outseam):
Shirt neck:	Sleeve:
Shoe size:	Width:
Fitting date #1:	Time:
Fitting date #2:	Time:
Pick-up date:	Time:
Date returned:	Time:
Notes:	

Name:	Height:
Weight:	Tuxedo style and color:
Coat size:	Arm inseam:
Pants waist:	Length (outseam):
Shirt neck:	Sleeve:
Shoe size:	Width:
Fitting date #1:	Time:
Fitting date #2:	Time:
Pick-up date:	Time:
Date returned:	Time:
Notes:	

Name: _____   Height: _____

Weight: _____   Tuxedo style and color: _____

Coat size: _____   Arm inseam: _____

Pants waist: _____   Length (outseam): _____

Shirt neck: _____   Sleeve: _____

Shoe size: _____   Width: _____

Fitting date #1: _____   Time: _____

Fitting date #2: _____   Time: _____

Pick-up date: _____   Time: _____

Date returned: _____   Time: _____

Notes: _____

Fathers:

Name: _____   Height: _____

Weight: _____   Tuxedo style and color: _____

Coat size: _____   Arm inseam: _____

Pants waist: _____   Length (outseam): _____

Shirt neck: _____   Sleeve: _____

Shoe size: _____   Width: _____

Fitting date #1: _____   Time: _____

Fitting date #2: _____   Time: _____

Pick-up date: _____   Time: _____

Date returned: _____   Time: _____

Notes: _____

Name: Height:

Weight: Tuxedo style and color:

Coat size: Arm inseam:

Pants waist: Length (outseam):

Shirt neck: Sleeve:

Shoe size: Width:

Fitting date #1:   Time:

Fitting date #2:   Time:

Pick-up date: Time:

Date returned: Time:

Notes:

Name of tailor: **Location:**

Telephone: Hours:

Description of alterations: Estimate:

Actual cost: Is pressing/steaming included?

If no, cost: Is delivery available?

Delivery charge (if any):   Deposit due:

Date: Ready date and time:

Delivery instructions/Pick-up date: Notes:

PHOTOGRAPHER WORKSHEET

Name of photographer/studio: Address:

Telephone: Contact:

Hours they can be reached: Directions:

Appointments: Date:

Time: Date:

Time: Date:

Time: Name of package (if applicable):

Date of hired services: Time:

Number of hours: Overtime cost:

Travel fee: Fee for custom pages:

Fee for black and white prints: Fee for sepia prints:

Fee for album inscription: Additional fees (if any):

Engagement session included?   ❐ Yes   ❐ No   Additional cost, if any:

Will attend rehearsal?   ❐ Yes   ❐ No   Additional cost, if any:

Cost of film, proofing, and processing included?   ❐ Yes   ❐ No

Additional cost, if any:

Type of wedding album included: Date proofs will be ready:

Date order will be ready: Additional services included:

Cost: Total amount due:

Amount of deposit: Date:

Balance due: Date:

Sales tax included?   ❐ Yes   ❐ No   Terms of cancellation:

Notes:

Included in Package:

Item	Number Included	Cost of Each Additional	Notes
8" x 10" engagement portraits			
5" x 7" engagement prints			
4" x 5" engagement prints			
Wallet-size engagement prints			
Wedding proofs			
Wallet-size prints			
3" x 5" prints			
4" x 5" prints			
5" x 7" prints			
8" x 10" prints			
11" x 14" portraits			
Other prints (list below)			
Preview album			
Wedding album			
Wedding album pages			
Parent albums			
Other (list below)			

PHOTOGRAPHER CHECKLIST

Give a copy of this completed form to your wedding photographer.

Name of bride and groom: _____ Address: _____

Telephone: _____ Wedding date: _____

Ceremony location: _____ Reception location: _____

Special instructions: _____

Portraits: _____

- ❏ You and the groom during the ceremony (if possible)
- ❏ An official wedding portrait of you and your groom
- ❏ The entire wedding party
- ❏ You, your groom, and family members
- ❏ You and your mother
- ❏ You and your father
- ❏ You with both parents
- ❏ You with your groom's parents (your new in-laws)
- ❏ The groom with his mother
- ❏ The groom with his father
- ❏ The groom with both parents
- ❏ The groom with your parents (his new in-laws)
- ❏ Combination photos of the attendants
- ❏ You and your groom with any special people in your lives, such as grandparents or godparents
- ❏ Other: _____

Photos from the ceremony (if possible):

- ❏ Each member of the wedding party as he or she comes down the aisle
- ❏ The mother of the bride as she is ushered down the aisle
- ❏ The groom's parents

- ☐ You and your father coming down the aisle
- ☐ Your father leaving you at the altar
- ☐ The wedding party at the altar
- ☐ The ring exchange
- ☐ The vows
- ☐ The lighting of any candles or special ceremony features
- ☐ Any relatives or friends who participate in the ceremony by doing a reading or lighting a candle
- ☐ The kiss
- ☐ The walk from the altar
- ☐ Other:

Candids:

- ☐ Getting ready for the ceremony; putting on the veil, the garter
- ☐ The bridesmaids, and you with them before the wedding
- ☐ You and your father leaving
- ☐ You and your father arriving at the ceremony
- ☐ Getting out of the limousine/car
- ☐ You and your groom getting in the car
- ☐ Toasting one another in the car
- ☐ Reception arrival
- ☐ The first dance
- ☐ The cutting of the cake
- ☐ Tossing the bouquet
- ☐ Removing/tossing the garter
- ☐ Going-away dance
- ☐ Leaving for the honeymoon (possibly with a "just married" sign on the car)
- ☐ Other:

VIDEOGRAPHER WORKSHEET

Name of videographer/studio: Address:

Telephone: Contact:

Hours they can be reached: Directions:

Appointments: Date:

Time: Date:

Time: Date:

Time: Name of package (if applicable):

Date of hired services: Time:

Number of hours: Number of cameras:

Overtime cost: Travel fee:

Additional fees (if any):

Will attend rehearsal?   ❐ Yes   ❐ No   Additional cost, if any:

Length of videotape:

Date tape will be ready:

Videotape will include:

Pre-wedding preparations: ❐ Yes   ❐ No   Notes:

Individual interviews with bride and groom prior to ceremony: ❐ Yes   ❐ No

Notes:

Ceremony: ❐ Yes   ❐ No   Notes:

Reception: ❐ Yes   ❐ No   Notes:

Photo montage: ❐ Yes   ❐ No   Notes:

Other:

Package includes:

Sound:	☐ Yes	☐ No	Notes:
Music:	☐ Yes	☐ No	Notes:
Unedited version of wedding events:	☐ Yes	☐ No	Notes:
Edited version of wedding events:	☐ Yes	☐ No	Notes:

Price of additional copies of videotape:

Other:

Additional services included: Cost:

Total amount due: Amount of deposit:

Date: Balance due:

Date: Sales tax included?   ☐ Yes   ☐ No

Terms of cancellation:

Notes:

CEREMONY MUSIC WORKSHEET

Organist's name:

Address:

Telephone: Fee:

Soloist's name:

Address:

Telephone: Fee:

Name of other musician, if applicable:

Address:

Telephone: Fee:

Part of Ceremony	Musical Selection	Performed By
Prelude		
Processional		
During the ceremony (list specific part below)		
Recessional		
Other		

RECEPTION MUSIC WORKSHEET

Name of band/DJ: ....

Address: ....

Telephone: ....

Manager/contact: ....

Hours he or she can be reached: ....

Number of performers: ....

Description of act: ....

Demo tape available? ❏ Yes ❏ No

Notes: ....

View live performance? ❏ Yes ❏ No

Date: .... Time: .... Location: ....

Appointments:

Date: ....

Time: ....

Date: ....

Time: ....

Date: ....

Time: ....

Date of hired services: ....

Time: ....

Number of hours: ....

Cocktail hour: ....

Overtime cost: ....

Includes the following services: ....

Equipment provided: ....

Equipment rented: ....

Rental costs: ....

Cost: ....

Total amount due: ....

Amount of deposit: ....

Date: ....

Balance due: ....

Date: ....

Terms of cancellation: ....

Notes: ....

FLORIST WORKSHEET

Name of florist: ....   Address: ....

Telephone: ....   Contact: ....

Hours: ....   Directions: ....

Appointments: ....   Date: ....

Time: ....   Date: ....

Time: ....   Date: ....

Time: ....   Services provided: ....

Date of delivery: ....   Time: ....

Location of bridal party: ....   Travel fee: ....

Additional fees (if any): ....   Cost: ....

Total amount due: ....   Amount of deposit: ....

Date: ....   Balance due: ....

Date: ....   Sales tax included?   ❐ Yes   ❐ No

Terms of cancellation: ....

Notes: ....

WEDDING PARTY FLOWERS WORKSHEET

PERSON/ITEM	DESCRIPTION	NUMBER	COST
Bride:			
Bouquet			
Headpiece			
Toss-away bouquet			
Going-away corsage			
Maid/Matron of honor:			
Bouquet			
Headpiece			
Bridesmaids:			
Bouquet			
Headpiece			
Flower Girls:			
Flowers			
Basket			
Headpiece			
Mothers of the bride and groom:			
Corsage			
Grandmothers of the bride and groom:			
Corsage			

PERSON/ITEM	DESCRIPTION	NUMBER	COST
Groom:			
Boutonniere			
Best man:			
Boutonniere			
Ushers:			
Boutonniere			
Ringbearer:			
Boutonniere			
Pillow			
Fathers of the bride and groom:			
Boutonniere			
Grandfathers (bride and groom):			
Boutonniere			
Readers:			
Corsage			
Boutonniere			
Other (list below)			
TOTAL			

CEREMONY FLOWERS AND DECORATIONS WORKSHEET

ITEM	DESCRIPTION	NUMBER	COST
Aisle runner			
Altar flowers			
Garland			
Potted flowers			
Potted plants			
Pews/chair flowers			
Pews/chair bows			
Candelabra			
Candle holders			
Candles			
Unity candle			
Wedding arch			
Columns			
Trellis			
Wreaths for church doors			
Other (list below)			
TOTAL			

RECEPTION FLOWERS AND DECORATIONS WORKSHEET

ITEM	DESCRIPTION	NUMBER	COST
Guest tables:			
Centerpieces			
Garland			
Candles			
Head table:			
Centerpieces			
Garland			
Candles			
Buffet table:			
Flowers			
Garland			
Decorations			
Cake table:			
Cake top			
Flowers			
Garland			
Decorations			
Guest book table:			
Flowers			
Decorations			

ITEM	DESCRIPTION	NUMBER	COST
Envelope table:			
Flowers			
Decorations			
Candelabra			
Candle holders			
Candles			
Archway			
Columns			
Trellis			
Wreaths			
Garlands			
Potted flowers			
Potted plants			
Hanging plants			
Other (list below)			
TOTAL			

BAKER WORKSHEET

Name of bakery: .... Address: ....

Telephone: .... Contact: ....

Hours: .... Directions: ....

Appointments: .... Date: ....

Time: .... Date: ....

Time: .... Date: ....

Time: .... Order date: ....

Delivery/Pick-up date: .... Time: ....

Delivery/Pick-up instructions: .... Cost: ....

Total amount due: .... Amount of deposit: ....

Date: .... Balance due: ....

Date: .... Sales tax included? ❏ Yes ❏ No

Terms of cancellation: .... Notes: ....

WEDDING CAKE WORKSHEET

ITEM	DESCRIPTION	COST
Wedding cake:		
Size		
Shape		
Number of tiers		
Number cake will serve		
Flavor of cake		
Flavor of filling		
Flavor of icing		
Icing decorations		
Cake top		
Cake decorations		
Other		
Groom's cake:		
Size		
Shape		
Number cake will serve		
Flavor		
Icing		
Cake top		
Cake decorations		
Other		
Cake serving set		
Cake boxes		
Delivery charge		
Other		
TOTAL		

TRANSPORTATION WORKSHEET

Name of company: .... Address: ....

Telephone: .... Contact: ....

Hours: .... Directions: ....

Services provided: .... Number of vehicles rented: ....

Description: .... Cost per hour: ....

Minimum number of hours: .... Overtime cost: ....

Hours of rental: .... Name of driver(s): ....

Cost: .... Total amount due: ....

Amount of deposit: .... Date: ....

Balance due: .... Date: ....

Sales tax included?   ❐ Yes   ❐ No

Terms of cancellation: ....

DRIVER'S CHECKLIST

Give a copy of this to each driver.

Vehicle: .... Driver: ....

Date: .... Name of bride and groom: ....

1. Place of pick-up:

Arrival time: .... Names of passenger(s): ....

Address: .... Telephone: ....

Directions: .... Special instructions: ....

2. Place of pick-up:

Arrival time: .... Names of passenger(s): ....

Address: .... Telephone: ....

Directions: .... Special instructions: ....

3. Place of pick-up:

Arrival time: .... Names of passenger(s): ....

Address: .... Telephone: ....

Directions: .... Special instructions: ....

4. Ceremony location:

Arrival time: .... Names of passenger(s): ....

Address: .... Telephone: ....

Directions: .... Special instructions: ....

5. Reception location:

Arrival time: .... Names of passenger(s): ....

Address: .... Telephone: ....

Directions: .... Special instructions: ....

STATIONERY WORKSHEET

Name of Stationer: .... Address: ....

Telephone: .... Contact: ....

Hours: .... Directions: ....

Appointments: ....

Time: .... Date: ....

Time: .... Date: ....

Time: .... Date: ....

Wedding Invitations:

Description: .... Manufacturer: ....

Style: .... Paper: ....

Paper color: .... Typeface: ....

Ink color: .... Printing process: ....

Tissue paper inserts: .... Printed outer envelopes: ....

Inner envelopes: .... Envelope liner: ....

Number ordered: .... Cost: ....

Reception Cards:

Description: .... Number ordered: ....

Cost: ....

Response Cards:

Description: .... Printed envelopes: ....

Envelope liner: .... Number ordered: ....

Cost: ....

Ceremony Cards:

Description: .... Number ordered: ....

Cost: ....

Pew Cards:

Description: .... Number ordered: ....

Cost: ....

Rain Cards:

Description: .... Number ordered: ....

Cost: ....

Travel Cards/Maps:

Description: .... Number ordered: ....

Cost: ....

Wedding Announcements:

Description: .... Printed envelopes: ....

Envelope liner: .... Number ordered: ....

Cost: ....

At-home Cards:

Description: .... Printed envelopes: ....

Envelope liner: .... Number ordered: ....

Cost: ....

Thank-you Notes:

Description: Printed envelopes:

Envelope liner: Number ordered:

Cost:

Ceremony Programs:

Description: Number ordered:

Cost:

Party Favors:

Description: Number ordered:

Cost:

Other:

Description: Number ordered:

Cost:

Order date: Ready date:

Time: Delivery/Pick-up instructions:

Cost: Total amount due:

Amount of deposit: Date:

Balance due: Date:

Sales tax included?   ❑ Yes   ❑ No   Terms of cancellation:

Notes:

INVITATION WORDING WORKSHEET

Wedding invitations:

Return address for invitation envelopes:

Reception cards:

Response cards:

Return address for response card envelopes:

Ceremony cards:

Pew cards:

Rain cards:

Travel cards:

At-home cards:

Return address for at-home card envelopes:

Thank-you notes:

Return address for thank-you note envelopes:

Ceremony programs:

Party favors:

Other:

Notes:

Honeymoon Budget Worksheet

Item	Description	Projected Cost	Actual Cost	Balance Due
Transportation				
Airfare				
Car rental				
Moped rental				
Bike rental				
Train pass				
Taxi				
Parking fees				
Other				
Accommodations				
Wedding night				
Honeymoon destination				
Other				
Food				
Meal plan				
Meals				
Drinks				
Entertainment				
Souvenirs				
Spending money				
Tips				
Other				
TOTAL				

TRAVEL SERVICES WORKSHEET

Travel Agency:

Address: Telephone:

Fax number: Contact:

Hours: Directions:

Car Rental Agency:

Address: Telephone:

Fax number: Contact:

Hours: Description of reserved vehicle (make/model):

Terms:

Transportation:

Destination: Carrier:

Flight/Route: Departure date:

Time: Arrival date:

Time: Confirmation number:

Date: Destination:

Carrier: Flight/Route:

Departure date: Time:

Arrival date: Time:

Confirmation number: Date:

Accommodations:

Hotel: Address:

Directions: Telephone:

Fax number: Check-in date:

Time: Check-out date:

Time: Type of room:

Daily rate: Total cost:

Confirmation number: Date:

Hotel: Address:

Directions: Telephone:

Fax number: Check-in date:

Time: Check-out date:

Time: Type of room:

Daily rate: Total cost:

Confirmation number: Date:

Hotel: Address:

Directions: Telephone:

Fax number: Check-in date:

Time: Check-out date:

Time: Type of room:

Daily rate: Total cost:

Confirmation number: Date:

PLANNING CHECKLIST

Six to twelve months before the wedding:

- ☐ Announce engagement
- ☐ Decide on type of wedding
- ☐ Decide on time of day
- ☐ Choose the location
- ☐ Set a date
- ☐ Set a budget
- ☐ Select bridal party
- ☐ Plan color scheme
- ☐ Select and order bridal gown
- ☐ Select and order headpiece
- ☐ Select and order shoes
- ☐ Select and order attendants' gowns
- ☐ Start honeymoon planning
- ☐ Go to bridal gift registry
- ☐ Start compiling the guest list
- ☐ Select caterer
- ☐ Select musicians
- ☐ Select florist
- ☐ Select photographer
- ☐ Start planning reception
- ☐ Reserve hall, hotel, etc., for reception
- ☐ Plan to attend pre-marital counseling at your church, if applicable
- ☐ Select and order wedding rings

Three months before the wedding:

- ❐ Complete guest list
- ❐ Make doctor's appointments
- ❐ Plan to have mothers select attire
- ❐ Select and order invitations
- ❐ Order personal stationery
- ❐ Start compiling trousseau
- ❐ Finalize reception arrangements (rent items now)
- ❐ Make reservations for honeymoon
- ❐ Confirm dress delivery
- ❐ Confirm time and date with florist
- ❐ Confirm time and date with caterer
- ❐ Confirm time and date with photographer
- ❐ Confirm time and date with musicians
- ❐ Confirm time and date with church
- ❐ Discuss transportation to ceremony and reception
- ❐ Order cake
- ❐ Select and order attire for groomsmen
- ❐ Schedule bridesmaids' dress and shoe fittings

Two months before the wedding:

- ❐ Mail all invitations to allow time for RSVPs
- ❐ Arrange for appointment to get marriage license
- ❐ Finalize honeymoon arrangements

One month before the wedding:

- ☐ Schedule bridal portrait
- ☐ Reserve accommodations for guests
- ☐ Begin to record gifts received and send thank-you notes
- ☐ Plan rehearsal and rehearsal dinner
- ☐ Purchase gifts for bridal party
- ☐ Purchase gift for fiancé if gifts are being exchanged
- ☐ Schedule final fittings, including accessories and shoes
- ☐ Schedule appointments at beauty salon for attendants
- ☐ Schedule bridesmaids' luncheon or party
- ☐ Arrange for placement of guest book
- ☐ Obtain wedding props, e.g., pillow for ringbearer, candles, etc.
- ☐ Get marriage license

Two weeks before the wedding:

- ☐ Mail bridal portrait with announcement to newspaper
- ☐ Finalize wedding day transportation
- ☐ Arrange to change name on license, Social Security card, etc.
- ☐ Confirm accommodations for guests
- ☐ Prepare wedding announcements to be mailed after the wedding

One week before the wedding:

- ☐ Start packing for honeymoon
- ☐ Finalize number of guests with caterer
- ☐ Double-check all details with those providing professional services (photographer, videographer, florist, etc.)
- ☐ Plan seating arrangements
- ☐ Confirm desired pictures with photographer
- ☐ Style your hair with headpiece
- ☐ Practice applying cosmetics in proper light
- ☐ Arrange for one last fitting of all wedding attire
- ☐ Make sure rings are picked up and fit properly
- ☐ Confirm receipt of marriage license
- ☐ Have rehearsal/rehearsal dinner (one or two days before wedding)
- ☐ Arrange to have the photographer and attendants arrive two hours before ceremony if there are to be pre-wedding pictures
- ☐ Arrange for music to start one half hour prior to ceremony
- ☐ Arrange to have the mother of the groom seated five minutes before ceremony
- ☐ Arrange to have the mother of the bride seated immediately before the processional
- ☐ Arrange for the aisle runner to be rolled out by the ushers immediately before the processional

On your wedding day:

- ☐ Try to relax and pamper yourself; take a long bath, have a manicure, etc.
- ☐ Eat at least one small meal; drink plenty of water
- ☐ Have your hair and makeup done a few hours before ceremony
- ☐ Start dressing one to two hours before ceremony

IMPORTANT ADDRESSES AND TELEPHONE NUMBERS

Bride:

Name: Address:

Telephone:

Groom:

Name: Address:

Telephone:

Family Members:

Name: Address:

Telephone:

Name: Address:

Telephone:

Name: Address:

Telephone:

Name: Address:

Telephone:

Wedding Party Members:

Name: Address:

Telephone:

Name: Address:

Telephone:

Name: Address:

Telephone:

Name: Address:

Telephone:

Wedding Party Members:

Name: Address:

Telephone:

Name: Address:

Telephone:

Name: Address:

Telephone:

Name: Address:

Telephone:

Wedding Consultant:

Name: Address:

Telephone:

Ceremony Officiant and Site:

Name: Address:

Telephone:

Reception Coordinator and Site:

Name: Address:

Telephone:

Jeweler:

Name: Address:

Telephone:

Important Addresses and Telephone Numbers (continued)

Bridal Salon:

Name: Address:

Telephone:

Men's Formalwear Shop:

Name: Address:

Telephone:

Caterer:

Name: Address:

Telephone:

Baker:

Name: Address:

Telephone:

Equipment Rental Company:

Name: Address:

Telephone:

Photographer:

Name: Address:

Telephone:

Videographer:

Name: Address:

Telephone:

Band, DJ, and Other Musicians:

Name: Address:

Telephone:

Name: Address:

Telephone:

Limousine Service:

Name: Address:

Telephone:

Travel Agent:

Name: Address:

Telephone:

Index

EVERYTHING

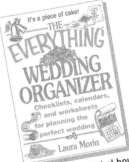

Trade paperback, Spiral bound
1-55850-828-7, $15.00

The Everything Wedding Organizer
by Laura Morin

The Everything Wedding Organizer features everything a frazzled bride- or groom-needs to get organized. Complete with dozens of worksheets, checklists, pockets, and loads of helpful hints, this handy planner can help you develop a working strategy to create the wedding of your dreams. Beginning with setting a date and creating a budget, every aspect of the wedding is covered, right to the last details, including the honeymoon. And it's small enough to carry around to appointments with florists, caterers, and other wedding professionals.

The Everything Jewish Wedding Book
by Helen Latner

The Everything Jewish Wedding Book includes absolutely everything you need to know to have the most wonderful Jewish ceremony and reception. It provides detailed information for every type of Jewish wedding. Your wedding will be a special and unique event. Whether you are planning a contemporary ceremony or a traditionally orthodox reception, there are Jewish traditions from all over the world that will suit your taste, lifestyle, and budget. Covering both religious and secular details, this is the one source that any Jewish bride and groom will need to plan the perfect wedding and get you ready for the most wonderful day of your life!

Trade paperback, 304 pages
1-55850-801-5, $12.95

Available Wherever Books Are Sold

If you cannot find these titles at your favorite retail outlet, you may order them directly from the publisher. BY PHONE: Call 1-800-872-5627. We accept Visa, MasterCard, and American Express. $4.95 will be added to your total order for shipping and handling. BY MAIL: Write out the full titles of the books you'd like to order and send payment, including $4.95 for shipping and handling, to: Adams Media Corporation, 260 Center Street, Holbrook, MA 02343. 30-day money-back guarantee.

We Have

EVERYTHING

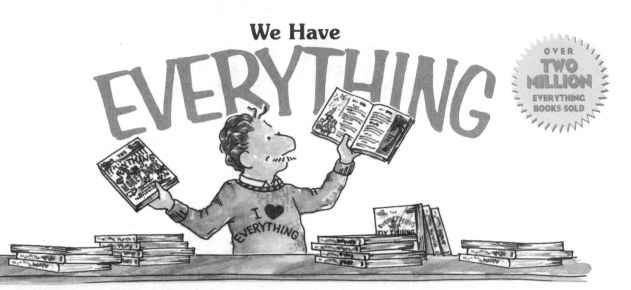

More Bestselling Everything Titles Available From Your Local Bookseller:

Everything **After College Book**
Everything **Astrology Book**
Everything **Baby Names Book**
Everything **Baby Shower Book**
Everything **Barbeque Cookbook**
Everything® **Bartender's Book**
Everything **Bedtime Story Book**
Everything **Beer Book**
Everything **Bicycle Book**
Everything **Bird Book**
Everything **Build Your Own
Home Page Book**
Everything **Casino Gambling Book**
Everything **Cat Book**
Everything® **Christmas Book**
Everything **College Survival Book**
Everything **Cover Letter Book**
Everything **Crossword and Puzzle Book**
Everything **Dating Book**
Everything **Dessert Book**
Everything **Dog Book**
Everything **Dreams Book**
Everything **Etiquette Book**
Everything **Family Tree Book**

Everything **Fly-Fishing Book**
Everything **Games Book**
Everything **Get-a-Job Book**
Everything **Get Published Book**
Everything **Get Ready For Baby Book**
Everything **Golf Book**
Everything **Guide to New York City**
Everything **Guide to Walt Disney
World®, Universal Studios®,
and Greater Orlando**
Everything **Guide to Washington D.C.**
Everything **Herbal Remedies Book**
Everything **Homeselling Book**
Everything **Homebuying Book**
Everything **Home Improvement Book**
Everything **Internet Book**
Everything **Investing Book**
Everything **Jewish Wedding Book**
Everything **Kids' Money Book**
Everything **Kids' Nature Book**
Everything **Kids' Puzzle Book**
Everything **Low-Fat High-Flavor
Cookbook**
Everything **Microsoft® Word 2000 Book**

Everything **Money Book**
Everything **One-Pot Cookbook**
Everything **Online Business Book**
Everything **Online Investing Book**
Everything **Pasta Book**
Everything **Pregnancy Book**
Everything **Pregnancy Organizer**
Everything **Resume Book**
Everything **Sailing Book**
Everything **Selling Book**
Everything **Study Book**
Everything **Tarot Book**
Everything **Toasts Book**
Everything **Total Fitness Book**
Everything **Trivia Book**
Everything **Tropical Fish Book**
Everything® **Wedding Book, 2nd Edition**
Everything® **Wedding Checklist**
Everything® **Wedding Etiquette Book**
Everything® **Wedding Organizer**
Everything® **Wedding Shower Book**
Everything® **Wedding Vows Book**
Everything **Wine Book**

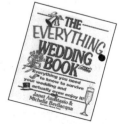
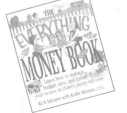
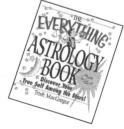
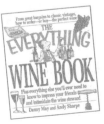
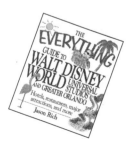